# Pharmacological Aspects of Essential Oils

*Pharmacological Aspects of Essential Oils: Current and Future Trends* provides a collection of therapeutic and pharmacological applications of the most researched essential oils of great importance derived from Clove, Cinnamon, Coriander, Turmeric, *Thymus zygis*, *Thyme vulgaris*, *Ocimum basilicum*, *Copaifera spp*, and *Nigella sativa* species. The new approach towards using a metal phenolic network with the essential oils as a tool of nanomedicine will surely open a new horizon for the research community. Treating disorders such as diabetes, insomnia, and obesity with essential oils will provide a new area of research. Aromatherapy, which is creating a market especially in the personal health care sector, is also discussed in the book. The relation between chemical composition and different biological properties is well discussed in respective chapters. The other practical topics related to the development of this industry of essential oils have been illustrated with elaborative figures and tables.

Providing such updated data on the pharmacological applications of essential oils is an asset to the community associated with the extraction and production of essential oils, biochemist, aromatherapist, agrotechnologists, and nutritionist fraternities.

Salient Features:

- Metal phenolic networks and essential oils as tool of nanomedicine
- Role of essential oils in aromatherapy
- Sophisticated development of various advanced techniques in the characterization of essential oils
- Pharmacological applications of Brazilian aromatic species
- Role of essential oils in management of diabetes, obesity, and insomnia

# EXPLORING MEDICINAL PLANTS

*Series Editor: Azamal Husen*
*Wolaita Sodo University, Ethiopia*

Medicinal plants render a rich source of bioactive compounds used in drug formulation and development; they play a key role in traditional or indigenous health systems. As the demand for herbal medicines increases worldwide, supply is declining as most of the harvest is derived from naturally growing vegetation. Considering global interests and covering several important aspects associated with medicinal plants, the *Exploring Medicinal Plants* series comprises volumes valuable to academia, practitioners, and researchers interested in medicinal plants. Topics provide information on a range of subjects including diversity, conservation, propagation, cultivation, physiology, molecular biology, growth response under extreme environment, handling, storage, bioactive compounds, secondary metabolites, extraction, therapeutics, mode of action, and healthcare practices.

Led by Azamal Husen, PhD, this series is directed to a broad range of researchers and professionals consisting of topical books exploring information related to medicinal plants. It includes edited volumes, references, and textbooks available for individual print and electronic purchases.

**Secondary Metabolites from Medicinal Plants**
Nanoparticles Synthesis and their Applications
*Rakesh Kumar Bachheti, Archana Bachheti*

**Aquatic Medicinal Plants**
*Archana Bachheti, Rakesh Kumar Bachheti, and Azamal Husen*

**Antidiabetic Medicinal Plants and Herbal Treatments**
*Azamal Husen*

**Ethnobotany and Ethnopharmacology of Medicinal and Aromatic Plants**
Steps Towards Drugs Discovery
*Adnan Mohd, Mitesh Patel and Mejdi Snoussi*

**Wild Mushrooms and Health Diversity, Phytochemistry, Medicinal Benefits, and Cultivation**
*Kamal Ch. Semwal, Steve L. Stephenson, and Azamal Husen*

**Medicinal Roots and Tubers for Pharmaceutical and Commercial Applications**
*Rakesh Kumar Bachheti and Archana Bachheti*

**Pharmacological Aspects of Essential Oils**
Current and Future Trends
*Sunita Singh, Pankaj Kumar Chaurasia, and Shashi Lata Bharati*

# Pharmacological Aspects of Essential Oils

## Current and Future Trends

Edited By

## Sunita Singh
Department of Chemistry, Navyug Kanya Mahavidyalaya,
University of Lucknow, Lucknow, Uttar Pradesh, India

## Pankaj Kumar Chaurasia
P.G. Department of Chemistry, L.S. College,
B.R. Ambedkar Bihar University, Muzaffarpur, Bihar, India

## Shashi Lata Bharati
Department of Chemistry, North Eastern Regional
Institute of Science and Technology, Arunachal Pradesh, India

**CRC Press**
Taylor & Francis Group
Boca Raton  London  New York

CRC Press is an imprint of the
Taylor & Francis Group, an **informa** business

First edition published 2024
by CRC Press
2385 NW Executive Center Drive, Suite 320, Boca Raton FL 33431

and by CRC Press
4 Park Square, Milton Park, Abingdon, Oxon, OX14 4RN

*CRC Press is an imprint of Taylor & Francis Group, LLC*

ISBN: 978-1-032-48590-4 (hbk)
ISBN: 978-1-032-48592-8 (pbk)
ISBN: 978-1-003-38977-4 (ebk)

DOI: 10.1201/9781003389774

Typeset in Times New Roman
by Apex CoVantage, LLC

# Contents

**Chapter 9**    Pharmacological Applications of Brazilian Aromatic
Species: *Aniba Rosaeodora* Ducke, *Casearia Sylvestris* Sw.,
*Spilanthes Acmella* Var. *Oleracea* (L.), and
*Xylopia Aromatica* (Lam.) Mart................................................ 126

*Sachin P. Bhatt, Popat Mohite, Abhijeet Puri,
Sudarshan Singh, Bhupendra G. Prajapati, Shruti Shiromwar,
and Vijay R. Chidrawar*

**Chapter 10**   Pharmacological Aspects and Chemical Characterization of
Syzygium Aromaticum: Current and Future Trends...................... 140

*Jigar Vyas, Nensi Raytthatha, and Bhupendra G. Prajapati*

**Chapter 13** Pharmacological Aspects of *Ocimum Basilicum* Essential Oil:
Current and Future Trends ............................................................. 175

*Yogita Ale, Shivani Rawat, Nidhi Nainwal, and Vikash Jakhmola*

**Chapter 14** Exploration of the Pharmacological Aspects of *Thyme
Vulgaris* Essential Oil (TEO).......................................................... 187

*Kiran Dobhal, Shalu Verma, Alka Singh, Ruchika Garg, and
Vikash Jakhmola*

**Chapter 19**  An Update of Anticancer Application of Essential Oils .................. 265

*Mohit Agrawal, Manmohan Singhal, Amit Kumar Nayak, and
Shailendra Bhatt*

# Editor Bios

**Dr. Sunita Singh** is an assistant professor of chemistry in the Navyug Kanya Mahavidyalaya, University of Lucknow since 2019. She pursued her Ph.D. in the year 2015 on the topic, "Chemistry, antioxidant and antimicrobial activities of essential oils and oleoresins of spices" from Deen Dayal Upadhyaya Gorakhpur University, Gorakhpur. She was awarded junior research and senior research fellowships from the University Grant Commission. She also worked as a research assistant (2010–2011) on the project sponsored by Council of Science & Technology, "Chemistry, Antioxidant and Antimicrobial activities of Oleoresins extracted from Cardamom, Black pepper and Caraway." She has published 25 research articles in journals of national and international repute. She has authored and coauthored 8 book chapters with national and international publishing houses. She has edited a book with sn international publisher. She has attended in total 30+ conferences and webinars of national and international repute and delivered more than 15 invited talks and oral presentations. She has presented her work in various global events. She is also an active member of the Association of Chemistry Teachers (India), International Clinical Aromatherapy Network, and Nutrition Working Group of the Global Harmonization Initiative.

**Dr. Pankaj Kumar Chaurasia**, Ph.D. is assistant professor in the Post Graduate Department of Chemistry, Langat Singh College, Muzaffarpur (Bhim Rao Ambedkar Bihar University, Muzaffarpur). He has experience teaching at post-graduate, under-graduate, and Inter Science level. He has a good academic as well as research career. He qualified by the National Eligibility Test in 2009 as Council of Science & Industrial Research-Junior Research Fellowship (CSIR-JRF) (NET) and was awarded Senior Research Fellow-National Eligibility Test in 2012. He received his Ph.D. degree in chemistry. He also worked as guest faculty (2016–2017) in the department of chemistry, University of Allahabad, Prayagraj (A Central University of India). He was awarded a research associateship by CSIR-New Delhi (India) in 2017 and worked as CSIR-Research Associate in Motilal Nehru National Institute of Technology, Allahabad/Prayagraj (India). In his research career, he has ~70 total publications, including ~43 journal publications, ~20 book chapters, and 6 books; many of the publications are in the pipeline. He is also guiding four Ph.D. research scholars. He has worked in different areas of chemistry and has research expertise in biological chemistry, biotechnology, microbiology, enzymology, organometallic chemistry, and environmental chemistry.

**Dr. Shashi Lata Bharati**, Ph.D. is working as an assistant professor in the department of chemistry, North Eastern Regional Institute of Science and Technology, Nirjuli, Arunachal Pradesh (India). She has a good academic as well as research career. She was awarded a University Grants Commission (UGC)-Department of Special Assistance fellowship for the meritorious students during her Ph.D. program.

She obtained her Ph.D. degree in chemistry. She was awarded a UGC post-doctoral fellowship for women in 2013 by UGC New Delhi and worked as a post-doctoral fellow in the department of chemistry of Deen Dayal Upadhyaya Gorakhpur University, Gorakhpur (India). She has published ~50 publications, including ~31 journal publications, ~14 book chapters, and 5 books in national and international journals/publishers of repute. She has guided many M.Sc. project students and one Ph.D. research scholar. She has expertise in the fields of inorganic chemistry, organometallic chemistry, biological chemistry, and enzymology.

# Contributors

**Mohit Agrawal**
Department of Pharmacology School of
Medical & Allied Sciences
K.R. Mangalam University
Gurugram, India

**Ms. Yogita Ale**
Uttaranchal Institute of Pharmaceutical
Sciences
Uttaranchal University
Dehradun, Uttarakhand, India

**Eswar Kumar Aouta**
University College of Pharmaceutical
Sciences
Palamuru University
Mahabubnagar, Telangana, India

**\*Sivakumar Arumugam**
(Protein Engineering Lab, School of
Biosciences and Technology, VIT
University
Vellore, India

**D. I. Arrieta Gamarra**
Instituto de Investigaciones Fisicoquímicas
Teóricas y Aplicadas (INIFTA)
CCT La Plata, CONICET, Facultad de
Ciencias Exactas
Argentina

**Kodiveri Muthukaliannan
Gothandam**
(High Throughput Lab, School of
Biosciences and Technology, VIT
University
Vellore, India

**Sachin P. Bhatt**
Gyanmanjari Pharmacy College
Gujarat Technological University
Bhavnagar, Gujarat, India

**Shailendra Bhatt**
School of Medical and Allied Sciences
G.D. Goenka University
Gurugram, Haryana, India

**Pankaj Kumar Chaurasia**
Post Graduate Department of
Chemistry, Langat Singh College
Bhim Rao Ambedkar Bihar University
Muzaffarpur, Bihar, India

**Vijay R. Chidrawar**
SVKM's NMIMS
School of Pharmacy and Technology
Management
Jadcharla 509301
Telangana, India

**Destaw Damtie**
Department of Biology
Bahir Dar University College of Science
Ethiopia

**Mrs. Kiran Dobhal**
College of Pharmacy
Shivalik campus
Dehradun, Uttarakhand, India

**Omayma A. Eldahshan**
Department of Pharmacognosy Faculty
of Pharmacy
Ain Shams University
Cairo, Egypt
Center for Drug Discovery Research
and Development
Ain Shams University
Cairo, Egypt

**Ahmed E. Elissawy**
Department of Pharmacognosy Faculty
of Pharmacy
Ain Shams University
Cairo, Egypt

Center for Drug Discovery Research
  and Development
Ain Shams University
Cairo, Egypt

**N. S. Fagali**
Instituto de Investigaciones
  Fisicoquímicas Teóricas y Aplicadas
  (INIFTA)
CCT La Plata, CONICET, Facultad de
  Ciencias Exactas
La Plata, Argentina.

**Janaki Ramaiah Mekala**
(Department of Biotechnology, Koneru
  Lakshmaiah Education Foundation,
  Green Fields, Vaddeswaram,
 Guntur, Andhra Pradesh, India

**M. A. Fernández Lorenzo de Mele**
Instituto de Investigaciones
  Fisicoquímicas Teóricas y Aplicadas
  (INIFTA)
CCT La Plata, CONICET, Facultad de
  Ciencias Exactas, UNLP
La Plata, Argentina

**M. R. Furlan**
Departamento de Ciências Agrárias
Universidade de Taubaté
São Paulo, Brazil

**D. Garcia**
Departamento de Ciências Agrárias
Universidade de Taubaté
São Paulo, Brazil

**Mrs. Ruchika Garg**
Maharaja Agrasen University
School of Pharmacy
Baddi, Solan, Himachal Pradesh, India

**Upendarrao Golla**
Department of Medicine
Penn State College of Medicine
Hershey, USA

**A. Gonzalez**
Instituto de Investigaciones
  Fisicoquímicas Teóricas y Aplicadas
  (INIFTA)
CCT La Plata, CONICET, Facultad de
  Ciencias Exactas, UNLP
La Plata, Argentina

**Jeena Gupta**
School of Bioengineering and
  Biosciences
Lovely Professional University
Phagwara, Punjab, India

**Prof. (Dr.) Vikash Jakhmola**
Uttaranchal Institute of Pharmaceutical
  Sciences (UIPS) Uttaranchal
  University
Dehradun - Uttarakhand, India

**Yash Jasoria**
School of Medical and Allied Sciences
K.R. Mangalam University
India

**Dr. Naveen Chandra Joshi**
Division of Research and Innovation
Uttaranchal University Dehradun
India

**Reena Kaushik**
Department of Pharmacy
Guru Ghasidas Central University
Bilaspur, Chhatisgarh, India

**Naveen Kumar**
Department of Chemistry
S.D. College Muzaffarnagar, Maa
  Shakumbhari University
Muzaffarnagar, Uttar Pradesh, India

**Pawan Kumar**
Department of Chemistry
S.D. College Muzaffarnagar, Maa
  Shakumbhari University
Muzaffarnagar, Uttar Pradesh, India

**Vipul Kumar**
Department of Pharmaceutical Chemistry
Delhi Institute of Pharmaceutical
   Sciences and Research, Delhi
   Pharmaceutical Sciences and
   Research University
New Delhi, India

**Rudra Awdhesh Kumar Mishra**
High Throughput Lab, School of
   Biosciences and Technology
VIT University
Vellore, India

**Popat Mohite**
St. Johns Institute of Pharmacy and
   Research,
Vevoor, Palghar (E), Maharashtra, India

**Debojyoti Mondal**
School of Bioengineering and Biosciences
   Lovely Professional University
Phagwara, Punjab, India

**Dr. Nidhi Nainwal**
Uttaranchal Institute of Pharmaceutical
   Sciences
Uttaranchal University
Dehradun, Uttarakhand, India

**Sharada Nalla**
University College of Pharmaceutical
   Sciences
Palamuru University
Mahabubnagar, Telangana, India

**Amit Kumar Nayak**
School of Medical & Allied Sciences
G. D. Goenka University
Gurugram, India

**Alev Önder**
Department of Pharmacognosy Faculty
   of Pharmacy
Ankara University
Ankara, Türkiye

**Sujatha Palatheeya**
University College of Pharmaceutical
   Sciences
Palamuru University
Mahabubnagar, Telangana, India

**Madhavi Patel**
Parul Institute of Pharmacy Faculty of
   Pharmacy
Parul University
Vadodara, Gujarat, India

**Bhupendra G. Prajapati**
Shree S. K. Patel College of
   Pharmaceutical Education and
   Research
Ganpat University
Mehsana, Gujarat, India

**Abhijeet Puri**
St. Johns Institute of Pharmacy and
   Research
Vevoor, Palghar (E), Maharashtra,
   India

**Miss Jaya Rautela**
Uttaranchal Institute of Pharmaceutical
   Sciences
Uttaranchal University
Dehradun, Uttarakhand, India

**Miss Shivani Rawat**
School of Pharmaceutical Sciences
Sardar Bhagwan Singh University
India

**Nensi Raytthatha**
Sigma Institute of Pharmacy
Sigma University
Vadodara, Gujarat, India

**Piyush Sharma**
Department of Zoology
S.D. College Muzaffarnagar, Maa
   Shakumbhari University
Muzaffarnagar, Uttar Pradesh, India

**Shruti Shiromwar**
Ph.D. Research Scholar
Universiti Sains Malaysia
Penang, Malaysia

**Abdel Nasser B. Singab**
Department of Pharmacognosy Faculty
    of Pharmacy
Ain Shams University
Cairo, Egypt
Center for Drug Discovery Research
    and Development
Ain Shams University
Cairo, Egypt

**Ms. Alka Singh**
Bhupal Nobles' Institute of
    Pharmaceutical Sciences
Bhupal Nobles' University
School of Pharmaceutical Sciences and
    Technology
Sardar Bhagwan Singh University
India

**Sudarshan Singh**
Department of Pharmaceutical Sciences
    Faculty of Pharmacy
Chiang Mai University
Thailand

**Sunita Singh**
Department of Chemistry
Navyug Kanya Mahavidyalaya
University of Lucknow
Lucknow, India

**Manmohan Singhal**
Faculty of Pharmacy
DIT University
Dehradun, Uttrakhand, India

**Hagar A. Sobhy**
Department of Pharmacognosy Faculty
    of Pharmacy
Ain Shams University
Cairo, Egypt

Center for Drug Discovery Research
    and Development
Ain Shams University
Cairo, Egypt

**A. D. de Souza**
Centro Universitário das Américas
FAM São Paulo
São Paulo, Brazil

**Ms. Jyotsana Suyal**
Uttaranchal Institute of Pharmaceutical
    Sciences
Uttaranchal University
School of Pharmaceutical and
    Population Health Informatics
DIT University
Dehradun, Uttarakhand, India

**Antoaneta Trendafilova**
Institute of Organic Chemistry with
    Centre of Phytochemistry
Bulgarian Academy of Sciences Sofia,
    Bulgaria

**V. C. Cajiao Checchin**
Instituto de Investigaciones
    Fisicoquímicas Teóricas y Aplicadas
    (INIFTA)
CCT La Plata, CONICET, Facultad de
    Ciencias Exactas, UNLP
La Plata, Argentina

**Ms. Shalu Verma**
Uttaranchal Institute of Pharmaceutical
    Sciences
Uttaranchal University
School of Pharmaceutical Sciences
Shri Guru Ram Rai University
Dehradun, Uttarakhand, India

**Jigar Vyas**
Sigma Institute of Pharmacy
Sigma University
Vadodara, Gujarat, India

# Preface

The global essential oils market size is going to expand in coming years due to their increasing demand from major end use industries such as cosmetics, food and beverages, personal care, and aromatherapy. Unlike most conventional medicines, drugs, essential oils have no major side effects. Such traits are projected to be the major driving factor for market growth. In recent years, a trend of green consumerism is evolving where products of natural origin get more acceptance than the chemical and synthetic ones. Properties from antioxidant to anticancer potentials of these essential oils are well studied in both *in vivo* and *in vitro* studies, providing a vast area of future research.

The book comprises 19 chapters which deal with various pharmacological aspects of essential oils and extracts obtained from different sources. **Chapter 1** describes the various sources and processes (production and post-production operations) involved in the production of essential oils. **Chapters 2** and **3** discuss the technological advancement involved in chemical characterization of essential oils and sophisticated development of various advanced techniques employed in the characterization of essential oils and their pharmaceutical preparation. **Chapter 4** deliberates the components of essential oils as building blocks of functional materials for nanomedicine using metal-phenolic networks and self-assembly approaches. **Chapters 5, 6,** and **7** discusses the application of essential oils in the management of diabetes and insomnia, and their role in Egyptian health industry. **Chapter 8** deals with important aspects of essential oils in aromatherapy while **Chapter 9** describes the pharmacological applications of Brazilian aromatic species. **Chapter 10** discusses the pharmacological aspects and chemical characterization of *Syzygium aromaticum* essential oil. **Chapter 11** describes the advanced application of *Thymus zygis* essential oil in treating cancer. **Chapter 12** gives an insight into the pharmacological and pharmaceutical potential of cinnamon oil. **Chapter 13** discusses the current and future trends involved in pharmacological aspects of *Ocimum basilicum* essential oil. **Chapter 14** explores the therapeutic potentials of *Thyme vulgaris* essential oils. **Chapter 15** elaborates the therapeutic potential of *Copaifera* oil-resin **Chapters 16** and **17** elaborate the pharmacological aspects of turmeric and coriander essential oils. **Chapter 18** discusses the phytochemistry and pharmacological activities and therapeutic potentials of *Nigella sativa* L. **Chapter 19** discusses the update information on the anticancer applications of essential oils.

This book provides a comprehensive compilation of past, present, and future perspectives of essential oils including their antioxidant, antimicrobial, and anticancer properties; toxicology; and chemical composition, along with effectual competency in treating disorders like diabetes, insomnia, depression, nausea, anxiety, and stress, and other practical topics obligatory for the development of this industry of essential oils.

# 1 Sources and Processes (Production and Post-Production Operations) Involved in the Production of Essential Oils

*Destaw Damtie*

## 1.1 INTRODUCTION

Essential oils (EO), also known as volatile oils, ethereal oils, aetheroleum, or simply oils which are extracted, such as oil of clove, are highly concentrated, aromatic, volatile liquids extracted from aromatic plants (Butnariu and Sarac 2018; Manion and Widder 2017) by steam distillation, hydrodistillation, solvent extraction, carbon dioxide ($CO_2$) and supercritical $CO_2$ extraction, maceration, enfleurage, cold press extraction, and turbo distillation (Hanif et al. 2019; Rios 2016).

The use of aromatic plants by ancient people as spices and remedies for the treatment of diseases and in religious ceremonies dates back to 10,000 BC (Baser and Buchbauer 2021). The history of essential oils including its distillation and industry begun in the Orient, especially in Egypt, Persia, and India (Guenther 2014). Essential oils are defined as mixtures of secondary metabolites from plants and typically exhibit a strong odor because they have more than one constituent substance (more than one constituent substances, MOCS), containing a variety of volatile terpenes, aldehydes, alcohols, ketones, and simple phenolics (Bunse et al. 2022).

The applications of essential oils are diverse (Chávez-González, Rodríguez-Herrera, and Aguilar 2016). They have good medicinal applications and are used in the treatment of different diseases including infectious diseases, depression, and anxiety, and have antifungal, antimicrobial, anticancer, and wound healing properties (Irshad et al. 2020). Essential oils are also used extensively in the perfume, cosmetics, and toiletries industries (Worwood and Worwood 2003), in agriculture, against plant pathogens and weeds (Raveau, Fontaine, and Lounès-Hadj Sahraoui 2020), and as promising alternatives to chemical insecticides (Campolo et al. 2018). For instance, they serve as ecofriendly tools for mosquito control (Muturi et al. 2019).

DOI: 10.1201/9781003389774-1

The broad bioactivities of essential oils go to the various active components in each essential oil. Interactions between these components may lead to synergistic, additive, or antagonist effects (Katiki et al. 2017). The synergistic effect can be defined as the ability of EO components to act together with the antibiotic component to increase the activity of the EO against multi-drug resistant (MDR) bacteria (Aljaafari et al. 2019).

Essential oils consist of a variety of antimicrobial and preservative active constituents (e.g., terpenes, terpenoids, carotenoids, coumarins, curcumins) that have great significance in the food industry (Pandey et al. 2017). Sections 1.1.1 to 1.1.8 which follow show the major constituents of essential oils with antimicrobial, antioxidant, antiviral, analgesic, anticancer, insecticidal, anti-parasitic, and anti-inflammatory properties, respectively.

### 1.1.1 ANTIMICROBIAL

Essential oils with major components of methyl disulfide, allyl sulfide, allyl disulfide, allyl trisulfide, trimethylene trisulfide, allyl tetrasulfide, cinnamaldehyde, eugenol, copaene, β-caryophyllene, caryophyllene, thymol, p-cymene, γ-terpinene, linalool, sabinyl monoterpenes, terpinen-4-ol, carvacrol, eugenyl acetate, methylchalvicol, methyl eugenol, methyl cinnamate, 1,8-cineole, 2(E)-decanal, 2(E)dodecenal, limonene, citral, α-terpinyl acetate, β-sesquiphellandrene, zingiberene, borneol, verbenone, camphor, a-pinene, menthol, menthone, menthyl acetate, menthofurane, β-pinene, eucalyptol, coronarin-E, α-pinene, 10-*epi*-γ-eudesmol, methyl salicylate, fenchol, 1,2-cyclohexanedione dioxime, 1,4-octadiene, germacrene D, spathulenol, caryophyllene oxide, iridodial, β-monoenol acetate, actinidine, anethole, estragole, geraniol, and cinnamyl alcohol have antimicrobial (antifungal and antibacterial) activities (Chouhan, Sharma, and Guleria 2017; Perricone et al. 2015; de Oliveira et al. 2018).

### 1.1.2 ANTIOXIDANT

Essential oils with the main active components like thymol, carvacrol, γ-terpinene, p-cymene, eugenol, α-terpinolene, 1,8-cineole, thymoquinone, D-limonene, α-pinene, bornyl acetate, β-caryophyllene, α-guaiene, germacrene D, linalool, methyl chavicol, carvone, trans-anethole, limonene, camphor, and camphene are reported for their antioxidant activities (de Oliveira et al. 2018; Amorati, Foti, and Valgimigli 2013; Rassem, Nour, and Yunus 2018).

### 1.1.3 ANTIVIRAL

Essential oils with caryophyllene oxide, guaiol, chrysanthenyl acetate, limonene oxide, α-thujone, cis-carveol, carvone, limonene, camphor, β-thujone, chamazulene, artemiseole, artemisia alcohol, borneol, τ-cadinol, 1,8-cineole, thymohydroquinone dimethyl ether, β-caryophyllene, α-copaene, himachalol, β-himachalene, α-himachalene, eugenol, linalool, (E)−cinnamaldehyde (E)−cinnamyl acetate, eugenyl acetate, benzyl benzoate, linalyl acetate, β-pinene, and γ-terpinene, sabinene, terpinen-4-ol, α-pinene, δ-3-carene, geranial, neral, geraniol, (2E,4E)-decadienal, γ-nonalactone, 5-pentyl-2(3H)-furanone, 3-isopropyl-1-pentanol, cis-ascaridole, m-cymene, trans-pinocarveol, globulol, p-cymene, α-terpinene, α-terpineol, camphene, cryptone, phellandral, cuminal, germacrene D, bicyclogermacrene, carveol, γ-muurolene, citronellal, β-eudesmol, α-muurolene, β-gurjunene, γ-eudesmol, (Z)-β-ocimene, spathulenol, decanal, decanol, 2-undecanone, decanoic acid, dodecanal, 2-tridecanone, fenchone, curzerene, cis-pinocamphone, trans-pinocamphone, β-phellandrene, (E)-anethole, myrcene, terpinene-4-ol, lavandulol, lavandulyl acetate, p-mentha-1(7),8-diene, 1-octen-3-ol, calamene, leptospermone, δ-cadinene, flavesone, viridiflorene, isoleptospermone, bicyclosesquiphellandrene, carvacrol, o-cymene, piperitenone oxide (= rotundifolone), thymol, α-bisabolol oxide A, α-bisabolol oxide B, bisabolone oxide A, cis-bicycloether (= (Z)-spiroether), (E)-β-farnesene, terpinolene, methyl eugenol, valencene, β-cubebene, α-cadinol, menthol, menthone, isomenthone, menthyl acetate, isopulegol, cis-piperitone epoxide, pulegone, α-bulnesene, α-humulene, trans-sabinene hydrate, carvacrol methyl ether, hexahydrofarnesyl acetone (= phytone), 2,4-di-t-butylphenol, phytol, hexadecene, octadecene, citronellol, citronellyl formate, geranyl formate, verbenone, 3-octanone, (Z)-α-santalol, (Z)-β-santalol, (Z)-trans-α-bergamotol, artemisia ketone, alloaromadendrene, (E)-β-damascenone, α-gurjunene, α-zingiberene, ar-curcumene, β-sesquiphellandrene, α-farnesene, α-phellandrene, and β-bisabolene as their main constituents have demonstrated antiviral activities (da Silva et al. 2020).

### 1.1.4 ANALGESIC

EOs possessing γ-terpinene, limonene, myrcene, geraniol, citronellal, eugenol, hexyl butyrate, hofmeisterin III, 1,8-cineole, α-pinene, β-caryophyllene, myristicin, thymol, carvacrol, α-bisabolol oxide B, piperitenone oxide, linalool, (E)-methyl cinnamate, neral, geranial, caryophyllene oxide, germacrene, 14-hydroxy-9-epicaryophyllene, δ-cadinene, δ-guaiene, γ-muurolene, α-bisabolol, zingiberene, and zerumbone as their main components have analgesic properties (Sarmento-Neto et al. 2015).

### 1.1.5 ANTICANCER

Essential oils reported for their anticancer activities possessed santolina alcohol, borneol, sabinol, methyl chavicol, α-thujone, terpinyl acetate, sabinene, α-pinene, α-thujene, myrcene, hexadecanoic acid, (z,z)-9,12-octadecadienoic acid, tetradecanoic acid, α-humulene, 7-epi-α-eudesmol, thymol, isopropyl isothiocyanate, γ-terpinene, trans-chrysanthenyl acetate, (E)-cinnamaldehyde, eugenol, β-caryophyllene, 2-decenoic acid, 2-methyl-5-hexenenitrile, 3-butenyl isothiocyanate, p-cymene, ascaridole, epicurzerenone, curdione, α-cadinol, caryophyllene oxide, α-muurolol, syn-7-hydroxy-7-anisylnorbornene, pregeijerene, cis-α-terpineol, 6,11-oxidoacor-4-ene, citronella, globulol, aromadendrene, limonene, 1,8-cineole, (E)-β-ionone, hexahydrofarnesylacetone, 1-p-menthen-8-ethyl acetate, (z)-citral, (E)-citral, eucalyptol, α-gurjunene, β-selinene, α-bisabololoxidea, (E)-β-farnesene, menthol, α-phellandrene, β-elemene, methyl cinnamate, (E)-nerolidol, carvacrol, citronellol, trans-geraniol, 10-epi-eudesmol, pinene, terpinen-4-ol, β-myrcene, santalol, bornyl acetate, camphene, thymoquinone, viridiflorene, β-terpineol, thujones, fenchone, nerol, kaempferol, geraniol, 4,5-dimetiltiazol-2-il, 2,5-difeniltetrazólio, d-limonene, perylic, 1-phenanthrenecarboxylic acid, α-caryophyllene, azulene benzenedicarboxylic acid, linalool, myrtenyl acetate, myrtenol, pulegol, citronellyl acetate, cinnamic aldehyde, cinnamyl aldehyde, betulinic acid, triterpenes, 2-cyclohexen-1-one, 4-ethynyl-4-hydroxy-3,5,5-trimethyl, monoterpenes, oxygenated (monoterpenes, sesquiterpenes, diterpenes), cis-β-ocimene, cis-tagetone, and trans-tagetenone as their major components (Bhalla, Gupta, and Jaitak 2013; de Oliveira et al. 2018).

### 1.1.6 INSECTICIDAL

The main constituents of essential oils with insecticidal properties include terpinen-4-ol, γ-terpinene, menthol, α-pinene, α-thujene, sabinene, β-pinene, bornyl acetate, camphene, limonene, diallyl disulfide, diallyl trisulfide, 1,8-cineole, β-caryophyllene, estragol, linalool, cuminaldehyde, p-cymene, eugenol, methyleugenol, citronellal, cis-thujanol, piperitone, α-phellandrene, camphor, methyl salicylate, geraniol, geranyl acetate, trans-anethole, khuenic acid, linalyl acetate, α-zingiberene, β-sesquiphellandrene, e-(trans)-β-farnesene, citral, and 2-tridecanone (Demeter et al. 2021; Bossou et al. 2013).

### 1.1.7 ANTI-PARASITIC

Ascaridole, carvacrol, caryophyllene oxide, (E)-cinnamaldehyde, eugenol, curzerene, γ-elemene, trans-β-elemenone, borneol, epi-d-muurolol, d-bisabolol, precocene I, eucalyptol, safrole, δ-cadinene, δ-cadinol, β-eudesmol, γ-gurjunene, and cedrene are among the major components of essential oils that have anti-parasitic properties (Bossou et al. 2013).

### 1.1.8 ANTI-INFLAMMATORY

Essential oils with anti-inflammatory activities contain active components mainly β-eudesmol, (E)-β-caryophyllene, caryophyllene oxide, t-muurolol, β-pinene, longiborneol, α-pinene, (E)-caryophyllene, iso-elemicin, α-cadinol, 2-isopropyl benzoic acid, 1,8-cineole, camphor, thymol, carvacrol, p-cymene, limonene, γ-terpinene, sabinene, geranial, neral, β-myrcene, geranyl acetate, α-phellandrene, dill ether, linalool, linalyl acetate, nerolidol, Z,E-farnesol, borneol, caryophyllene, and ledol (Kushwah and Gupta 2019).

## 1.2 SOURCES OF ESSENTIAL OILS

Essential oils involve a large range of plant oils which are highly aromatic. They are found mainly in the flowers, buds, leaves, twigs, bark, wood, roots, rhizomes, bulbs, fruits, peels, seeds, and resin of plants. A few of them are obtained from animal sources or are produced by microorganisms (Lawal and Ogunwande 2013). Typically, essential oils are found in superior plants (about 50 families) belonging to orders of angiosperms (Asterales, Laurales, Magnoliales, Zimgiberales, etc.) or ginsenosides (Pinales), but also known as sesquiterpenic lactone sesquiterpene volatile, or algae that produce halogenated sesquiterpenes (Butnariu and Sarac 2018). *Agavaceae, Anacardiaceae, Annonaceae, Apiaceae, Asteraceae, Burseraceae, Canellaceae, Cannabaceae, Cistaceae, Cupressaceae, Dipterocarpaceae, Ericaceae, Fabaceae, Geraniaceae, Illiciaceae, Lamiaceae, Lauraceae, Malvaceae, Myristicaceae, Myrtaceae, Oleaceae, Orchidaceae, Parmeliaceae, Pinaceae, Piperaceae, Poaceae, Rosaceae, Rubiaceae, Rutaceae, Santalaceae, Solanaceae, Styracaceae, Tiliaceae, Valerianaceae, Verbenaceae, Violaceae,* and *Zingiberaceae* are among the essential oil-producing plant families (Tisserand and Young 2013). The aromatic plants biosynthesize essential oils in specialized cell types, such as osmophores, glandular trichomes, and ducts and cavities, present on different parts of these plants (Rehman et al. 2016).

Osmophores are specialized scent glands on floral organs in the form of flaps, hairs, or brushes that have the fragrance-producing properties to attract pollinators. Trichomes (hairs) are various extensions of the epidermis, some of which are glandular, such as terpenes (essential oils, carotenoids, saponins, or rubber), tannins, or crystals (such as salt) (Glimn-Lacy and Kaufman 2006). Secretory ducts are elongated cavities. Some cells of the cavity are secretory epithelial cells where the oils are biosynthesized. They are found in all of the families *Apiaceae, Asteraceae, Clusiaceae,* and *Pinaceae* (Svoboda, Svoboda, and Syred 2001).

The major constituents of *Agavaceae* are mono-2-ethylhexyl phthalate, 1,2-benzene dicarboxylic acid, n-docosane, and eicosane (Rizwan et al. 2012). *Anacardiaceae* EOs possess β-phellandrene, limonene (17.5%), methyl chavicol, germacrene B, trans-α-bergamotene, germacrene D, β-copaene, linalool, α-cadinol, β-caryophyllene, 9-epi-(E)-caryophyllene, β-phellandrene, α-phellandrene, hexadecanoic acid, epi-α-cadinol, β-bisabolene, epi-α-muurolol, α-pinene, (E)-β-ocimene, α-terpinolene, δ-3-carene, α-gurjunene, β-selinene, α-selinene, β-sesquiphellandrene, α-zingiberene, myrcene, β-gurjunene, muurolene, α-humulene, epi- bicyclosesquiphellandrene, and β-pinene (Kossouoh et al. 2008; Montanari et al. 2012; Damić et al. 2010; Zoghbi et al. 2014; Amhamdi et al. 2009).

The most abundant components of *Annonaceae* EOs are α-pinene, β-pinene, limonene, (E)-caryophyllene, bicyclogermacrene, caryophyllene oxide, germacrene D, spathulenol, and β-elemene, β-caryophyllene, p-cymene, g-elemene, δ-cadinene, bicycloelemene, α-zingiberene aromadendrene, β-selinene, α-terpinene, α-santalene, terpinen-4-ol, trans-α-bergamotene, and allo-ocimene (Cascaes et al. 2021; Fournier, Leboeuf, and Cavé 1999; Thang et al. 2013).

The main constituents of *Apiaceae* EOs are (E)-anethole, thymol, D-limonene, carotol, δ-3-carene, methyl isoeugenol, estragole, limonene, dillapiole, pulegone, (Z)-sec-butyl propenyl disulfide, (E)-sec-butyl propenyl disulfide, carvone, γ-terpinene, α-phellandrene, myristicin, 2-dodecen-1-al, (Z)-sec-butylpropenyl disulphide, (Z)-β-ocimene, p-cymene, 2-methylbutyrate, curzerene, β-pinene, anethole, perillaldehyde, p-cumin aldehyde, β-selinene, germacrone, disulfide methyl 1-(methylthio)propyl, cuminaldehyde, ρ-cymene, germacrene B, α-pinene, 1,3,8-p-menthatriene, myrcene, cis-ocimene, lavandulyl acetate, o-cymene, carvacrol, fenchone, β-myrcene, β-bisabolene, α-methyl-benzenemethanol, caprinic alcohol, sabinene, bicyclogermacrene, β-phellandrene, terpinolene, thymol methyl ether, borneol, 1,8-cineole, and geijerene (Spinozzi et al. 2021).

The main components of *Asteraceae* EOs β-caryophyllene, germacrene-D, α-copaene, β-pinene, α-Bisabolol, terpinolene, spathulenol, caryophyllene oxide, bicyclogermacrene, 5-indanol, p-cymen-8-ol, limonene, germacrene A, α-humulene, *trans*-nerolidol, β-farnesene, β-sesquiphellandrene, p-methoxy-β-cyclopropylstyrene, heptadecane, p-methoxy-humulene oxide, benzene acetaldehyde, (*E*)-chrysanthenyl acetate, 1,4-hydroxy-α-humulene, santolina triene, 1,8-cineole, *δ*-cadinene, (*E*)-caryophyllene, Sabinene, α-phellandrene, (Z)-*β*-ocimene, (E)-*β*-ocimene, dihydrotagetone, allo-ocimene, (Z)-tagetone, (E)-tagetone, (Z)-ocimenone, and (E)-ocimenone. Camphor, borneol, camphene, intermedeol, α-pinene, (E)-pinocarveol (Silvério et al. 2013; Pires et al. 2006; Kasim et al. 2014; Cazella et al. 2019; Chehregani et al. 2010; Riccobono et al. 2017; Gakuubi et al. 2016; El Yaagoubi et al. 2021)

The main components of *Burseraceae* Eos are α-pinene, α-phellandrene, p-cymene, 1,8-cineole, p-acetyl anisole, δ-3-carene, limonene, terpinolene, α-terpineol, β-pinene, β-phellandrene, 3-carene, eucalyptol, (E)-2,3-epoxycarene, 1,5-isopropyl-2-methylbicyclo[3.1.0]hex-3-en-2-ol, (3E,5E)-2,6-dimethyl-1,3,5,7-octatetraene, 1-(2,4-dimethylphenyl)ethanol, 3,4-dimethylstyrene, α-campholenal, α-terpineol, isoincensole, isoincensole acetate, verticilla-4(20),7,11-triene, α-terpinene, α-thujene, verticiol, caryophyllene, methyl cycloundecanecarboxylate, incensol, terpinen-4-ol, along with n-octanol, n-octyl acetate, trans-verbenol, terpinen-4-ol, hydrocarbon, E-β-ocimene, E-caryophyllene, boswellic acids, acymene, 2-hydroxy-5-methoxyacetophenone, camphor, germacrene D, β-caryophyllene, myrcene, β-caryophyllene, α-humulene, 2-phenylethanol, γ-terpinene, terpinen-4-ol, nerolidol, (E)-β-farnesene, δ-cadinene, α-copaene, β-elemene, bisabolol, β-sesquiphellandrene, α-oxobisabolene, γ-bisabolene, α-selinene, cadina-1,4-diene, germacrene B, t-muurolol, caryophyllene oxide, α-cadinol, dl-Limonene, isofuranogermacrene, lindestrene, furanoeudesma-1,3-diene, furanodiene, curzerene, germacrone, 2–0-acetyl-8,12-epoxygermacra1(10),4,7,11-tetraene, sabinene, α-, β-amyrin, hop-22(29)-en-3β-ol, furanoeudesma-1,4-diene-6-one, trans-dihydro-α-terpineol, aromadendrene, benzenoids, trans-caryophyllene, spathulenol, trans-α-bergamotene, 9-epi-caryophyllene, trans-isolongifolanone, 14-hydroxi-9-epi-caryophyllene, α-terpinolene, γ-elemene, selin-11-en-4-α-ol, and khusimone (Murthy et al. 2016).

The main components of *Canellaceae* essential oils are 1,8-cineole, terpinen-4-ol, α-terpinyl acetate, α-terpineol, linalool, caryophyllene oxide, (E)-caryophyllene, myrcene, α-pinene, β-pinene, sabinene, limonene, β-phellandrene, bicyclogermacrene, spathulenol, drimenol, E-nerolidol, (E)-β-ocimene, (Z)-β-ocimene, α-humulene, and β-caryophyllene (Abaul et al. 1995; de Castro Oliveira et al. 2019; Khumalo et al. 2019; Lawal et al. 2014; Andrade et al. 2013). *Cannabaceae* essential oils contain β-caryophyllene, β-myrcene, α-humulene, caryophyllene oxide, decane, α-pinene, myrcene, terpinolene, limonene, (*E*)-*β*-ocimene, *β*-pinene, 9-epi-caryophyllene, cannabidiol, caryophyllene, and humulene as their major components (El Bakali et al. 2022; Gulluni et al. 2018; Pieracci et al. 2021; Vuerich et al. 2019). The essential oils of the *Cistaceae* family include major components like viridiflorol, myristicin, γ-gurjunene, bornyl acetate, pinocarveol, labdane diterpenoid

13-epi-manoyl oxide, trans-pinocarveol, p-cymene, ledol, sclareol, τ-cadinol, myrtenol, borneol, hexadecanoic acid, terpinen-4-ol, and α-pinene, spathulenol, and decanoic acid (Benali et al. 2020; Oller-López et al. 2005; El Karkouri et al. 2021; Baldemir et al. 2014).

The main components of the EOs of *Cupressaceae* are α-pinene, β-pinene, δ-3-carene, 3-carene, α-cedrol, caryophyllene, α-humulene, limonene, dl-limonene, α-terpinolene, α-terpinyl acetate, (-)-bornyl acetate, isobornyl acetate, α-cadinol, τ-muurolol, α-terpinene, γ-terpinene, terpinen-4-ol, γ-elemene, linalool, cuparene, δ-cadinene, α-cedrene, cedrol, α-cedrol, β-cedrene, umbellulone, sabinene, myr-cene, β-myrcene, elemol, and 3-cyclohexen-1-ol (Park and Woo 2022; Guleria, Kumar, and Tiku 2008; Carroll et al. 2011; Asgary et al. 2013; Muhizi et al. 2021; Yohana et al. 2022; Khamis and Chai 2021; Hashemi and Safavi 2012).

The main components of *Dipterocarpaceae* essential oils include α-gurjunene, γ-gurjunene, (-)-isoledene, alloaromadendrene, β-caryophyllene, spathulenol, terpinen-4-ol, α-terpineol, α-pinenes, β-pinenes, globulol, myrcene, limonene, α-thujene, sabinene, bicyclogermacrene, eugenol, and γ-terpinene (Kuspradini, Putri, and Mitsunaga 2018; Yongram et al. 2019).

*Ericaceae* essential oils contain α-pinene, δ-cadinene, β-pinene, limonene, δ-amorphene, α-muurolene, (E)-caryophyllene, decenal, α-terpineol, caryophyl-lene, and palmitic acid (Dosoky et al. 2016; Al-Mijalli, Mrabti, Ouassou, et al. 2022; Castrillón Cardona et al. 2015). *Fabaceae* essential oils have major com-ponents like camphor, β-caryophyllene, δ-cadinene, α-muurolene, α-calacorene, caryophyllene oxide, incensole, phytone, pentadecanal, α-pinene, and *iso*-phytol, phytol, hexadecanoic acid, octadecenoic, hexadecanoic acids, etc. (Khallouki et al. 2002; Owolabi et al. 2020; Moronkola and Oladosu 2013). *Geraniaceae* essential oils contain menthol, menthene, eremophilene, isoborneol, isogeraniol, α-pinene, linalyl acetate, 3-carene, citronellol, citronellyl formate, L-menthone, linalool, geraniol, β-citronellol, δ-selinene, etc. (Al-Mijalli, Mrabti, Assaggaf, et al. 2022; Yohana et al. 2022; Boukhris et al. 2013). *Illiciaceae* essential oils possess euca-lyptol, α-terpineol, carvone, d-limonene, trans-carveol, linalool, linalyl acetate, safrole, methyl eugenol, and so on (Wang et al. 2011; Kim et al. 2009; Tucker and Maciarello 1999).

*Lamiaceae* essential oils' main components include menthol, menthone, isom-enthone, 1,8-cineole, eugenol, terpineol-4; 4- terpineol, sabinene hydrate, thymol, α-thujene, α-pinene, sabinene, β-pinene, 1-octen3-ol, 3-carene, (E)-β-ocimene, α-terpinyl acetate, β-caryophyllene, germacrene D, carvacrol, p-cymene, and c-terpi-nene (Ramos da Silva et al. 2021). The major components of *Lauraceae* essen-tial oils are 1,8-cineole, safrole, trans-cinnamaldehyde, and β-caryophyllene (Damasceno et al. 2019); the *Malvaceae* EOs are β-bisabolol, myrtenal, trans-2-cis-6-nonadienal, cineole, hexatriacontane, tetratetracontane, 2,5-Di-tert-octyl-p-benzoquinone, α-selinene, β-pinene, butyl phthalate, Z-8-octadecen-1-ol acetate, 9-hexyl heptadecane, arachidic acid, tetracosane, 1-hexacosanol, phytol; α-farnesene, n-hexadecanoic acid, farnesol, 2-methylheptadecane, heptacosane, 2,6,10,14-tetramethyl, etc. (Hasimi et al. 2017; Akwu et al. 2021; Thompson et al. 1971). The major components of *Myristicaceae* essential oils are sabinene, α-pinene, α-phellandrene, terpinen-4-ol, and β-pinene (Kapoor et al. 2013; Ogunwande et al.

2003); the *Myrtaceae* are α-pinene, 1,8-cineole, p-menth-1-en-8-ol, and caryophyllene (Siddique et al. 2015).

*Oleaceae*'s EOs have major components of benzyl acetate, benzyl benzoate, phytol, linalool, isophytol, geranyl linalool, methyl linoleate, eugenol, α-farnesene, β-maaliene, n-hexadecanoic acid, etc. (Temraz et al. 2009; Yangui et al. 2021) and that of *Orchidaceae* essential oils are methyl-(E)-p-methoxycinnamate, 13-heptadecyn-1-ol, 2,5-dimethoxybenzyl alcohol, 4-(1,1,3,3-tetramethylbutyl)-phenol, etc. (Mokni et al. 2016).

*Pinaceae* are sources of α-pinene, β-pinene, limonene, camphene, myrcene β-phellandrene, bornyl acetate, *trans-(E)*-caryophyllene, germacrene D, δ-cadinene, α-terpineol, borneol, terpinen-4-ol, camphene hydrate, *cis*-3-hexen-1-ol, Δ³-carene, hydrosol, maltol, etc. (Hmamouchi et al. 2001; Tumen et al. 2010; Karapandzova et al. 2014; Garneau et al. 2012). *Piperaceae* serve as sources of safrole, terpinolene, α-(E)-ocimene, bicyclogermacrene, trans-β-caryophyllene, germacrene D, α-selinene, β-pinene, β-selinene, α-cubebene, trans-nerolidol, caryophyllene oxide, β-elemene, curzerene, germacrene B, 1-butyl-3,4-methylenedioxybenzene, *trans*-caryophyllene, α-pinene, δ-cadinene, limonene, spathulenol, (E)-nerolidol, β-caryophyllene, borneol, α-amorphene, benzyl benzoate, myrcene, bicycloelemene, α-copaene, 1, 8-cineole (5.7%), etc. (Sauter et al. 2012; Benitez, Meléndez León, and Stashenko 2009; da Silva et al. 2016; Bezerra et al. 2020; Salleh, Ahmad, and Yen 2014).

The *Poaceae* family essential oils also serve as a source of geraniol, piperitone, elemol, limonene, 5-epi-7-epi-α-eudesmol, eudesmanediol, hinesol, cis-p-menth-2-en-1-ol, trans-p-menth-2-en-1-ol, β-eudesmol, agarospirol, 7-epi-α-eudesmol, α-eudesmol, γ-eudesmol, shyobunol, selina-6-en-4-ol, p-menth-2-en-1-ols, citral (a and b), borneol, isopulegol, 6-methyl hept-5-en-2- one, geranyl acetate, γ-terpinene, α-thujene, α-pinene, sabinene, n-decanol, α-terpinyl acetate, β-caryophyllene, α-humulene, germacrene D, β-bisabolene, γ-cadinene, and 1,8-cineole (Verma et al. 2019; Ganjewala 2009; Kumar et al. 2013). The essential oils of *Rosaceae* contain citronellol, geraniol, nonadecane, elemol, α-eudesmol, methyl myrtenate, limonene, α-thujone, myrtenyl acetate, linolenic acid, and others (Almasirad et al. 2007; Hudifa et al. 2013; Dhami et al. 2018; Schultze and Vollmann 1995).

*Rubiaceae* essential oils contain main components such as β-caryophyllene, β-elemene, farnesyl butanoate, myrcene, trans-nerolidol, α-caryophyllene, *trans-β*-caryophyllene, caryophyllene oxide, τ-cadinol, pentadecanal, methyl (7Z, 10Z, 13Z)-hexadecatrienoate, 2,3- dimethylnaphthoquinone, α-pinene, geranial, ar-turmerone, 10-epi-γ-eudesmol, trans-α-bergamotene, transcalamenene, δ-cadinene, oxygenated sesquiterpenoids, spathulenol, and τ-muurolol, α-cadinol (Rao, Lai, and Gao 2017; Rasoarivelo et al. 2011; Owolabi et al. 2013; Avoseh et al. 2020; Owolabi et al. 2022).

*Rutaceae* essential oils have 2-undecanone, 2-nonanone, octyl acetate, limonene, sabinene, citronellal, linalool, hedycaryol, β-caryophyllene, α-humulene, α-pinene, β-phellandrene, α-terpinene, (E)-β-ocimene, λ-terpinene, germacrene D, and β-selinene as main components (Krayni et al. 2018; Md Othman et al. 2016; Orlanda and Nascimento 2015; Dai et al. 2012). *Santalaceae* are sources of α- and β-santalol, (Z)-α-santalol, and (Z)-β-santalol (Xin-Hua et al. 2012; Braun et al.

2014). On the other hand, *Solanaceae* essential oils can be sources of (E)-phytol, pentadecanal, pentadecane, α-humulene, β-caryophyllene, ethyl palmitate, methyl salicylate, *β*-elemol, germacrene D, dillapiole, α-cadinol, *p*-cymene, (E)-1-(2,6,6-trimethyl-1,3-cyclohexadien-1-yl)-2-buten-1-one, *β*-damascenone, α-phellandrene, *β*-pinene, α-bisabolol acetate, (Z,E)-4,6,8-megastigmatriene, linalyl butanoate, 8-methylene-tricyclo[3.2.1.0(2,4)]octane, limonene, etc. (Essien et al. 2012; Kouao et al. 2021; Taherpour et al. 2017). *Styracaceae* essential oils also contain (E)-2-hexenal, linalool, geranial, tridecanal, dodecane, α-terpineol, and eugenol (9.9%) (Tayoub et al. 2006).

The main components of *Tiliaceae* essential oils are hexadecanoic acid, 2-phenethyl benzoate, β-ionone, geranyl acetone, farnesyl acetone, hexahydrofarnesyl acetone, 6,10,14-trimethyl-2-pentadecanone, tricosane, heneicosane, nonanal, octadeca-9,12-dienoic acid (Toker et al. 1999; Kowalski et al. 2017). *Valerianaceae* essential oils are rich sources of patchouli alcohol, maaliol, seychellene, bornyl acetate, α-guaiene, α-bulnesene/δ-guaiene, 7-epi-α-selinene, kessane, viridiflorol, α-patchoulene, β-guaiene, valeranone, spathulenol, calarene/ß-gurjunene, α-santalene, and ß-patchoulene (Raina and Negi 2015; Georgiev, St. Stojanova, and At. Tchapkanov 1999).

*Verbenaceae* essential oils possess geranial, neral, limonene, geraniol, germacrene D, α-curcumene, bicyclogermacrene, β-caryophyllene, (Z)-β-ocimene, geranyl acetate, isoborneol, bornyl acetate, α-humulene, α-fenchene, 1.8-cineole, carvone, carvacrol, and *p*-cymene as their main components (Argyropoulou et al. 2007; de Morais et al. 2016; Majolo et al. 2022). *Violaceae* essential oils can be the main sources of 1-phenyl butanone, linalool, benzyl alcohol, α-cadinol, globulol, viridiflorol, pulegone, epi-α-cadinol, terpinen-4-ol, germacrene A, paramethyl anisole, Bis (2- ethylhexyl) maleate, 2, 4, 4, 6-tetramethyl-2-heptene, hexen-3-ol, and Cis verbenol (Chandra et al. 2015, 2017). The *Zingiberaceae* family essential oils can also be sources of components like zingiberene, turmerone, methyl chavicol, and γ-terpinene, β-pinene, borneol, α-pinene, myrtenal, dihydroedulan I, n-hexadecanol, α-copaene, β-caryophyllene, 1,8-cineole, β-myrcene, camphor, *p*-cymene, geraniol, α-fenchyl acetate, ocimene, and methyl cinnamate (Norajit, Laohakunjit, and Kerdchoechuen 2007; Tuan et al. 2022; Santos et al. 2012; Van et al. 2021).

## 1.3 PLANT MATERIAL PREPARATION AND ESSENTIAL OIL EXTRACTION

### 1.3.1 HARVESTING AND PREPARATION OF PLANTS FOR ESSENTIAL OIL EXTRACTION

Essential oils are complex blends of volatile compounds produced by living organisms and isolated from a whole plant or a plant part of known taxonomic origin (Franz and Novak 2020). It is advisable to collect plants during the flowering phenophase in the case of flowers, semi-mature leaves (when they are tender, before flowering), and roots (after plants complete their life cycles) in order to have a high essential oil content (Tripathi and Hazarika 2014; Détár et al. 2021). Furthermore, early morning is the best time to harvest plant parts for maximum quality and yield of essential oils (Younis et al. 2009). The collected plant or plant parts must be identified by a taxonomist into its species, genus, family, order, class levels and pressed specimens should be deposited in a herbarium for future reference (Bulugahapitiya 2013).

Before drying, the plant parts collected should be washed with water to remove dirt particles (Ghaffar et al. 2015). The collected parts of aromatic plants are often dried before extraction to reduce moisture content (Ashafa, Grierson, and Afolayan 2008). "Drying" is the phase of the post-harvest system during which the product is rapidly dried until it reaches the "safe moisture" level, i.e., 10%. Proper drying extends the shelf life, conserves the fresh characteristics, impedes the growth of fungi and molds, reduces transportation costs, and maximizes storage space (Al-Hamdani et al. 2022). The use of different drying techniques has an impact on essential oil composition and yield. For instance, a study conducted by Hazrati et al. (2021) compared the EO yield and composition of *Salvia lavandulifolia* from fresh, shade-dried, sunlight-dried, freeze-dried, microwave-dried, and oven-dried (40, 60, and 80°C). Shade-, sun-, and oven-drying (40°C) were found to be the most important techniques for attaining maximum yields of EO, in descending order (Hazrati et al. 2021).

### 1.3.2 EXTRACTION OF ESSENTIAL OILS

Hydrodistillation (water distillation, water and steam distillation, and steam distillation) and solvent extraction are used to extract essential oils (Elyemni et al. 2019; Aramrueang, Asavasanti, and Khanunthong 2019). In water distillation, fresh or dried raw plant materials are soaked in a container containing water. The essential oils are extracted by the diffusion mechanism by heating the water with plants until the steam comes out (AL-Hilphy 2017). Water and steam distillation involves immersion of plant material in water in a distiller that has a heat source and is fed with live steam into the water and plant material mixture (Handa et al. 2008). Steam distillation is the most popular method used to extract and isolate essential oils from plants for use in natural products. Steam is generated outside the still in a satellite steam generator generally referred to as a boiler (Handa et al. 2008). The steam from the boiling water and steam carries the vapor of the volatiles to a condenser; both are cooled and return to the liquid or solid state, while the non-volatile residues remain behind the boiling container. The volatiles are not miscible with water, which will spontaneously form a distinct phase after condensation, allowing them to be separated by decantation or with a separatory funnel.

For plant parts that are too delicate for distillation (such as flowers), solvent extraction is used to extract essential oils. Solvent extraction uses solvents such as methanol, ethanol, hexane, or petroleum ether (SonomaPress 2014). The resulting mixture of solvent, plant oils, and botanical solids is typically filtered and vacuum distilled to remove as much solvent as possible (FocusHerb 2022). Essential oils can also be extracted with liquid $CO_2$ under pressure. $CO_2$ behaves similar to all other extraction solvents except that it can be used as a subcritical liquid or as a supercritical liquid (De Silva 1999). *Expression* (cold press extraction) is the method employed to extract essential oils from the oil sacs contained in the rinds of fruit such as orange, lemon, bergamot, mandarin, and tangerine. This was a very labor-intensive process, involving pressing the rind into the sponges, which absorbed the essential oil, and were then squeezed out. Today it is done by machines (Worwood and Worwood 2003).

### 1.3.3  POST-PRODUCTION OPERATIONS OF ESSENTIAL OILS

Essential oils extracted through distillation may contain some dissolved water. If the water is not removed, it can cause turbidity and unwanted aging reactions in the oil. Therefore, the water needs to be removed either by storing the oil in a cold environment so that the water will come out of the solution and be separated or, more preferably, it should be filtered through a bed of anhydrous sodium sulfate (De Silva 1995). The essential oils should be stored in a refrigerator (4°C) until use to retain their primary quality (Mehdizadeh, Ghasemi Pirbalouti, and Moghaddam 2017). They should be kept in dark, glass bottles to protect the contents from the sun's rays (Worwood and Worwood 2003).

## 1.4  CONCLUSIONS

Essential oils of aromatic plants are composed of an arsenal of chemical constituents which possess biological activities. Essential oil components may result in antagonistic, additive, or synergistic activities. The biological activities of the essential oils of aromatic plants include antimicrobial, antioxidant, antiviral, analgesic, anticancer, insecticidal, anti-parasitic, anti-inflammatory, etc. The sources of EOs are different plant families such as *Agavaceae, Anacardiaceae, Annonaceae, Apiaceae, Asteraceae, Burseraceae, Canellaceae, Cannabaceae, Cistaceae, Cupressaceae, Dipterocarpaceae, Ericaceae, Fabaceae, Geraniaceae, Illiciaceae, Lamiaceae, Lauraceae, Malvaceae, Myristicaceae, Myrtaceae, Oleaceae, Orchidaceae, Parmeliaceae, Pinaceae, Piperaceae, Poaceae, Rosaceae, Rubiaceae, Rutaceae, Santalaceae, Solanaceae, Styracaceae, Tiliaceae, Valerianaceae, Verbenaceae, Violaceae,* and *Zingiberaceae.* To have a high essential oil content, it is advisable to collect plants during the flowering phenophase in the case of flowers, semi-mature leaves (when they are tender, before flowering), and roots (after plants complete their life cycles). The best drying condition for the collected medicinal plants is shade drying, followed by sun drying and oven drying (40°C) in descending order. The dried plant parts should be powdered and subjected to hydrodistillation (water distillation, water and steam distillation, and steam distillation) and solvent extraction of the essential oils. Essential oils extracted through distillation may contain some dissolved water. If the water is not removed, it can cause turbidity and unwanted aging reactions in the oil. The extracted essential oils should be free of water, either by storing the oil in a cold environment or by filtering through a bed of anhydrous sodium sulfate. The essential oils should be stored in a refrigerator (4°C) until use to retain their primary quality. They should be kept in dark, glass bottles to protect the contents from the sun's rays.

## REFERENCES

Abaul, Jacqueline, Lyn Udino, Paul Bourgeois, and Jean-Marie Bessière. 1995. "Composition of the essential oils of Canella winterana (L.) Gaertn." *Journal of Essential Oil Research* no. 7 (6):681–683.

Akwu, Nneka Augustina, Yougasphree Naidoo, Sadashiva Thimmegowda Channangihalli, Moganavelli Singh, Nirasha Nundkumar, and Johnson Lin. 2021. "The essential oils of Grewia Lasiocarpa E. Mey. Ex Harv.: Chemical composition, in vitro biological activity and cytotoxic effect on Hela cells." *Anais da Academia Brasileira de Ciências* no. 93.

Al-Hamdani, Anfal, Hemanatha Jayasuriya, Pankaj B Pathare, and Zahir Al-Attabi. 2022. "Drying characteristics and quality analysis of medicinal herbs dried by an indirect solar dryer." *Foods* no. 11 (24):4103.

AL-Hilphy, Asaad Rehman Saeed. 2017. "Engineering interventions for extraction of essential oils from plants." In *Engineering interventions in foods and plants*, 51–85. Apple Academic Press.

Aljaafari, Mariam, Maryam Sultan Alhosani, Aisha Abushelaibi, Kok-Song Lai, and Swee-Hua Erin Lim. 2019. "Essential oils: Partnering with antibiotics." In *Essential oils-oils of nature*. IntechOpen.

Almasirad, Ali, Yaghoob Amanzadeh, Ali Taheri, and Mehrdad Iranshahi. 2007. "Composition of a historical rose oil sample (Rosa damascena Mill., Rosaceae)." *Journal of Essential Oil Research* no. 19 (2):110–112.

Al-Mijalli, Samiah Hamad, Hanae Naceiri Mrabti, Hamza Assaggaf, Ammar A Attar, Munerah Hamed, Aicha EL Baaboua, Nasreddine El Omari, Naoual El Menyiy, Zakaria Hazzoumi, and Ryan A Sheikh. 2022. "Chemical profiling and biological activities of pelargonium graveolens essential oils at three different phenological stages." *Plants* no. 11 (17):2226.

Al-Mijalli, Samiah Hamad, Hanae Naceiri Mrabti, Hayat Ouassou, Rachid Flouchi, Emad M Abdallah, Ryan A Sheikh, Mohammed Merae Alshahrani, Ahmed Abdullah Al Awadh, Hicham Harhar, and Nasreddine El Omari. 2022. "Chemical composition, antioxidant, anti-diabetic, anti-acetylcholinesterase, anti-inflammatory, and antimicrobial properties of arbutus unedo L. and Laurus nobilis L. essential oils." *Life* no. 12 (11):1876.

Amhamdi, Hassan, Fatima Aouinti, Jean Paul Wathelet, and Ali Elbachiri. 2009. "Chemical composition of the essential oil of pistacia lentiscus L. from Eastern Morocco." *Records of Natural Products* no. 3 (2).

Amorati, Riccardo, Mario C Foti, and Luca Valgimigli. 2013. "Antioxidant activity of essential oils." *Journal of Agricultural and Food Chemistry* no. 61 (46):10835–10847.

Andrade, Milene Aparecida, Maria das Graças Cardoso, Juliana De Andrade, Lucilene Fernandes Silva, Maria Luisa Teixeira, Juliana Maria Valério Resende, Ana Cristina da Silva Figueiredo, and José Gonçalves Barroso. 2013. "Chemical composition and antioxidant activity of essential oils from Cinnamodendron dinisii Schwacke and Siparuna guianensis Aublet." *Antioxidants* no. 2 (4):384–397.

Aramrueang, Natthiporn, Suvaluk Asavasanti, and Aphinya Khanunthong. 2019. "Leafy vegetables." In *Integrated processing technologies for food and agricultural by-products*, 245–272. Elsevier.

Argyropoulou, Catherine, Dimitra Daferera, Petros A Tarantilis, Costas Fasseas, and Moschos Polissiou. 2007. "Chemical composition of the essential oil from leaves of Lippia citriodora HBK (Verbenaceae) at two developmental stages." *Biochemical Systematics and Ecology* no. 35 (12):831–837.

Asgary, Sedigheh, Gholam Ali Naderi, Mohammad Reza Shams Ardekani, Amirhossein Sahebkar, Atousa Airin, Sanaz Aslani, Taghi Kasher, and Seyed Ahmad Emami. 2013. "Chemical analysis and biological activities of Cupressus sempervirens var. horizontalis essential oils." *Pharmaceutical Biology* no. 51 (2):137–144.

Ashafa, AOT, DS Grierson, and AJ Afolayan. 2008. "Effects of drying methods on the chemical composition of." *Asian Journal of Plant Sciences* no. 7 (6):603–606.

Avoseh, Nudewhenu Opeyemi, Oladipupo Adejumobi Lawal, Isiaka Ajani Ogunwande, Roberta Ascrizzi, Guido Flamini, and Elizabeth Amoo. 2020. "In vivo anti-inflammatory and anti-nociceptive activities, and chemical constituents of essential oil from the leaf of Gardenia jasminoides J. Ellis (Rubiaceae)." *Trends in Phytochemical Research* no. 4 (4):203–212.

Baldemir, Ayşe, Betül Demirci, Neslihan Şam, and Müberra Koşar. 2014. "The composition of the essential oil of *Helianthemum canum* (L.) Baumg growing in Turkey". Paper read at Natural Volatiles & Essential Oils.

Baser, K Husnu Can, and Gerhard Buchbauer. 2021. *Handbook of essential oils: Science, technology, and applications.* CRC Press.

Benali, Taoufiq, Abdelhakim Bouyahya, Khaoula Habbadi, Gokhan Zengin, Abdelmajid Khabbach, and Khalil Hammani. 2020. "Chemical composition and antibacterial activity of the essential oil and extracts of Cistus ladaniferus subsp: Ladanifer and Mentha suaveolens against phytopathogenic bacteria and their ecofriendly management of phytopathogenic bacteria." *Biocatalysis and Agricultural Biotechnology* no. 28:101696.

Benitez, Nayive Pino, Erika M Meléndez León, and Elena E Stashenko. 2009. "Essential oil composition from two species of Piperaceae family grown in Colombia." *Journal of Chromatographic Science* no. 47 (9):804–807.

Bezerra, José Weverton Almeida, Felicidade Caroline Rodrigues, Rafael Pereira da Cruz, Luiz Everson da Silva, Wanderlei do Amaral, Ricardo Andrade Rebelo, Ieda Maria Begnini, Camila Fonseca Bezerra, Marcello Iriti, and Elena Maria Varoni. 2020. "Antibiotic potential and chemical composition of the essential oil of Piper caldense C. DC. (Piperaceae)." *Applied Sciences* no. 10 (2):631.

Bhalla, Yashika, Vinay Kumar Gupta, and Vikas Jaitak. 2013. "Anticancer activity of essential oils: A review." *Journal of the Science of Food and Agriculture* no. 93 (15):3643–3653.

Bossou, Annick D, Sven Mangelinckx, Hounnankpon Yedomonhan, Pelagie M Boko, Martin C Akogbeto, Norbert De Kimpe, Félicien Avlessi, and Dominique CK Sohounhloue. 2013. "Chemical composition and insecticidal activity of plant essential oils from Benin against Anopheles gambiae (Giles)." *Parasites & Vectors* no. 6 (1):1–17.

Boukhris, Maher, Mouhiba Ben Nasri-Ayachi, Imed Mezghani, Mohamed Bouaziz, Makki Boukhris, and Sami Sayadi. 2013. "Trichomes morphology, structure and essential oils of Pelargonium graveolens L'Hér. (Geraniaceae)." *Industrial Crops and Products* no. 50:604–610.

Braun, Norbert A, Sherina Sim, Birgit Kohlenberg, and Brian M Lawrence. 2014. "Hawaiian sandalwood: Oil composition of Santalum paniculatum and comparison with other sandal species." *Natural Product Communications* no. 9 (9):1934578X1400900936.

Bulugahapitiya, Vajira P. 2013. *Plants based natural products.* University of Ruhuna.

Bunse, Marek, Rolf Daniels, Carsten Gründemann, Jörg Heilmann, Dietmar R Kammerer, Michael Keusgen, Ulrike Lindequist, Matthias F Melzig, Gertrud E Morlock, and Hartwig Schulz. 2022. "Essential oils as multicomponent mixtures and their potential for human health and well-being." *Frontiers in Pharmacology:*2645.

Butnariu, Monica, and Ioan Sarac. 2018. "Essential oils from plants." *Journal of Biotechnology and Biomedical Science* no. 1 (4):35.

Campolo, Orlando, Giulia Giunti, Agatino Russo, Vincenzo Palmeri, and Lucia Zappalà. 2018. "Essential oils in stored product insect pest control." *Journal of Food Quality* no. 2018.

Carroll, John F, Nurhayat Tabanca, Matthew Kramer, Natasha M Elejalde, David E Wedge, Ulrich R Bernier, Monique Coy, James J Becnel, Betul Demirci, and Kemal Husnu Can Başer. 2011. "Essential oils of Cupressus funebris, Juniperus communis, and J. chinensis (Cupressaceae) as repellents against ticks (Acari: Ixodidae) and mosquitoes (Diptera: Culicidae) and as toxicants against mosquitoes." *Journal of Vector Ecology* no. 36 (2):258–268.

Cascaes, Márcia Moraes, Odirleny dos Santos Carneiro, Lidiane Diniz do Nascimento, Ângelo Antônio Barbosa de Moraes, Mozaniel Santana de Oliveira, Jorddy Neves Cruz, Giselle Maria Skelding Pinheiro Guilhon, and Eloisa Helena de Aguiar Andrade. 2021. "Essential oils from annonaceae species from Brazil: A systematic review of their phytochemistry, and biological activities." *International Journal of Molecular Sciences* no. 22 (22):12140.

Castrillón Cardona, William Fernando, Javier Andrés Matulevich Peláez, Laura Ximena Díaz Barrera, and Soranlly Paola Vasco Zamudio. 2015. "Chemical composition of the essential oils Cavendishia compacta and Cavendishia guatapeensis (Ericaceae)." *Tecnura* no. 19 (spe):153–157.

Cazella, Luciane Neris, Jasmina Glamoclija, Marina Soković, José Eduardo Gonçalves, Giani Andrea Linde, Nelson Barros Colauto, and Zilda Cristiani Gazim. 2019. "Antimicrobial activity of essential oil of Baccharis dracunculifolia DC (Asteraceae) aerial parts at flowering period." *Frontiers in Plant Science* no. 10:27.

Chandra, Deepak, Gunjan Kohli, Kundan Prasad, G Bisht, Vinay Deep Punetha, KS Khetwal, Manoj Kumar Devrani, and HK Pandey. 2015. "Phytochemical and ethnomedicinal uses of family Violaceae." *Current Research in Chemistry* no. 7 (2):44–52.

Chandra, Deepak, Gunjan Kohli, Kundan Prasad, G Bisht, Vinay Deep Punetha, and HK Pandey. 2017. "Chemical composition of the essential oil of Viola seedrpens from Bageshwar (Shama), Uttarakhad, India." *Journal of Medicinal Plants Research* no. 11 (32):513–517.

Chávez-González, ML, R Rodríguez-Herrera, and CN Aguilar. 2016. "Essential oils: A natural alternative to combat antibiotics resistance." In *Antibiotic resistance-mechanisms and new antimicrobial approaches*; Kon, K., Rai, M., Eds: 227–237. Elsevier.

Chehregani, Abdolkarim, Fariba Mohsenzadeh, Naser Mirazi, Somayeh Hajisadeghian, and Zahra Baghali. 2010. "Chemical composition and antibacterial activity of essential oils of Tripleurospermum disciforme in three developmental stages." *Pharmaceutical Biology* no. 48 (11):1280–1284.

Chouhan, Sonam, Kanika Sharma, and Sanjay Guleria. 2017. "Antimicrobial activity of some essential oils: Present status and future perspectives." *Medicines* no. 4 (3):58.

da Silva, Joyce Kelly R, Pablo Luis Baia Figueiredo, Kendall G Byler, and William N Setzer. 2020. "Essential oils as antiviral agents, potential of essential oils to treat SARS-CoV-2 infection: An in-silico investigation." *International Journal of Molecular Sciences* no. 21 (10):3426.

da Silva, Marcelo Felipe Rodrigues, Patrícia Cristina Bezerra-Silva, Camila Soledade de Lira, Bheatriz Nunes de Lima Albuquerque, Afonso Cordeiro Agra Neto, Emmanuel Viana Pontual, Jefferson Rodrigues Maciel, Patrícia Maria Guedes Paiva, and Daniela Maria do Amaral Ferraz Navarro. 2016. "Composition and biological activities of the essential oil of Piper corcovadensis (Miq.) C. DC (Piperaceae)." *Experimental Parasitology* no. 165:64–70.

Dai, Do Ngoc, Ngo Xuan Luong, Tran Dinh Thang, Leopold Jirovetz, Martina Höferl, and Erich Schmidt. 2012. "Chemical composition of the essential oil of Zanthoxylum avicennae (Lam.) DC leaves (Rutaceae) from Vietnam." *Journal of Essential Oil Bearing Plants* no. 15 (1):7–11.

Damasceno, Carolina Sette Barbosa, Natasha Tiemi Fabri Higaki, Josiane de Fátima Gaspari Dias, Marilis Dallarmi Miguel, and Obdulio Gomes Miguel. 2019. "Chemical composition and biological activities of essential oils in the family Lauraceae: A systematic review of the literature." *Planta Medica* no. 85 (13):1054–1072.

Damić, Ana M, Petar D Marin, Adebayo A Gbolade, and Mihailo S Ristić. 2010. "Chemical composition of Mangifera indica essential oil from Nigeria." *Journal of Essential Oil Research* no. 22 (2):123–125.

de Castro Oliveira, Júlia Assunção, Rafaela Karin de Lima, Erica Alves Marques, and Manuel Losada Gavilanes. 2019. "phytochemical aspects and biological activities of essential oil of species of the family Canellaceae: A review." *Plant Science Today* no. 6 (3):315–320.

de Morais, Sandra Ribeiro, Thiago Levi Silva Oliveira, Lanussy Porfiro de Oliveira, Leonice Manrique Faustino Tresvenzol, Edemilson Cardoso da Conceição, Maria Helena Rezende, Tatiana de Sousa Fiuza, Elson Alves Costa, Pedro Henrique Ferri, and José Realino de Paula. 2016. "Essential oil composition, antimicrobial and pharmacological activities of Lippia sidoides Cham. (Verbenaceae) from Sao Goncalo do Abaete, Minas Gerais, Brazil." *Pharmacognosy Magazine* no. 12 (48):262.

de Oliveira, Mozaniel Santana, Marcos Martins Almeida, MLAR Salazar, Flávia Cristina Seabra Pires, Fernanda Wariss Figueiredo Bezerra, Vânia Maria Borges Cunha, Renato Macedo Cordeiro, Glides Rafael Olivo Urbina, Marcilene Paiva da Silva, and Ana Paula Souza e Silva. 2018. "Potential of medicinal use of essential oils from aromatic plants." *Potential of Essential Oils*:1–21.

De Silva, Tuley. 1995. *A manual on the essential oil industry*. United Nations Industrial Development Organization.

De Silva, Tuley. 1999. A manual on the essential oil industry/editor, K. Tuley De Silva. Paper read at UNIDO Workshop on Essential Oil and Aroma Chemical Industries (3rd: 1995: Anadolu Universitesi) TBAM-ICS/UNIDO Training Course on Quality Improvement of Essential Oils, Eskişehir, Turkey.

Demeter, Sébastien, Olivier Lebbe, Florence Hecq, Stamatios C Nicolis, Tierry Kenne Kemene, Henri Martin, Marie-Laure Fauconnier, and Thierry Hance. 2021. "Insecticidal activity of 25 essential oils on the stored product pest, Sitophilus granarius." *Foods* no. 10 (2):200.

Détár, E, É Zámbori-Németh, B Gosztola, A Harmath, M Ladányi, and Zs Pluhár. 2021. "Ontogenesis and harvest time are crucial for high quality lavender: Role of the flower development in essential oil properties." *Industrial Crops and Products* no. 163:113334.

Dhami, DS, GC Shah, Vinod Kumar, Yogesh Joshi, Manish Tripathi, and M Bisht. 2018. "Essential oil composition and antibacterial activity of Agrimonia Pilosa Ledeb (Rosaceae)." *Chemical Science* no. 7 (3):499–505.

Dosoky, Noura S, Prabodh Satyal, Suraj Pokharel, and William N Setzer. 2016. "Chemical composition, enantiomeric distribution, and biological activities of rhododendron anthopogon leaf essential oil from nepal." *Natural Product Communications* no. 11 (12):1934578X1601101230.

El Bakali, Ismail, Aboubakr Boutahar, Mohamed Kadiri, and Abderrahmane Merzouki. 2022. "A comparative phytochemical profiling of essential oils isolated from three hemp (Cannabis sativa L.) cultivars grown in central-northern Morocco." *Biocatalysis and Agricultural Biotechnology* no. 42:102327.

El Karkouri, Jamila, Mohamed Bouhrim, Omkulthom Mohamed Al Kamaly, Hamza Mechchate, Amal Kchibale, Imad Adadi, Sanae Amine, Souâd Alaoui Ismaili, and Touriya Zair. 2021. "Chemical composition, antibacterial and antifungal activity of the essential oil from cistus ladanifer L." *Plants* no. 10 (10):2068.

El Yaagoubi, Mohamed, Sergio Ortiz, Hicham Mechqoq, Carlos Cavaleiro, Marylin Lecsö-Bornet, Maria João Rodrigues, Luísa Custódio, Abdelhamid El Mousadik, Raphaël Grougnet, and Noureddine El Aouad. 2021. "Chemical composition, antibacterial screening and cytotoxic activity of Chiliadenus antiatlanticus (Asteraceae) essential oil." *Chemistry & Biodiversity* no. 18 (6):e2100115.

Elyemni, Majda, Bouchra Louaste, Imane Nechad, Taha Elkamli, Abdelhak Bouia, Mustapha Taleb, Mahdi Chaouch, and Noureddine Eloutassi. 2019. "Extraction of essential oils of Rosmarinus officinalis L. by two different methods: Hydrodistillation and microwave assisted hydrodistillation." *The Scientific World Journal* no. 2019.

Essien, EE, IA Ogunwande, WN Setzer, and O Ekundayo. 2012. "Chemical composition, antimicrobial, and cytotoxicity studies on S. erianthum and S. macranthum essential oils." *Pharmaceutical Biology* no. 50 (4):474–480.

FocusHerb. 2022. *The benefits of various essential oils and extracts for skin care* [cited 25 January 2023]. Available from www.focusherb.com/blog/essential-oils-and-extracts/

Fournier, Gilbert, Michel Leboeuf, and André Cavé. 1999. "Annonaceae essential oils: A review." *Journal of Essential Oil Research* no. 11 (2):131–142.

Franz, Chlodwig, and Johannes Novak. 2020. "Sources of essential oils." In *Handbook of essential oils*, 41–83. CRC Press.

Gakuubi, Martin Muthee, John M Wagacha, Saifuddin F Dossaji, and Wycliffe Wanzala. 2016. "Chemical composition and antibacterial activity of essential oils of Tagetes minuta (Asteraceae) against selected plant pathogenic bacteria." *International Journal of Microbiology* no. 2016.

Ganjewala, D. 2009. "Cymbopogon essential oils: Chemical compositions and bioactivities." *International Journal of Essential Oil Therapeutics* no. 3 (2–3):56–65.

Garneau, François-Xavier, Guy Collin, Hélène Gagnon, and André Pichette. 2012. "Chemical composition of the hydrosol and the essential oil of three different species of the pinaceae family: Picea glauca (Moench) Voss., Picea mariana (Mill.) BSP, and Abies balsamea (L.) Mill." *Journal of Essential Oil Bearing Plants* no. 15 (2):227–236.

Georgiev, Evgenii V, Albena St. Stojanova, and Vesko At. Tchapkanov. 1999. "On the Bulgarian valerian essential oil." *Journal of Essential Oil Research* no. 11 (3):352–354.

Ghaffar, Abdul, Muhammad Yameen, Shumaila Kiran, Shagufta Kamal, Fatima Jalal, Bushra Munir, Sadaf Saleem, Naila Rafiq, Aftab Ahmad, and Iram Saba. 2015. "Chemical composition and in-vitro evaluation of the antimicrobial and antioxidant activities of essential oils extracted from seven Eucalyptus species." *Molecules* no. 20 (11):20487–20498.

Glimn-Lacy, Janice, and Peter B Kaufman. 2006. *Botany illustrated: Introduction to plants, major groups, flowering plant families*. Springer.

Guenther, Ernest. 2014. *The essential oils-Vol 1: History-origin in plants-production-analysis*. Read Books Ltd.

Guleria, Sanjay, Ashok Kumar, and Ashok Kumar Tiku. 2008. "Chemical composition and fungitoxic activity of essential oil of Thuja orientalis L. grown in the north-western Himalaya." *Zeitschrift für Naturforschung C* no. 63 (3–4):211–214.

Gulluni, Nadia, Tania Re, Idalba Loiacono, Giovanni Lanzo, Luigi Gori, Claudio Macchi, Francesco Epifani, Nicola Bragazzi, and Fabio Firenzuoli. 2018. "Cannabis essential oil: A preliminary study for the evaluation of the brain effects." *Evidence-Based Complementary and Alternative Medicine: eCAM* no. 2018.

Handa, Sukhdev Swami, Suman Preet Singh Khanuja, Gennaro Longo, and Dev Dutt Rakesh. 2008. "Extraction technologies for medicinal and aromatic plants (United Nations Industrial Development Organisation and the International Centre for Science and High Technology)." *International Centre for Science and High Technology-United Nations Industrial Development Organization, Area Science Park Padriciano* no. 99:34012.

Hanif, Muhammad Asif, Shafaq Nisar, Ghufrana Samin Khan, Zahid Mushtaq, and Muhammad Zubair. 2019. "Essential oils." In *Essential oil research*, 3–17. Springer.

Hashemi, Seyed Mehdi, and Seyed Ali Safavi. 2012. "Chemical constituents and toxicity of essential oils of oriental arborvitae, Platycladus orientalis (L.) Franco, against three stored-product beetles." *Chilean Journal of Agricultural Research* no. 72 (2):188.

Hasimi, Nesrin, Abdulselam Ertaş, Elif Varhan Oral, Hüseyin Alkan, Mehmet Boğa, Mustafa Abdullah Yılmaz, İsmail Yener, Işıl Gazioğlu, Cumali Özaslan, and Mehmet Akdeniz. 2017. "Chemical profile of Malva neglecta and Malvella sherardiana by Lc-MS/MS, GC/MS and their anticholinesterase, antimicrobial and antioxidant properties with aflatoxin-contents." *Marmara Pharmaceutical Journal* no. 21 (3):471–484.

Hazrati, Saeid, Kazem Lotfi, Mostafa Govahi, and Mohammad-Taghi Ebadi. 2021. "A comparative study: Influence of various drying methods on essential oil components and biological properties of Stachys lavandulifolia." *Food Science & Nutrition* no. 9 (5):2612–2619.

Hmamouchi, M, J Hamamouchi, M Zouhdi, and JM Bessiere. 2001. "Chemical and antimicrobial properties of essential oils of five Moroccan Pinaceae." *Journal of Essential Oil Research* no. 13 (4):298–302.

Hudifa, Lobna K, Ahmad S Alnouri, Talal A Aburjai, and Mohammad M Hudaib. 2013. "Chemical composition of the essential oil from roots of Sarcopoterium spinosum (L.) (Rosaceae) grown in Syria." *Journal of Essential Oil Bearing Plants* no. 16 (3):412–416.

Irshad, Muhammad, M Ali Subhani, Saqib Ali, and Amjad Hussain. 2020. "Biological importance of essential oils." *Essential Oils-Oils of Nature*:1.

Kapoor, IPS, Bandana Singh, Gurdip Singh, Carola S De Heluani, MP De Lampasona, and Cesar AN Catalan. 2013. "Chemical composition and antioxidant activity of essential oil and oleoresins of nutmeg (Myristica fragrans Houtt.) fruits." *International Journal of Food Properties* no. 16 (5):1059–1070.

Karapandzova, Marija, Gjose Stefkov, Ivana Cvetkovikj, Elena Trajkovska-Dokik, Ana Kaftandzieva, and Svetlana Kulevanova. 2014. "Chemical composition and antimicrobial activity of the essential oils of Pinus peuce (Pinaceae) growing wild in R. Macedonia." *Natural Product Communications* no. 9 (11):1934578X1400901124.

Kasim, Lateef S, Kafayat O Olaleye, AB Fagbohun, SF Ibitoye, and OE Adejumo. 2014. "Chemical composition and antibacterial activity of essential oils from Struchium sparganophora Linn. ktze asteraceae." *Advances in Biological Chemistry* no. 2014.

Katiki, LM, AME Barbieri, RC Araujo, CJ Veríssimo, H Louvandini, and JFS Ferreira. 2017. "Synergistic interaction of ten essential oils against Haemonchus contortus in vitro." *Veterinary Parasitology* no. 243:47–51.

Khallouki, Farid, Chafique Younos, Rachid Soulimani, and Jean Marie Bessiere. 2002. "Chemical composition of the essential oil of Ononis natrix L. Fabaceae." *Journal of Essential Oil Research* no. 14 (6):431–432.

Khamis, Al-Dhafri S, and Lay Ching Chai. 2021. "Chemical and antimicrobial analyses of juniperus chinensis and juniperus seravschanica essential oils and comparison with their methanolic crude extracts." *International Journal of Analytical Chemistry* no. 2021.

Khumalo, GP, NJ Sadgrove, S Van Vuuren, and B-E Van Wyk. 2019. "Antimicrobial activity of volatile and non-volatile isolated compounds and extracts from the bark and leaves of Warburgia salutaris (Canellaceae) against skin and respiratory pathogens." *South African Journal of Botany* no. 122:547–550.

Kim, Ji-Young, Sang-Suk Kim, Tae-Heon Oh, Jong Seok Baik, Gwanpil Song, Nam-Ho Lee, and Chang-Gu Hyun. 2009. "Chemical composition, antioxidant, anti-elastase, and anti-inflammatory activities of Illicium anisatum essential oil." *Acta Pharmaceutica* no. 59 (3):289–300.

Kossouoh, Cosme, Mansour Moudachirou, Victor Adjakidje, Jean-Claude Chalchat, and Gilles Figuérédo. 2008. "Essential oil chemical composition of Anacardium occidentale L. leaves from Benin." *Journal of Essential Oil Research* no. 20 (1):5–8.

Kouao, Toffe Alexis, Bosson Antoine Kouame, Zana A Ouattara, Janat Akhanovna Mamyrbekova-Bekro, Ange Bighelli, Felix Tomi, and Yves-Alain Bekro. 2021. "Chemical characterisation of essential oils of leaves of two Solanaceae: Solanum rugosum and Solanum erianthum from Côte d'Ivoire." *Natural Product Research* no. 35 (14):2420–2423.

Kowalski, Radoslaw, Tomasz Baj, Klaudia Kalwa, Grazyna Kowalska, and Monika Sujka. 2017. "Essential oil composition of Tilia cordata flowers." *Journal of Essential Oil Bearing Plants* no. 20 (4):1137–1142.

Krayni, Hanen, Nahed Fakhfakh, Mohamed Kossentini, and Sami Zouari. 2018. "Fruits of ruta chalepensis L. (Rutaceae) as a source of 2-undecanone." *Journal of Essential Oil Bearing Plants* no. 21 (3):789–795.

Kumar, Peeyush, Sapna Mishra, Anushree Malik, and Santosh Satya. 2013. "Housefly (Musca domestica L.) control potential of Cymbopogon citratus Stapf. (Poales: Poaceae) essential oil and monoterpenes (citral and 1, 8-cineole)." *Parasitology Research* no. 112 (1):69–76.

Kushwah, Ritika, and MK Gupta. 2019. "Anti-inflammatory potential of some essential oils: A review." *Asian Journal of Pharmaceutical Research and Development* no. 7 (6):68–71.

Kuspradini, H, AS Putri, and T Mitsunaga. 2018. "Chemical composition, antibacterial and antioxidant activities of essential oils of Dryobalanops lanceolata Burck. Leaf." *Research Journal of Medicinal Plants* no. 12 (1):19–25.

Lawal, Oladipupo A, and Isiaka A Ogunwande. 2013. "Essential oils from the medicinal plants of Africa." In *Medicinal Plant Research in Africa*, 203–224. Elsevier.

Lawal, Oladipupo A, Isiaka A Ogunwande, Andy R Opoku, Adeleke A Kasali, and Adebola O Oyedeji. 2014. "Chemical composition and antibacterial activities of essential oil of Warburgia salutaris (Bertol. F.) Chiov: From South Africa." *Journal of Biologically Active Products from Nature* no. 4 (4):272–277.

Majolo, Cláudia, Humberto Ribeiro Bizzo, Franmir Rodrigues Brandão, Ana Maria Souza da Silva, Edsandra Campos Chagas, Francisco Célio Maia Chaves, and Aleksander Westphal Muniz. 2022. "Chemical composition of Lippia Linn. (Verbenaceae) essential oils and their antibacterial potential against Aeromonas spp. isolates from Colossoma macropomum." *Journal of Essential Oil Research*:1–11.

Manion, Chelsea R, and Rebecca M Widder. 2017. "Essentials of essential oils." *American Journal of Health-System Pharmacy* no. 74 (9):e153–e162.

Md Othman, Siti Nur Atiqah, Muhammad Aizam Hassan, Lutfun Nahar, Norazah Basar, Shajarahtunnur Jamil, and Satyajit D Sarker. 2016. "Essential oils from the Malaysian Citrus (Rutaceae) medicinal plants." *Medicines* no. 3 (2):13.

Mehdizadeh, Leila, Abdollah Ghasemi Pirbalouti, and Mohammad Moghaddam. 2017. "Storage stability of essential oil of cumin (Cuminum cyminum L.) as a function of temperature." *International Journal of Food Properties* no. 20 (sup2):1742–1750.

Mokni, Ridha El, Saoussen Hammami, Stefano Dall'Acqua, Gregorio Peron, Khaled Faidi, Jeremy Phillip Braude, Houcine Sebei, and Mohamed Hédi El Aouni. 2016. "Chemical composition, antioxidant and cytotoxic activities of essential oil of the inflorescence of Anacamptis coriophora subsp. fragrans (Orchidaceae) from Tunisia." *Natural Product Communications* no. 11 (6):1934578X1601100640.

Montanari, Ricardo M, Luiz CA Barbosa, Antonio J Demuner, Cleber J Silva, Nelio J Andrade, Fyaz MD Ismail, and Maria CA Barbosa. 2012. "Exposure to Anacardiaceae volatile oils and their constituents induces lipid peroxidation within food-borne bacteria cells." *Molecules* no. 17 (8):9728–9740.

Moronkola, Dorcas Olufunke, and Ibrahim Adebayo Oladosu. 2013. "Chemical compositions of Lonchocarpus cyanescens Benth., (Fabaceae): Case study of its volatile oils, and two triterpenoids." *American Journal of Plant Sciences* no. 2013.

Muhizi, Théoneste, Jacqueline Makatiani, Jackson Cherutoi, and Papias Nteziyaremye. 2021. "Variation of yield and chemical composition of essential oil from Cupressus lusitanica growing in different Agro-ecological zones of Rwanda." *Asian Journal of Applied Chemistry Research* no. 9 (2):42–56.

Murthy, K Sri Rama, M Chandrasekhara Reddy, S Sandhya Rani, and T Pullaiah. 2016. "Bioactive principles and biological properties of essential oils of Burseraceae: A review." *Journal of Pharmacognosy and Phytochemistry* no. 5 (2):247.

Muturi, Ephantus J, Kenneth Doll, Mark Berhow, Lina B Flor-Weiler, and Alejandro P Rooney. 2019. "Honeysuckle essential oil as a potential source of ecofriendly larvicides for mosquito control." *Pest Management Science* no. 75 (7):2043–2048.

Norajit, Krittika, Natta Laohakunjit, and Orapin Kerdchoechuen. 2007. "Antibacterial effect of five Zingiberaceae essential oils." *Molecules* no. 12 (8):2047–2060.

Ogunwande, IA, NO Olawore, KA Adeleke, and O Ekundayo. 2003. "Chemical composition of essential oil of myristica fragrans houtt (nutmeg) from nigeria." *Journal of Essential Oil Bearing Plants* no. 6 (1):21–26.

Oller-López, Juan L, Ricardo Rodríguez, Juan M Cuerva, J Enrique Oltra, Btissam Bazdi, Abdelaziz Dahdouh, Ahmed Lamarti, and Ahmed Ibn Mansour. 2005. "Composition of the essential oils of Cistus ladaniferus and C. monspeliensis from Morocco." *Journal of Essential Oil Research* no. 17 (5):553–555.

Orlanda, JF França, and AR Nascimento. 2015. "Chemical composition and antibacterial activity of Ruta graveolens L. (Rutaceae) volatile oils, from São Luís, Maranhão, Brazil." *South African Journal of Botany* no. 99:103–106.

Owolabi, Moses S, Oladipupo A Lawal, Noura S Dosoky, Prabodh Satyal, and William N Setzer. 2013. "Chemical composition, antimicrobial, and cytotoxic assessment of Mitracarpus scaber Zucc. (Rubiaceae) essential oil from southwestern Nigeria." *American Journal of Essential Oils and Natural Products* no. 1 (1):4–6.

Owolabi, Moses S, Akintayo Ogundajo, Nelly Ndukwe, Noura S Dosoky, and William N Setzer. 2020. "Antimicrobial activities and chemical compositions of Daniellia oliveri and Leptoderris micrantha (Fabaceae) essential oils from Nigeria." *Natural Product Communications* no. 15 (10):1934578X20965462.

Owolabi, Moses S, Lanre Akintayo Ogundajo, Balogun Olaoye Solomon, Ambika Poudel, and William N Setzer. 2022. "Chemical composition of Gardenia ternifolia Schumach & Thonn (Rubiaceae) leaf essential oil." *American Journal of Essential Oils and Natural Products* no. 10 (1):6–9.

Pandey, Abhay K, Pradeep Kumar, Pooja Singh, Nijendra N Tripathi, and Vivek K Bajpai. 2017. "Essential oils: Sources of antimicrobials and food preservatives." *Frontiers in Microbiology* no. 7:2161.

Park, Chanjoo, and Heesung Woo. 2022. "Development of native essential oils from forestry resources in South Korea." *Life* no. 12 (12):1995.

Perricone, Marianne, Ersilia Arace, Maria R Corbo, Milena Sinigaglia, and Antonio Bevilacqua. 2015. "Bioactivity of essential oils: A review on their interaction with food components." *Frontiers in Microbiology* no. 6:76.

Pieracci, Ylenia, Roberta Ascrizzi, Valentina Terreni, Luisa Pistelli, Guido Flamini, Laura Bassolino, Flavia Fulvio, Massimo Montanari, and Roberta Paris. 2021. "Essential oil of Cannabis sativa L: Comparison of yield and chemical composition of 11 hemp genotypes." *Molecules* no. 26 (13):4080.

Pires, Andreza Maria L, Maria Rose Jane R Albuquerque, Edson P Nunes, Vânia MM Melo, Edilberto R Silveira, and Otília Deusdênia L Pessoa. 2006. "Chemical composition and antibacterial activity of the essential oils of Blainvillea rhomboidea (Asteraceae)." *Natural Product Communications* no. 1 (5):1934578X0600100510.

Raina, Archana P, and KS Negi. 2015. "Essential oil composition of Valeriana jatamansi Jones from Himalayan regions of India." *Indian Journal of Pharmaceutical Sciences* no. 77 (2):218.

Ramos da Silva, Luiz Renan, Oberdan Oliveira Ferreira, Jorddy Nevez Cruz, Celeste de Jesus Pereira Franco, Tainá Oliveira dos Anjos, Marcia Moraes Cascaes, Wanessa Almeida da Costa, Eloisa Helena de Aguiar Andrade, and Mozaniel Santana de Oliveira. 2021. "Lamiaceae essential oils, phytochemical profile, antioxidant, and biological activities." *Evidence-Based Complementary and Alternative Medicine* no. 2021.

Rao, Huijuanzi, Pengxiang Lai, and Yang Gao. 2017. "Chemical composition, antibacterial activity, and synergistic effects with conventional antibiotics and nitric oxide production inhibitory activity of essential oil from Geophila repens (L.) IM Johnst." *Molecules* no. 22 (9):1561.

Rasoarivelo, Sylvia Tiana Ralambonirina, Raphaël Grougnet, Philippe Vérité, Marylin Lecsö, Marie-José Butel, François Tillequin, Christiane Rakotobe Guillou, and Brigitte Deguin. 2011. "Chemical composition and antimicrobial activity of the essential oils of Anthospermum emirnense and Anthospermum perrieri (Rubiaceae)." *Chemistry & Biodiversity* no. 8 (1):145–154.

Rassem, Hesham Hussein, Abdurahman Hamid Nour, and Rosli Mohammed Yunus. 2018. "Biological activities of essential oils: A review." *Pacific International Journal* no. 1 (2):1–14.

Raveau, Robin, Joël Fontaine, and Anissa Lounès-Hadj Sahraoui. 2020. "Essential oils as potential alternative biocontrol products against plant pathogens and weeds: A review." *Foods* no. 9 (3):365.

Rehman, Rafia, Muhammad Asif Hanif, Zahid Mushtaq, Bereket Mochona, and Xin Qi. 2016. "Biosynthetic factories of essential oils: The aromatic plants." *Natural Products Chemistry & Research* no. 2016.

Riccobono, Luana, Antonella Maggio, Maurizio Bruno, Vivienne Spadaro, and Francesco Maria Raimondo. 2017. "Chemical composition and antimicrobial activity of the essential oils of some species of Anthemis sect: Anthemis (Asteraceae) from Sicily." *Natural Product Research* no. 31 (23):2759–2767.

Rios, Jose-Luis. 2016. "Essential oils: What they are and how the terms are used and defined." In *Essential oils in food preservation, flavor and safety*, 3–10. Elsevier.

Rizwan, Komal, Muhammad Zubair, Nasir Rasool, Muhammad Riaz, Muhammad Zia-Ul-Haq, and Vincenzo De Feo. 2012. "Phytochemical and biological studies of Agave attenuata." *International Journal of Molecular Sciences* no. 13 (5):6440–6451.

Salleh, Wan Mohd Nuzul Hakimi Wan, Farediah Ahmad, and Khong Heng Yen. 2014. "Chemical compositions and antimicrobial activity of the essential oils of Piper abbreviatum, P. erecticaule and P. lanatum (Piperaceae)." *Natural Product Communications* no. 9 (12):1934578X1400901235.

Santos, Geanne KN, Kamilla A Dutra, Rosângela A Barros, Claudio AG da Câmara, Diana D Lira, Norma B Gusmão, and Daniela MAF Navarro. 2012. "Essential oils from Alpinia purpurata (Zingiberaceae): Chemical composition, oviposition deterrence, larvicidal and antibacterial activity." *Industrial Crops and Products* no. 40:254–260.

Sarmento-Neto, José Ferreira, Lázaro Gomes Do Nascimento, Cícero Francisco Bezerra Felipe, and Damião Pergentino De Sousa. 2015. "Analgesic potential of essential oils." *Molecules* no. 21 (1):20.

Sauter, Ismael Pretto, Guilherme Evaldt Rossa, Aline Machado Lucas, Samuel Paulo Cibulski, Paulo Michel Roehe, Luiz Antônio Alves da Silva, Marilise Brittes Rott, Rubem Mário Figueiró Vargas, Eduardo Cassel, and Gilsane Lino von Poser. 2012. "Chemical composition and amoebicidal activity of Piper hispidinervum (Piperaceae) essential oil." *Industrial Crops and Products* no. 40:292–295.

Schultze, W, and C Vollmann. 1995. "Composition of the essential oil from the underground parts of Geum reptans L. (Rosaceae)." *Flavour and Fragrance Journal* no. 10 (4):249–253.

Siddique, Saima, Zahida Perveen, Shaista Nawaz, Khurram Shahzad, and Zeeshan Ali. 2015. "Chemical composition and antimicrobial activities of essential oils of six species from family Myrtaceae." *Journal of Essential Oil Bearing Plants* no. 18 (4):950–956.

Silvério, Marcelo S, Glauciemar Del-Vechio-Vieira, Míriam AO Pinto, Maria S Alves, and Orlando V Sousa. 2013. "Chemical composition and biological activities of essential oils of Eremanthus erythropappus (DC) McLeisch (Asteraceae)." *Molecules* no. 18 (8):9785–9796.

SonomaPress. 2014. *Essential oils & aromatherapy, an introductory guide: More than 300 recipes for health, home and beauty.* Sonoma Press.

Spinozzi, Eleonora, Filippo Maggi, Giulia Bonacucina, Roman Pavela, Maria C Boukouvala, Nickolas G Kavallieratos, Angelo Canale, Donato Romano, Nicolas Desneux, and André BB Wilke. 2021. "Apiaceae essential oils and their constituents as insecticides against mosquitoes: A review." *Industrial Crops and Products* no. 171:113892.

Svoboda, K, T Svoboda, and Andrew Syred. 2001. "A closer look: Secretory structures of aromatic and medicinal plants." *Herbal Gram* no. 53:34–43.

Taherpour, Avat Arman, Mohammad Mehdi Khodaei, Baram Ahmed Hama Ameen, Majid Ghaitouli, Nosratollah Mahdizadeh, Hamid Reza Amjadian, and Kambiz Larijani. 2017. "Chemical composition analysis of the essential oil of Solanumn nigrum L. by HS/SPME method and calculation of the biochemical coefficients of the components." *Arabian Journal of Chemistry* no. 10:S2372–S2375.

Tayoub, Ghaleb, Isabelle Schwob, Jean-Marie Bessière, Jacques Rabier, Véronique Masotti, Jean-Philippe Mévy, Martine Ruzzier, Gabriel Girard, and Josette Viano. 2006. "Essential oil composition of leaf, flower and stem of Styrax (Styrax officinalis L.) from south-eastern France." *Flavour and Fragrance Journal* no. 21 (5):809–912.

Temraz, Abeer, Pier Luigi Cioni, Guido Flamini, and Alessandra Braca. 2009. "Chemical composition of the essential oil from Jasminum pubescens leaves and flowers." *Natural Product Communications* no. 4 (12):1934578X0900401223.

Thang, Tran D, Do N Dai, Tran M Hoi, and Isiaka A Ogunwande. 2013. "Essential oils from five species of Annonaceae from Vietnam." *Natural Product Communications* no. 8 (2):1934578X1300800228.

Thompson, AC, Barbara W Hanny, PA Hedin, and RC Gueldner. 1971. "Phytochemical studies in the family Malvaceae. I: Comparison of essential oils of six species by gas-liquid chromatography." *American Journal of Botany* no. 58 (9):803–807.

Tisserand, Robert, and Rodney Young. 2013. *Essential oil safety: A guide for health care professionals.* Elsevier Health Sciences.

Toker, Gülnur, KHC Baser, M Kürkçüoglu, and Temel Özek. 1999. "The composition of essential oils from Tilia L. species growing in Turkey." *Journal of Essential Oil Research* no. 11 (3):369–374.

Tripathi, YC, and P Hazarika. 2014. "Impact of harvesting cycle, maturity stage, drying and storage on essential oil content of patchouli leaves grown in northeast region of India." *Journal of Essential Oil Bearing Plants* no. 17 (6):1389–1396.

Tuan, Doan Quoc, Dien Dinh, Thang Nam Tran, Ty Viet Pham, Duc Viet Ho, Nhan Trong Le, Anh Tuan Le, and Hoai Thi Nguyen. 2022. "Chemical composition of essential oil from the Zingiber monophyllum (Zingiberaceae) from Vietnam." *Journal of Essential Oil Bearing Plants* no. 25 (5):987–993.

Tucker, Arthur O, and Michael J Maciarello. 1999. "Volatile oils of Ilucium floridanum and I. parviflorum (Illiciaceae) of the southeastern United States and their potential economic utilization." *Economic Botany* no. 53 (4):435–438.

Tumen, Ibrahim, Harzemsah Hafizoglu, Ayben Kilic, Ilhami Emrah Dönmez, Huseyin Sivrikaya, and Markku Reunanen. 2010. "Yields and constituents of essential oil from cones of Pinaceae spp. natively grown in Turkey." *Molecules* no. 15 (8):5797–5806.

Van, Hong Thien, Tran Dinh Thang, Thao Nguyen Luu, and Van Dat Doan. 2021. "An overview of the chemical composition and biological activities of essential oils from Alpinia genus (Zingiberaceae)." *RSC Advances* no. 11 (60):37767–37783.

Verma, Ram Swaroop, Swati Singh, Rajendra Chandra Padalia, Sudeep Tandon, KT Venkatesh, and Amit Chauhan. 2019. "Essential oil composition of the sub-aerial parts of eight species of Cymbopogon (Poaceae)." *Industrial Crops and Products* no. 142:111839.

Vuerich, Marco, Claudio Ferfuia, Fabio Zuliani, Barbara Piani, Angela Sepulcri, and Mario Baldini. 2019. "Yield and quality of essential oils in hemp varieties in different environments." *Agronomy* no. 9 (7):356.

Wang, Cheng Fang, Peng Liu, Kai Yang, Yan Zeng, Zhi Long Liu, Shu Shan Du, and Zhi Wei Deng. 2011. "Chemical composition and toxicities of essential oil of Illicium fragesii fruits against Sitophilus zeamais." *African Journal of Biotechnology* no. 10 (79):18179–18184.

Worwood, Susan E, and Valerie Ann Worwood. 2003. *Essential aromatherapy: A pocket guide to essential oils and aromatherapy*. New World Library.

Xin-Hua, Zhang, Jaime A Teixeira da Silva, Jia Yong-Xia, Yan Jian, and Ma Guo-Hua. 2012. "Essential oils composition from roots of Santalum album L." *Journal of Essential Oil Bearing Plants* no. 15 (1):1–6.

Yangui, Thabèt, Hanen Chakroun, Abdelhafidh Dhouib, and Mohamed Bouaziz. 2021. "Biological properties and chemical composition of essential oils from fresh and shade dried olive leaves of olea europaea L. Chemlali cultivar." *Journal of Essential Oil Bearing Plants* no. 24 (6):1389–1401.

Yohana, Revocatus, Paulo S Chisulumi, Winifrida Kidima, Azar Tahghighi, Naseh Maleki-Ravasan, and Eliningaya J Kweka. 2022. "Anti-mosquito properties of Pelargonium roseum (Geraniaceae) and Juniperus virginiana (Cupressaceae) essential oils against dominant malaria vectors in Africa." *Malaria Journal* no. 21 (1):1–15.

Yongram, Chawalit, Bunleu Sungthong, Ploenthip Puthongking, and Natthida Weerapreeyakul. 2019. "Chemical composition, antioxidant and cytotoxicity activities of leaves, bark, twigs and oleo-resin of Dipterocarpus alatus." *Molecules* no. 24 (17):3083.

Younis, Adnan, Atif Riaz, M Aslam Khan, and Asif Ali Khan. 2009. "Effect of time of growing season and time of day for flower harvest on flower yield and essential oil quality and quantity of four Rosa cultivars." *Floriculture and Ornamental Biotechnology* no. 3:98–103.

Zoghbi, Maria das Graças Bichara, Raimunda Alves Pereira, Giselle do Socorro Luz de Lima, and Maria de Nazaré do Carmo Bastos. 2014. "Variation of essential oil composition of Tapirira guianensis Aubl. (Anacardiaceae) from two sandbank forests, north of Brazil." *Química nova* no. 37:1188–1192.

# 2 Technological Advancement for the Chemical Characterization of Essential Oils

*Naveen Kumar, Pawan Kumar,
and Piyush Sharma*

## 2.1 INTRODUCTION

Essential oils are produced by living organisms, separated only by physical means (pressing and distillation) from whole plants or plant parts of known taxonomic origin. The essential oil components mainly belong to the majority of the terpene family (Šilha et al. 2020; Dhifi et al. 2016). The classification of terpenoids is established by the number of isoprene units (molecules with 5 carbon atoms). The smallest terpenes contain a single isoprene unit and are known as hemiterpenes (C5). The monoterpenes (C10), sesquiterpenes (C15), diterpenes (C20), triterpenes (C30) and polyterpenes (>C30) are the special different kinds of terpenes (Croteau, Kutchan, and Lewis 2000). Thousands of compounds belonging to the terpene family have been identified in essential oils to date and the composition of essential oils is mainly composed of mono- and sesquiterpene hydrocarbons and their oxygenated (hydroxyl and carbonyl) derivatives, along with aliphatic, alcohols, aldehydes and esters (Modzelewska et al. 2005; Zwenger and Basu 2008) (Figure 2.1). Essential oils have excellent medicinal properties (Dhifi et al. 2016; Popa et al. 2021; Guerra-Boone et al. 2015) and help protect the body from the onslaught of pathogens due to the presence of phytochemicals such as flavonoids, alkaloids, terpenoids and tannins. Interest in essential oils has been revived in recent decades with the popularity of aromatherapy, a branch of alternative medicine that claims healing properties in essential oils and other aromatic compounds (Ogwuche and Edema 2020). The chemical composition of essential oils is influenced by extraction methods, refinement, geographic and climatic factors (Barra 2009). Additionally, many natural and/ or synthetic compounds are added to increase the market value of the oil (Radulović and Blagojević 2012). Therefore, confirming the identity of essential oils and detecting contamination is a complex issue. Due to the volatile nature of constituents

DOI: 10.1201/9781003389774-2

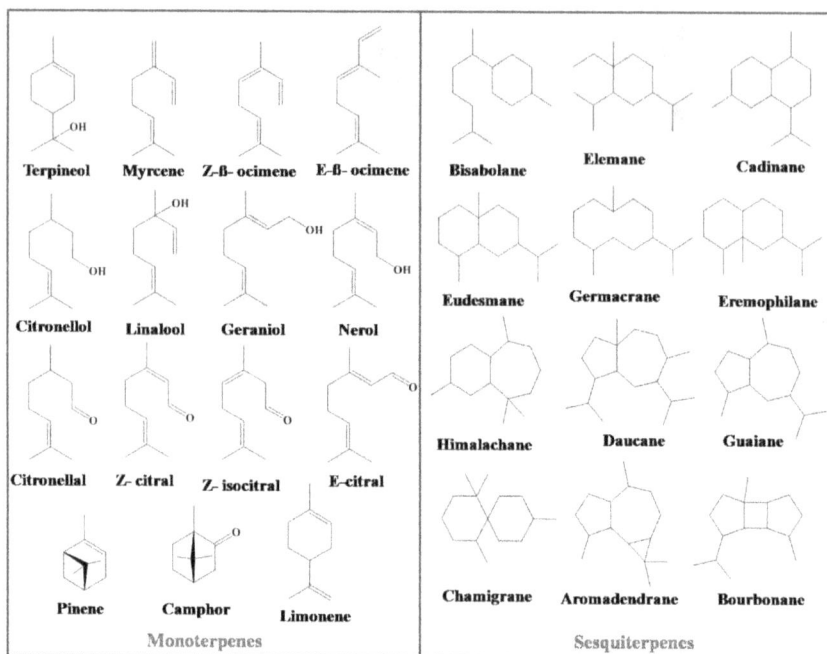

**FIGURE 2.1**  Structures of some monoterpenes and sesquiterpenes.

present in essential oil, they are preferably analyzed by gas chromatography (GC) (Tholl et al. 2006). Nowadays, many hyphenated and advanced variants of GC and HPLC are available for the chemical analysis of essential oils. Moreover, chemometrics has become a popular method for analyzing complex systems because it can solve peak overlapping and embedding problems and can provide a large amount of information (Li, Kong, and Wu 2013).

## 2.1.1 Techniques Applied to the Analysis of Essential Oils

At one time, thin-layer chromatography (TLC), gas chromatography (GC) and various liquid column chromatographies (LC) were available as analytical methods for essential oils analysis. Additionally, several spectroscopic techniques such as UV, IR, $^1$H and $^{13}$C NMR spectroscopy and MS spectrometry are available. In the years that followed, several additional techniques were developed and applied to the analysis of essential oils such as high-performance liquid chromatography (HPLC), supercritical fluid chromatography (SFC) and spectroscopy techniques combined with chemometric tools. Also, their identification has been made possible by various so-called hyphenation techniques (GC-MS, LC-MS, GC-FTIR, etc.) and multidimensional analysis techniques which provide valuable information about individual separated components (Kelani et al. 2020; Cagliero et al. 2022; Bouriah et al. 2021). Some techniques used for EO are shown in Table 2.1.

**TABLE 2.1**

**Some Techniques Used for Essential Oil Analysis**

| Chromatographic Techniques | Spectroscopic Techniques | Hyphenated Techniques |
|---|---|---|
| TLC | FTIR | GC-MS |
| GC | UV | HPLC-GC |
| LC | NMR | GC-FTIR |
| HPLC | MS | GC-UV |
| SFC | | SFC-GC |
| | | HPLC-MS |
| | | LC-NMR |
| | | GC-MS-MS |
| | | GC×GC-MS |

## 2.1.1.1 Chromatographic Techniques

*Thin-Layer Chromatography (TLC)*

TLC has been used for the analysis of essential oils for many years and provides valuable information compared to simple measurements of chemical and physical values. Therefore, this method has been adopted by many pharmacopoeias as a standard laboratory method for characterizing essential oils (Reitsema 1954; Pothier et al. 2001). This method is efficient and fast, and combines sensitivity and simplicity at low cost. However, nowadays this technique is rarely used for the analysis of complex mixtures such as essential oils due to its low resolution.

*Gas Chromatography (GC)*

The volatility and polarity of essential oil components made gas chromatography the method of choice. The heart of any chromatography system is the column. Many efforts have been made to improve separations in GC using very long columns, small diameter columns or selective stationary phases. Column efficiency and selectivity depend on column properties and quality, as well as the chemistry of stationary phase. The most commonly used non-polar stationary phases for essential oil analysis are methylpolysiloxanes (DB-1, OV-1, OV 101, HP-1, etc.) and methyl-phenylpolysiloxanes (DB-5, SBP-5, HP-5, CPSil-5 etc.). The polar phases are primarily based on various polyethylene glycols (Carbowax®, DB-Wax, HP-20M, etc.) and cyanopropylphenylpolysiloxanes (e.g., OV-1701, DB-1701, DB-1701, SPB-1701, etc.) (Sgorbini et al. 2006). Mass spectrometry (MS) detectors are the most common detector type for routine GC analysis of volatiles in plants. Sensitive mass spectrometer detection limits are in the pictogram and femtogram range. Besides mass spectrometry, FID, Fourier transform infrared spectroscopy (FTIR), ultraviolet spectroscopy (UV) and atomic emission spectroscopy (AES) have also been proposed as GC detectors for volatiles analysis. GG-FTIR method has been used to identify closely related isomers with very similar EI mass spectra and provide information about the complete molecule. Difficulties in quantification and time-consuming data interpretation limit the usefulness of the technique due to the lack of commercially available IR spectral libraries. Also the chromatography-ultraviolet spectroscopy (GC-UV) and gas chromatography-atomic emission spectroscopy (GC-AES) methods have gained little importance in the field of essential oil research (Smelcerovic et al. 2013). The similarity of retention indices for many related components indicates that component duplication is a common expectation. The presence of unsaturated bonds, various branched and cyclic compounds and oxygen-containing analogues (such as alcohols and ketones) further complicates matters. Therefore, essential oil analysts will very quickly adopt new separation techniques to improve their analyses.

*High Speed GC: Fast GC (F-GC) and Ultra-Fast Module GC (UFM-GC)*

The use of fast GCs can reduce the cost per analysis by shortening analysis times. The important parameters affecting the speed of GC analysis are GC column length and diameter, mobile phase speed, and oven temperature programming (Table 2.2). The most effective way to speed up GC separations without sacrificing separation efficiency is to use short, narrow internal diameter columns with thin coatings, high carrier gas flow rates and fast heating ramps (Korytár et al. 2002; Blumberg and Klee 1998).

When F-GC is used for routine analysis of EO, it is usually coupled with a quadrupole mass spectrometer (F-GC-qMS) as the analytical instrument. Mondello et al. studied the application of an F-GC to the analysis of five citrus essential oils: bergamot (*Citrus bergamia*[L.] Osbeck), sweet and bitter orange (*aurantium* L. × Citrus), mandarin (*Citrus reticulata* Blanco) and lemon (*Citrus limon*[L.] Osbeck). The F-GC procedure employed required optimization of the experimental conditions (high inlet pressure, accelerated temperature programming speed and split ratio) and thus the adoption of appropriate equipment. The analysis time was reduced to 3.3 minutes, approximately 14 times faster than conventional GC analysis, and excellent results were obtained with little loss of peak resolution (Cagliero et al. 2022; Mondello et al. 2004). Tranchida et al. analyzed basil essential oil (*Ocimumbasilicum* L.) using the

---

**TABLE 2.2**
**Key Parameters that Affect the Speed of Analysis of GC**

| Parameter | GC Type | | |
|---|---|---|---|
| | Conventional | Fast | Ultra-Fast |
| Heating rate (°C/min) | 1–20 | 20–60 | 60–1200 |
| Column length (m) | 60–15 | 15–5 | 5–2 |
| Column internal diameter (μm) | 320–250 | 250–100 | 100–50 |
| Peak width (s) | 10–5 | 5–0.5 | 0.2–0.05 |

F-GC-qMS method. They observed that analysis time was reduced from 25 minutes for conventional GC-MS to 5.3 minutes for F-GC. The overall resolution was similar and the number of compounds positively identified was the same, demonstrating the reliability of F-GC in the field of essential oils analysis (Tranchida et al. 2008).

## Gas Chromatography-Olfactometry (GC-O)

GC-O allows the evaluation of odorant active ingredients in complex mixtures based on the correlation between chromatographic peaks of the eluting material recognized simultaneously by two detectors, one of which is the human olfactory system. GC-O based on electronic sensors (e-nose) is increasingly being used to identify complex volatiles. An electronic nose is a series of chemical sensors connected to a pattern recognition system that responds to smells that are inhaled. In addition to being subjective like sensory evaluation, it is cheaper and can be analyzed in a shorter time than conventional gas chromatography (Wardencki, Chmiel, and Dymerski 2013). Nie et al. used an e-nose coupled with ultra-fast gas chromatography for rapid screening of antioxidant active components in essential oils from rosemary (EOR). The proposed method can identify the chemical constituents of EOR and rapidly screen for antioxidants by comparing the changes in the chromatographic peak areas of each component. The reliability and feasibility of using an e-nose to identify the chemical constituents of EOR was validated by gas chromatography-mass spectrometry (GC-MS/MS). GC-MS/MS results indicated that the main components of EOR were α-pinene, p-cymene, camphor, verbenone and eucalyptol (Nie et al. 2020).

## Chiral GC or Enantioselective Gas Chromatography (ES-GC)

One of the most important developments in GC in the past was the introduction of enantioselective capillary columns with high separation efficiency, so that we were able to separate and identify a large number of chiral substances. The development of stable chiral phases for GC, mainly based on cyclodextrins, has enabled detailed studies of the enantiomeric composition of volatile compounds (Smelcerovic et al. 2013). A number of essential oils have already been studied by ES-GC using various chiral stationary phases, with certain chiral stationary phases preferentially separating certain enantiomers. For example 2,3-di-O-ethyl-6-O-tert-butyldimethylsilyl-β-CD on a polymethylphenylsiloxane (PS086) phase allowed the characterization of lavender and citrus oils containing linalool, linalyl oxides, linalyl acetate, α-terpineol, borneol, bornyl acetate and cis- and trans-nerolidol. Peppermint oil, on the other hand, has been analyzed using 2,3-di-O-methyl-6-O-tert-butyldimethylsilyl-β-CD in the PS086 phase, and especially for α- and β-pinene, limonene, menthol, isomenthol, menthone and isomenthone (Bicchi et al. 1997). Carlo Bicchi et al. used a rapid enantioselective gas chromatography method to analyze various chiral components in lavender essential oil such as α- and β-pinene, camphene, β-phellandrene, limonene, 1-octen-3-ol, camphor, linalool, borneol, linalyl acetate, terpinen-4-ol, lavandulyl acetate, lavandulol and α-terpineol. In this study, analysis conditions were first optimized for conventional 25 m × 0.25 mm inner diameter column (dc) coated with $6^{I-VII}$-O-tert-butyldimethylsilyl-$2^{I-VII}$-$3^{I-VII}$-O-ethyl-β-cyclodextrin (CD) as chiral stationary phase diluted at 30% in PS086 (polymethylphenylpolysiloxane, 15% phenyl), starting from routine analysis (Bicchi et al. 2010).

*High Performance Liquid Chromatography*

HPLC is usually the method of choice for analyzing less volatile components of essential oils, and its versatility, selectivity and sensitivity make it a potential alternative for analyzing volatile oils. In addition, HPLC analysis has several advantages when thermostable compounds are difficult to analyze by GC. HPLC-MS provides excellent information on the content and nature of essential oil constituents. Limiting factors in the application of HPLC for the analysis of terpenoids are the inherent limitations of commonly available detectors and the relatively narrow range of k' values of liquid chromatography systems. Reversed-phase HPLC was used for analysis of non-volatile components found in essential oils of major citrus fruits (orange, tangerine, mandarin, lemon oil). A Phenomenex Luna 3 μm PFP (2), 150 mm × 4.6 mm liquid chromatography column with guard column and UV detector was selected for this study. They reported that PMF was found only in orange, tangerine and mandarin oils, and that furocoumarins and coumarins were found only in lemon oil. Thus, HPLC analysis is superior to GC analysis in citrus oil authenticity studies (Fan et al. 2015). Bouriah et al. used HPLC-MS together with GC-MS and ¹H NMR, to determine the chemical composition of the of *Micromeriainodora* growing in western Algeria. Overall, the main components in this study were the monoterpenes α-terpinyl acetate (29.1%) and camphor (7.0%), and the sesquiterpene cis-14-nor-muurol-5-en-4-one (13.8%). Other minor monoterpene components were α-pinene (0.2%), limonene (0.3%) and borneol (0.2%). Finally, other representative sesquiterpenes were caryophyllene oxide and α-cadinol (3.1 and 2.6%, respectively). HPLC-MS analysis of *M. inodora* methanol extracts allowed preliminary identification of 38 components. Of the components, 19 have been identified as flavonoids. The most representative compounds in this class were luteolin derivatives, followed by quercetin, kaempferol and apigenin derivatives (Bouriah et al. 2021). The issue of chirality is paramount, because EO can be considered a sustainable source of valuable optically pure compounds. High-performance liquid chromatography (HPLC) on a chiral stationary phase with polarimetric detection has proven useful for separating pure enantiomers of terpenes from crude EO without sample pretreatment. Chiral high-performance liquid chromatography (HPLC) with polarization detection and vibrational circular dichroism (VCD) was used to separate the major chiral compounds from *Bubonium graveolens* essential oil (Said et al.). In this study, three major chiral compounds, namely (−) cis-chrysanthenyl acetate, (+) oxocyclonerolidol and (−) cis-acetyloxychrysanthenylacetate, were isolated by preparative HPLC (Said et al. 2017).

### 2.1.1.2 Spectroscopic Techniques

Some of the methods described in the foregoing section suffer from long analysis times, high cost and lack of portable equipment, which limit their broad application to routine control analysis. Chromatographic separation conditions often need to be significantly optimized for each type of essential oil. Additionally, reading GC/MS chromatograms requires skill and experience. To meet these challenges, non-destructive and easy-to-use analytical spectroscopy methods such as IR, UV and NMR have been used for the analysis of EOs.

## UV Spectroscopy

UV spectroscopy is the method of choice for testing the presence of furanocoumarins in various citrus oils. The presence of these components can be easily determined based on their characteristic UV absorption. Frerot et al. quantifies total furocoumarins in citrus oils by HPLC coupled with UV, and then carefully examines the UV spectral data to avoid misleading interpretation of peaks. They identified 15 furocoumarins (namely psoralen, epoxybergamottin, oxypeucedanin, bergamottin, bergapten, isoimperatorin, oxypeucedanin hydrate, 8-geranyloxypsoralen, imperatorin, byakangelicin, xanthotoxin, heraclenin, isopimpinellin, byakangelicol and phelloterin) and reported UV at 310 nm wavelength was the detection method of choice for quantification (Frérot and Decorzant 2004). To separate and characterize the chemical composition of essential oils and the furanocoumarin profiles of $CH_2Cl_2$ extracts from underground parts and fruits of nine *Heracleum* taxa (*Apiaceae*), Petrović et al. used GC-MS and LC-MS together with UV, MS, $^1$H and ROESY NMR. Analyzed furanocoumarins had characteristic UV spectra of 8-monosubstituted furanocoumarins (at $\lambda_{max}$ = 218; 248; 302 nm), 5-monosubstituted ($\lambda_{max}$ = 222; 250; 266; 312 nm) or 5,8- disubstituted ($\lambda_{max}$= 222; 242; 270; 314 nm) linear furanocoumarins, as well as of angular furanocoumarins ($\lambda_{max}$= 224; 254; 306 nm) (Ušjak et al. 2018).

## FTIR Spectroscopy

FTIR spectroscopy allows fast, green, non-destructive and cost-effective assessment of quality of essential oils. Mid-infrared spectroscopy was mainly used as a qualitative method to identify unknown pure substances by providing structural characterization based on functional groups vibration (Agatonovic-Kustrin et al. 2020). For example four essential oils were isolated by Maria et al. from dried leaves of aromatic plants (parsley, lovage, basil and thyme) and analyzed by FTIR spectroscopy. FTIR spectra were recorded in the range 4000–650 cm$^{-1}$ and spectral regions containing useful molecular structural information were identified in the ranges 640–1840 and 2770–3070 cm$^{-1}$ (Morar et al. 2017). Lorena et al. extracted essential oils from *Salvia officinalis* L. and characterized by FTIR spectroscopy. In this study, spectra were recorded in the range 4000–400 cm$^{-1}$ and indicated the presence of thujone, camphor, 1,8-cineole and pinene monoterpenes. They reported that the IR peak at 1734 cm$^{-1}$ due to the C=O stretch was attributed to thujone and camphor, while pinene was confirmed by the presence of an IR peak at 1640 cm$^{-1}$ due to the –C=C– stretch (Ciko et al. 2016). Infrared spectra recorded from plant extracts are usually very complex, because plant extracts are composed of multiple components. Moreover, since each functional group on an individual molecule contributes to the spectral pattern, complexity in the final spectrum due to peak overlap and vibrational mixing make band assignment difficult. Chemometrics has become a popular method for analyzing complex systems because it can solve peak overlapping and embedding problems and can provide a large amount of information. In this sense Li et al. analyzed essential oil components of cinnamon barks using FTIR spectroscopy combined with chemometrics. Yields of essential oils and major components such as cinnamaldehyde, eugenol and α-guayene have been obtained for cinnamon bark, and these data are useful for rational use and cultivation of cinnamon resources

(Li, Kong, and Wu 2013). Recently, GC-MS and FTIR, and Raman spectra were used in combination with chemometrics to identify various volatile oil constituents of the famous Turkish *Rosa damascena* essential oil. Findings show that FTIR and Raman spectroscopy combined with chemometrics are fast, reliable, robust, accurate, simple, inexpensive and non-destructive for the quality assessment of *R. damascena* essential oil and therefore, it may be recommended as an important analytical technique (Cebi, Arici, and Sagdic 2021).

## Nuclear Magnetic Resonance (NMR) Spectroscopy

The application of NMR spectroscopy to investigate complex mixtures without prior separation of individual components is relatively rare due to the low sensitivity, large number of signals and their superposition. However, the application of NMR spectroscopy to the analysis of essential oils offers special advantages such as quick, reproducible, low-temperature operation, robust structural predictions and short data acquisition times. It operates at ambient temperature which prevents decomposition of heat-labile analytes. Additionally, qNMR is a method that does not require the generation of calibration curves or the use of reference standards that are identical to the analytes, making it more advantageous compared to chromatography and other spectroscopic techniques. Qualitative analysis of essential oils is based on the comparison of oil spectra using broad band decoupling and pure oil components that need to be obtained under identical conditions such as solvent, temperature, etc. to confirm that the difference in chemical shifts of the individual NMR lines of the mixture and the reference compound is negligible (Kemprai et al. 2020; Cerceau, Barbosa, Filomeno, et al. 2016). A fast and efficient $^1$H-NMR method for the quantification of terpenes in eucalyptus, pink pepper and turpentine oils has been developed and validated. The limits of detection (LOD) and limits of quantification (LOQ) were 0.1 mg and 2.5 mg, respectively. Statistical tests show that the results obtained with the $^1$H-NMR method are similar to those obtained with the GC-FID technique using external and internal standardization and normalization at 95% confidence level. Repeatability and reproducibility (R&R) values displayed that the $^1$H-NMR method has the lowest R&R value (1.81) and is suitable for the quantification of α-pinene in essential oil (Kemprai et al. 2020). Recently Kemprai et al. used the $^1$H-qNMR method for the quantification of propenylbenzenes in eugenol and related seven analogues in essential oils. Specificity (methoxy/acetate signal), linearity (ranging from 0.05 to 5.00 mg per assay), sensitivity (detection and quantification limits of 4.4 and 14.9 µg/mL, respectively), accuracy and precision are validated. The developed method was reported to be fast, sensitive and reliable with better structural authentication of the analytes of interest (Cerceau, Barbosa, Filomeno, et al. 2016). Cerceau et al. also developed a $^1$H-NMR method for the quantification of α-bisabolol in *E. erythropappus* (Candea) essential oil and compared the results with a gas chromatography (GC) method. Quantification of α-bisabolol by $^1$H-NMR was successfully performed on most *E. erythropappus* essential oil samples evaluated, except for those with more complex compositions. The limits of detection (LOD) and limits of quantification (LOQ) were 0.26 mg and 2.59 mg, respectively. The result obtained by the $^1$H-NMR method was SD = 0.59%, which was smaller than that obtained by GC (SD = 1.18%) (Cerceau, Barbosa, Alvarenga, et al. 2016). Moreover, the powerful combination of NMR and chemometrics enables qualitative and quantitative characterization of whole organic products without expensive and laborious sample preparation processes or prior chemical separations. For example, GC-MS and $^1$H-qNMR spectroscopy coupled with chemometrics were used to study the variability of major organic compounds in seven *Ocimum* essential oils. Despite the confirmatory results, chemometric analysis indicated a more robust (better fit) of the $^1$H-NMR model compared to the GC-MS method with respect to certain statistical parameters (Freitas et al. 2018). Therefore, qNMR spectroscopy may be a promising technique for quality control of essential oils.

### 2.1.1.3 Hyphenated and Multidimensional Techniques

Hyphenation is the combination of two chromatographic techniques or one chromatographic technique with spectroscopy, or the application of different analytical approaches in unrelated (orthogonal) dimensions of analysis to improve analytical resolution or quality of data from an analysis. Collectively, these can be called multidimensional methods. The combination of these technology results in a highly effective system for extensive profiling of complex mixtures. However, the performance of different approaches is highly dependent on the detectors used. Use of the detector allows for prior peak labeling or de-replication and additional online structural data on the separated compounds. For example, mass spectrometry (MS), nuclear magnetic resonance (NMR), photodiode array (PDA) and electrospray ionization (ESI) are commonly used for liquid-based separations. On the other hand, GC is mainly used in combination with MS, flame ionization detector (FID), infrared (IR) spectroscopy, near infrared (NIR) detector, etc. Diode array detector (DAD) or MS is mainly applied to the SFC approach. To date, MS remains the detector of choice due to its high specificity and sensitivity, regardless of the applied MS (quadrupole [Q], time-of-flight [TOF], ion trap [IT] or matrix-assisted laser desorption/ionization [MALDI]) (Masondo and Makunga 2019).

*Gas Chromatography-Mass Spectrometry (GC-MS)*

Combining gas chromatography and mass spectrometry has led to the development of easy-to-use and high-performance systems in terms of sensitivity, data acquisition and processing, and the relatively low cost of these systems make them the most widely used methods for analyzing essential oils (Popa et al. 2021; Fan et al. 2015). In these techniques the compounds were identified by comparing their mass spectra with the GC-MS spectral library (Figure 2.2) and comparing their retention indices to literature values (Wangchuk et al. 2013). For volatile compounds, GC-MS analysis followed by library screening has long been an accepted method of identification in complex mixtures. For each acquired spectrum, this method finds the most similar spectra in the reference library and displays the compounds that produced them in a "hit list" sorted by similarity to the acquired spectrum (Stein 2012). Li et al. was used GC-MS to evaluate the chemical composition of flower and leaf essential oils of four salvia species (*Salvia miltiorrhiza*, *Salvia przewalskii*, *Salvia officinalis*, and *Salvia deserta*). This study successfully identified 63, 51, 69 and 72 compounds in the flower oil and 62, 68, 71 and 63 compounds in the leaf oil of *Salvia*

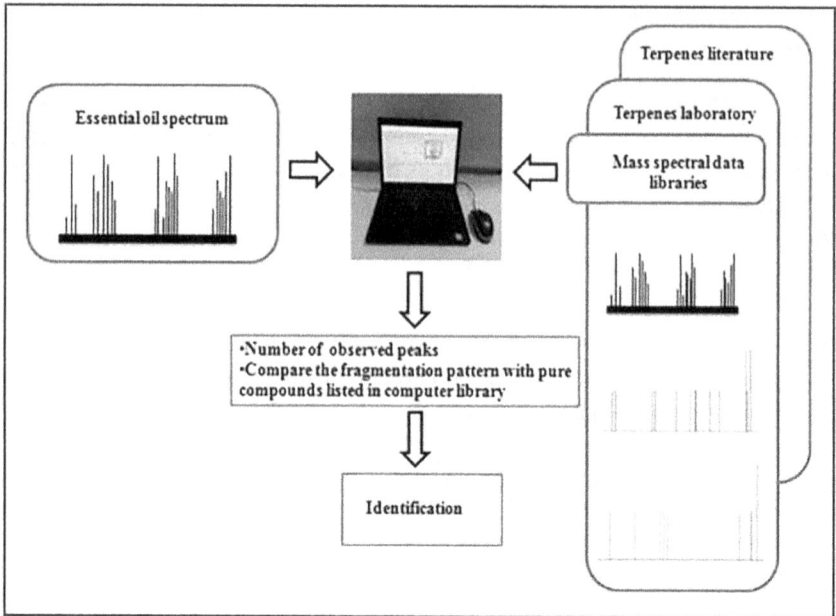

**FIGURE 2.2** Computer-Aided Identification of the Individual Constituents of Essential Oils

*miltiorrhiza, Salvia przewalskii, Salvia officinalis,* and *Salvia deserta,* respectively (Li et al. 2015). Recently, the chemical compositions of essential oils and corresponding hydrolysates from six species of the *Lamiaceae* family were determined by GC-MS, and a total of 161 compounds were successfully identified (Popa et al. 2021). Unfortunately, the mass spectra of essential oil components are often very similar. This is because within the broad class of monoterpenes there are numerous isomers with the same molecular formula but different structures and their mass spectra are often very similar. Therefore, the availability of high-resolution MS tools is the need of the hour to confirm the molecular formulas of the unknown components detected. One of the recent methods proposed to enable improved analysis of complex mixtures is known as fast GC-coupled time-of-flight mass spectrometry (GC-TOF-MS). TOF-MS can generate instantaneous spectra. Therefore, there is no bias occurring from the mismatch between scan rates and the peak abundance changes in the ion source. Recently, better separations of essential oils were reported with GC-TOF-MS (Li et al. 2021; Lin and Long 2023). Lin et al. used GC-TOF-MS-based metabolomics to evaluate the seasonal effects on the chemical composition (sesquiterpene hydrocarbons, oxygenated sesquiterpenes and esters) and bioactivity of 118 essential oils (EOs) from the leaves of *G. xanthochymus* and *G. yunnanensi* (Lin and Long 2023). GC-TOF-MS was also used by Molele et al. to investigated the cytotoxicity, anti-mycotoxigenic and antioxidant activity of some medicinal plants. In this study organic extracts of *M. aethiopicum* and *S. africana* were subjected to GC-MS analysis to identify and determine the presence of phytocompounds in the extracts which can then further be associated to the biological activity of plant extract. The plants were selected based on their potential antifungal and antioxidant activity. *M. aethiopicum* and *S. africana* revealed the total of 66 and 127 phytocompounds, respectively (Molele, Makhafola, and Mongalo 2023).

### *HPLC-MS, HPLC-NMR Spectroscopy*

Online coupling of HPLC with MS and NMR spectroscopy is another important technique that combines high performance separation with structure elucidation spectroscopy, but it is mainly applied to non-volatile mixtures. LC-NMR analysis is often performed independently of LC-MS analysis. LC-MS is used as the first dereplication step in chemical profiling of mixtures, and compounds are tentatively identified by molecular weight and fragment information after manual searching of libraries. LC-NMR is then used in the second step of more detailed structural studies of compounds that exhibit unique structural features. Recently, Bouriah et al. used high-performance liquid chromatography coupled with an integrated nuclear magnetic resonance (NMR) and mass spectrometry (HPLC-MS) approach to determine the chemical composition of the essential oil, volatile and crude extract components of *Micromeria inodora*. Analysis of the essential oil identified 66 components, mainly oxidized monoterpenes and sesquiterpenes (38.2% and 32.0%, respectively) and sesquiterpene hydrocarbons (10.8%). NMR and LC-MSn analyses revealed the presence of aglyconic and glycosylated flavonoids, phenylpropanoid derivatives and tri terpenoid acids, mainly in the $CH_4$, $CH_2Cl_2$ and n-hexane extracts (Bouriah et al. 2021). Formisano et al. used UPLC-DAD-MS followed by NMR characterization of compounds isolated from the bergamot polyphenol fraction (BPF). In this study, a combination of these techniques was found to be highly efficient in identifying 39 components (32 flavanone/flavone/flavonol derivatives, 3 coumarins, 3 limonoids and 1 phenylpropanoid) (Formisano et al. 2019). A hyphenated chromatography (UHPLC-qTOF-MS) technique was used with UV-Vis and FTIR spectroscopy to analyze bioactive compounds in a methanol extract of *M. balsamina* leaves and confirmed that it contains a wide variety of compounds such ascardiac glycosides, flavonoids, saponins, tannins and terpenoids (Mabasa et al. 2021).

### *Supercritical Fluid and Gas Chromatography (SFC-GC)*

Supercritical fluid chromatography (SFC) is a chromatographic technique that uses supercritical fluid, a low-viscosity solvent, as the mobile phase. The most commonly used supercritical fluid is carbon dioxide ($scCO_2$). This is because $CO_2$ is cheaper and less toxic, allowing for a "greener" analytical method. As an advanced application of gas chromatography (GC), cSFC is typically combined with a flame ionization detector (FID) and requires pure supercritical fluids as the mobile phase. Capillary SFC using carbon dioxide as the mobile phase and FID as the detector has been applied to the analysis of several essential oils and appears to provide more reliable quantization than GC, especially notably for oxygen compounds. Compared to GC, SFC permits for a much broader variety of working situations and green separation of thermally labile compounds. In addition, SFC requires less organic solvent and the peak expansion of SFC is narrower than that of LC (Chen et al. 2022). SFC and GC pairing strategies have been applied to a variety of sample types. Modern applications of SFC in conjunction with GC have focused on the analysis of complex samples, with the most advanced strategies using SFC-GC×GC and SFC×GC×GC instruments developed to facilitate removal of $CO_2$ from $^1D$ fractions with minimal loss of analyte prior to GC×GC analysis (Kaplitz et al. 2021).

### 2.1.1.4   Multidimensional Gas Chromatographic Techniques (MDGC)

Complex samples require extremely high-resolution analytical methods for in-depth analysis of sample components. Multidimensional chromatography is a method capable of providing higher resolution. Many different chromatographic combinations have been successfully deployed to produce multidimensional separation set-ups. Such configurations ensure higher peak power for the analytes by using two or more mutually independent separation steps in the analytical system. Of all these combinations, two-dimensional gas chromatography and two-dimensional gas-liquid chromatography are considered to be the most effective multidimensional with practical value, especially in the profiling of volatile substances (Rasheed et al. 2021). Multidimensional gas chromatography (MDGC) systems offer higher peak power and separation capabilities than standard GC systems, which can help in the identification and quantification of trace compounds that can be detected and co-eluted with other compounds in higher amounts. In a typical MDGC system, a second column with a different stationary phase is connected to the first dimensional column (1D) by a transmitter and increases peak resolution and peak capacitance. Analysis can be performed either in heart-cut (GC-GC) or in comprehensive mode (GC×GC). In GC-GC, selected discrete fractions of the eluate from the 1D column are sent to the second dimensional (2D) column while in comprehensive two-dimensional gas chromatography (GC×GC), there is continuous (fractional) modulation of the eluate, where each fraction is transferred to a short 2D column with a narrow path. Lebanov et al. reported and discussed the technical developments and application of MDGC in essential oil analysis (Lebanov et al. 2019a, 2019b). MDGC supports much more comprehensive chemical profiling, for example, Gabetti et al. recently adopted the GC×GC ToF MS platform combined with offline 1D-GC-OAEDA (flavor extraction dilution analysis) to study both fingerprints and profiles of Piemonte peppermint essential oil (*M. × piperita* L.) essential oils of different varieties and geographical origin. They report that the UT chromatographic fingerprint provides high chemical dimensionality by mapping more than 350 peak regions at 70 eV and 135 at 12 eV, and from these 95 components identified by responses compared with the existing literature (Gabetti et al. 2021). The separation efficiency of the MDGC technique can be best seen in the example of investigation of the chemical composition of the essential oils of *M. obtusa* and *P. cubataonum* In *M. obtusa* essential oil, 80 compounds were identified by GC×GC-qMS, while only 22 compounds were identified by GC-MS. For essential oils from the branches and leaves of *P. cubataonum*, 66 and 57 compounds were determined by GC×GC-qMS, respectively, compared with 20 and 14 compounds by GC-MS, respectively (Santos et al. 2014). In another example, Ray et al., by applying GC×GC-Time of Flight (TOF)-MS for the first time, successfully identified 53 terpenoids in rhizome oil of *Hedychium coronarium* (Ray et al. 2017). Therefore, GC×GC-ToF-MS chromatographic fingerprinting proved to be a powerful and reliable method to identify the characteristic chemical signature of EOs and to identify and quantify trace components.

*Multidimensional Liquid-Gas Chromatography (LC-GC)*

Unlike multidimensional gas chromatography (MDGC), the LC-GC coupling exploits more separation mechanisms by combining the selectivity of LC separation with the high efficiency and sensitivity of GC separation. The LC-GC technique has been extensively exploited to study unique types of constituents, such as the mono- and industrial sesquiterpene hydrocarbons of citrus oils, the composition of aldehydes in sweet orange oil, and the enantiomeric distribution of monoterpene alcohols in lemon, tangerine, sweet orange and bitter orange oil. Connecting an LC-GC system to a mass spectrometer (LC-GC-MS) increases the potential of the technique; preliminary LC separation, reducing the mutual interference of components, greatly simplifies MS identification (Smelcerovic et al. 2013). There are several reports devoted to interface design for LC and GC coupling. These include on-column, loop-type and vaporization interfaces for conventional phase separation, phase transition and oven transfer desorption for reverse-phase LC-GC analysis (Rasheed et al. 2021). Much more useful is the use of comprehensive 2D GC, which can be combined with an online LC pre-separation step, thus, forming an LC-GCxGC system, which is technically not different from the LC-GC process. In fact, no special requirements are needed to implement the LC-GCxGC system. Zoccali et al. described the analysis of volatile oxygenated fractions of four genuine mandarin (*Citrus deliciosa* Ten.) essential oils (green, yellow, red and Mexican), by using the offline combination of high-performance liquid chromatography (HPLC) and comprehensive two-dimensional gas chromatography-quadrupole mass spectrometry (GCxGC-qMS). Considering the four types of samples subjected to LC-GCxGC-qMS analysis, 179 different compounds were identified; of these, 110 are reported here for the first time in mandarin oils (Zoccali et al. 2017). Furthermore, Zoccali et al. investigated the chemical composition of three lemon essential oils using an off-line combination of normal-phase high-performance liquid chromatography (NP-HPLC) and comprehensive 2D gas chromatography – quadrupole mass spectrometry (GCxGC-QMS). In this study of both hydrocarbons and oxygen, a total of 153 components were identified in the three oils (Zoccali et al. 2019). Therefore, multidimensional liquid – gas chromatography techniques can be a powerful analytical tool for essential oil analysis.

## 2.2   CONCLUDING REMARKS AND FUTURE PERSPECTIVES

GC and GC-MS have played an important role in determining the chemical composition of essential oils and have provided unique identification of known compounds in a very complex mixture. HPLC is also an important technique for the examination of essential oils and has advantages over gas chromatography because it is suitable for the analysis of thermally unstable compounds present in essential oils. Furthermore, analysis time is becoming an important issue nowadays and hence fast GC and HPLC methods are needed. If shorter columns are used, with smaller particle sizes, good performance can be achieved in shorter analysis times. Multidimensional chromatography technique plays an important role in the analysis of essential oils in different substrates. Due to the ability of multidimensional chromatography in the detection of new compounds, one can expect new technical improvements in this technology. In the future, multidimensional chromatography will continue to play an important role in the validation and quality assurance of essential oil and essential oil-based products. NMR spectroscopy has had wide applications in determining the components of essential oils. For the complete identification of small compounds requiring 2D-NMR measurements, either LC-SPE-NMR or cap LC-NMR techniques are required. In addition, the use of hyphenation techniques, such as GC-MS, LC-MS and LC-NMR, provides important insights into the structure of essential oil components. Therefore, in the future, the combination of different chromatographic and spectroscopic methods will certainly be optimal for the structural determination of the components of essential oils.

## REFERENCES

Agatonovic-Kustrin, Snezana, Petar Ristivojevic, Vladimir Gegechkori, Tatiana M Litvinova, and David W. Morton. 2020. "Essential oil quality and purity evaluation via ft-ir spectroscopy and pattern recognition techniques." *Applied Sciences* 10 (20):7294.

Barra, Andrea. 2009. "Factors affecting chemical variability of essential oils: A review of recent developments." *Natural Product Communications* 4 (8):1934578X0900400827.

Bicchi, Carlo, Leonid Blumberg, Cecilia Cagliero, Chiara Cordero, Patrizia Rubiolo, and Erica Liberto. 2010. "Development of fast enantioselective gas-chromatographic analysis using gas-chromatographic method-translation software in routine essential oil analysis (lavender essential oil)." *Journal of Chromatography A* 1217 (9):1530–1536.

Bicchi, Carlo, Angela D'Amato, Valeria Manzin, and Patrizia Rubiolo. 1997. "Cyclodextrin derivatives in GC separation of racemic mixtures of volatiles. Part XI: Some applications of cyclodextrin derivatives in GC enantioseparations of essential oil components." *Flavour and Fragrance Journal* 12 (2):55–61.

Blumberg, LM, and MS Klee. 1998. "Theory and practice of fast capillary GC: Efficiency and speed of analysis." Proceedings of 20th International Symposium of Capillary Chromatography, Riva del Garda, Italy and References Cited Therein.

Bouriah, Nacéra, Hamdi Bendif, Gregorio Peron, Mohamed Djamel Miara, Stefano Dall'Acqua, Guido Flamini, and Filippo Maggi. 2021. "Composition and profiling of essential oil, volatile and crude extract constituents of Micromeria inodora growing in western Algeria." *Journal of Pharmaceutical and Biomedical Analysis* 195:113856.

Cagliero, Cecilia, Carlo Bicchi, Arianna Marengo, Patrizia Rubiolo, and Barbara Sgorbini. 2022. "Gas chromatography of essential oil: State-of-the-art, recent advances, and perspectives." *Journal of Separation Science* 45 (1):94–112.

Cebi, Nur, Muhammet Arici, and Osman Sagdic. 2021. "The famous Turkish rose essential oil: Characterization and authenticity monitoring by FTIR, Raman and GC-MS techniques combined with chemometrics." *Food Chemistry* 354:129495.

Cerceau, Cristiane I, Luiz CA Barbosa, Elson S Alvarenga, Antonio G Ferreira, and Sérgio S Thomasi. 2016. "A validated 1H NMR method for quantitative analysis of α-bisabolol in essential oils of Eremanthus erythropappus." *Talanta* 161:71–79.

Cerceau, Cristiane I, Luiz CA Barbosa, Claudinei A Filomeno, Elson S Alvarenga, Antônio J Demuner, and Paulo H Fidencio. 2016. "An optimized and validated 1H NMR method for the quantification of α-pinene in essentials oils." *Talanta* 150:97–103.

Chen, Min, Shan-Shan Wen, Rui Wang, Qing-Xuan Ren, Chen-Wan Guo, Ping Li, and Wen Gao. 2022. "Advanced development of supercritical fluid chromatography in herbal medicine analysis." *Molecules* 27 (13):4159.

Ciko, Lorena, Adelaida Andoni, Fatos Ylli, Ervisjana Plaku, Krenaida Taraj, and Armand Çomo. 2016. "Extraction of essential oil from Albanian Salvia officinalis L. and its characterization by FTIR Spectroscopy." *Asian Journal of Chemistry* 28 (6):1401.

Croteau, Rodney, Toni M Kutchan, and Norman G Lewis. 2000. "Natural products (secondary metabolites)." *Biochemistry and Molecular Biology of Plants* 24:1250–1319.

Dhifi, Wissal, Sana Bellili, Sabrine Jazi, Nada Bahloul, and Wissem Mnif. 2016. "Essential oils' chemical characterization and investigation of some biological activities: A critical review." *Medicines* 3 (4):25.

Fan, Hao, Qingli Wu, James E Simon, Shyi-Neng Lou, and Chi-Tang Ho. 2015. "Authenticity analysis of citrus essential oils by HPLC-UV-MS on oxygenated heterocyclic components." *Journal of Food and Drug Analysis* 23 (1):30–39.

Formisano, Carmen, Daniela Rigano, Annalisa Lopatriello, Carmina Sirignano, Giuseppe Ramaschi, Lolita Arnoldi, Antonella Riva, Nicola Sardone, and Orazio Taglialatela-Scafati. 2019. "Detailed phytochemical characterization of bergamot polyphenolic fraction (BPF) by UPLC-DAD-MS and LC-NMR." *Journal of Agricultural and Food Chemistry* 67 (11):3159–3167.

Freitas, João Vito B, Elenilson G Alves Filho, Lorena Mara A Silva, Guilherme J Zocolo, Edy S de Brito, and Nilce V Gramosa. 2018. "Chemometric analysis of NMR and GC datasets for chemotype characterization of essential oils from different species of Ocimum." *Talanta* 180:329–336.

Frérot, Eric, and Erik Decorzant. 2004. "Quantification of total furocoumarins in citrus oils by HPLC coupled with UV, fluorescence, and mass detection." *Journal of Agricultural and Food Chemistry* 52 (23):6879–6886.

Gabetti, Elena, Barbara Sgorbini, Federico Stilo, Carlo Bicchi, Patrizia Rubiolo, Franco Chialva, Stephen E Reichenbach, Valentina Bongiovanni, Chiara Cordero, and Andrea Cavallero. 2021. "Chemical fingerprinting strategies based on comprehensive two-dimensional gas chromatography combined with gas chromatography-olfactometry to capture the unique signature of Piemonte peppermint essential oil (Mentha x piperita var Italo-Mitcham)." *Journal of Chromatography A* 1645:462101.

Guerra-Boone, Laura, Rocío Alvarez-Román, Ricardo Salazar-Aranda, Anabel Torres-Cirio, Verónica Mayela Rivas-Galindo, Noemí Waksman de Torres, Gloria González, and Luis Alejandro Pérez-López. 2015. "Antimicrobial and antioxidant activities and chemical characterization of essential oils of Thymus vulgaris, Rosmarinus officinalis, and Origanum majorana from northeastern México." *Pakistan Journal of Pharmaceutical Sciences* 28.

Kaplitz, Alexander S, Mahmoud Elhusseiny Mostafa, Samantha A Calvez, James L Edwards, and James P Grinias. 2021. "Two-dimensional separation techniques using supercritical fluid chromatography." *Journal of Separation Science* 44 (1):426–437.

Kelani, Khadiga M, Mamdouh R Rezk, Hany H Monir, Menna S ElSherbiny, and Sherif M Eid. 2020. "FTIR combined with chemometric tools (fingerprinting spectroscopy) in comparison to HPLC: Which strategy offers more opportunities as a green analytical chemistry technique for pharmaceutical analysis." *Analytical Methods* 12 (48):5893–5907.

Kemprai, Phirose, Bhaskar Protim Mahanta, Pranjit Kumar Bora, Deep Jyoti Das, Jyoti Lakshmi Hati Boruah, Siddhartha Proteem Saikia, and Saikat Haldar. 2020. "A 1H NMR spectroscopic method for the quantification of propenylbenzenes in the essential oils: Evaluation of key odorants, antioxidants and post-harvest drying techniques for Piper betle L." *Food Chemistry* 331:127278.

Korytár, Peter, Hans-Gerd Janssen, Eva Matisová, and A Th Udo. 2002. "Practical fast gas chromatography: Methods, instrumentation and applications." *TrAC Trends in Analytical Chemistry* 21 (9–10):558–572.

Lebanov, Leo, Laura Tedone, Massoud Kaykhaii, Matthew R Linford, and Brett Paull. 2019a. "Multidimensional gas chromatography in essential oil analysis. Part 1: Technical developments." *Chromatographia* 82:377–398.

Lebanov, Leo, Laura Tedone, Massoud Kaykhaii, Matthew R Linford, and Brett Paull. 2019b. "Multidimensional gas chromatography in essential oil analysis. Part 2: Application to characterisation and identification." *Chromatographia* 82:399–414.

Li, Bo, Chenlu Zhang, Liang Peng, Zongsuo Liang, Xijun Yan, Yonghong Zhu, and Yan Liu. 2015. "Comparison of essential oil composition and phenolic acid content of selected Salvia species measured by GC-MS and HPLC methods." *Industrial Crops and Products* 69:329–334.

Li, Yan-qun, De-xin Kong, and Hong Wu. 2013. "Analysis and evaluation of essential oil components of cinnamon barks using GC-MS and FTIR spectroscopy." *Industrial Crops and Products* 41:269–278.

Li, Ying, Guangyao Dong, Xi Bai, Aoken Aimila, Xiaohui Bai, Maitinuer Maiwulanjiang, and HA Aisa. 2021. "Separation and qualitative study of Ruta graveolens L. essential oil components by prep-GC, GC-QTOF-MS and NMR." *Natural Product Research* 35 (21):4202–4205.

Lin, Fengke, and Chunlin Long. 2023. "GC-TOF-MS-based metabolomics correlated with bioactivity assays unveiled seasonal variations in leaf essential oils of two species in Garcinia L." *Industrial Crops and Products* 194:116356.

Mabasa, XE, LM Mathomu, NE Madala, EM Musie, and MT Sigidi. 2021. "Molecular spectroscopic (FTIR and UV-Vis) and hyphenated chromatographic (UHPLC-qTOF-MS) analysis and in vitro bioactivities of the Momordica balsamina leaf extract." *Biochemistry Research International* 2021.

Masondo, NA, and NP Makunga. 2019. "Advancement of analytical techniques in some South African commercialized medicinal plants: Current and future perspectives." *South African Journal of Botany* 126:40–57.

Modzelewska, Aneta, Surojit Sur, Srinivas K Kumar, and Saeed R Khan. 2005. "Sesquiterpenes: Natural products that decrease cancer growth." *Current Medicinal Chemistry-Anti-Cancer Agents* 5 (5):477–499.

Molele, PK, TJ Makhafola, and NI Mongalo. 2023. "GC-ToF-MS based phytochemical analysis and anti-mycotoxigenic activity of South African medicinal plants, Mystroxylon aethiopicum (Thunb.) Loes. and Spirostachys africana Sond." *South African Journal of Botany* 153:11–20.

Mondello, Luigi, Alessandro Casilli, Peter Quinto Tranchida, Rosaria Costa, Paola Dugo, and Giovanni Dugo. 2004. "Fast GC for the analysis of citrus oils." *Journal of Chromatographic Science* 42 (8):410–416.

Morar, Maria-Ioana, Florinela Fetea, Ancuţa Mihaela Rotar, Melinda Nagy, and CA Semeniuc. 2017. "Characterization of essential oils extracted from different aromatic plants by FTIR spectroscopy." *Bulletin of University of Agricultural Sciences and Veterinary Medicine Cluj-Napoca Food Science and Technology* 74:37–38.

Nie, Ji-Yu, Rong Li, Zi-Tao Jiang, Ying Wang, Jin Tan, Shu-Hua Tang, and Yi Zhang. 2020. "Antioxidant activity screening and chemical constituents of the essential oil from rosemary by ultra-fast GC electronic nose coupled with chemical methodology." *Journal of the Science of Food and Agriculture* 100 (8):3481–3487.

Ogwuche, CE, and MO Edema. 2020. "GC-MS and FTIR characterization of essential oil from the fresh leaves of Pandanus candalabrum obtained from Bayelsa state, Nigeria." *Nigerian Journal of Chemical Research* 25 (1):1–10.

Popa, Cristina Laura, Andreea Lupitu, Maria Daniela Mot, Lucian Copolovici, Cristian Moisa, and Dana Maria Copolovici. 2021. "Chemical and biochemical characterization of essential oils and their corresponding hydrolats from six species of the Lamiaceae family." *Plants* 10 (11):2489.

Pothier, Jacques, Nicole Galand, Mohamed El Ouali, and Claude Viel. 2001. "Comparison of planar chromatographic methods (TLC, OPLC, AMD) applied to essential oils of wild thyme and seven chemotypes of thyme." *Il Farmaco* 56 (5–7):505–511.

Radulović, Niko S, and Polina D Blagojević. 2012. "The most frequently encountered volatile contaminants of essential oils and plant extracts introduced during the isolation procedure: fast and easy profiling." *Phytochemical Analysis* 23 (2):131–142.

Rasheed, Dalia M, Ahmed Serag, Zeinab T Abdel Shakour, and Mohamed Farag. 2021. "Novel trends and applications of multidimensional chromatography in the analysis of food, cosmetics and medicine bearing essential oils." *Talanta* 223:121710.

Ray, Asit, Biswabhusan Dash, Ambika Sahoo, Noohi Nasim, Pratap Chandra Panda, Jeetendranath Patnaik, Biswajit Ghosh, Sanghamitra Nayak, and Basudeba Kar. 2017. "Assessment of the terpenic composition of Hedychium coronarium oil from Eastern India." *Industrial Crops and Products* 97:49–55.

Reitsema, Robert H. 1954. "Characterization of essential oils by chromatography." *Analytical Chemistry* 26 (6):960–963.

Said, Mohammed El-Amin, Isabelle Bombarda, Jean-Valère Naubron, Pierre Vanloot, Marion Jean, Abdelkrim Cheriti, Nathalie Dupuy, and Christian Roussel. 2017. "Isolation of the major chiral compounds from Bubonium graveolens essential oil by HPLC and absolute configuration determination by VCD." *Chirality* 29 (2):70–79.

Santos, Thalita G, Karina Fukuda, Massuo J Kato, Adilson Sartorato, Marta CT Duarte, Ana Lúcia TG Ruiz, João E de Carvalho, Fabio Augusto, Francisco A Marques, and Beatriz Helena LN Sales Maia. 2014. "Characterization of the essential oils of two species of Piperaceae by one-and two-dimensional chromatographic techniques with quadrupole mass spectrometric detection." *Microchemical Journal* 115:113–120.

Sgorbini, Barbara, Cecilia Cagliero, Chiara Cordero, Erica Liberto, Patrizia Rubiolo, and Carlo Bicchi. 2006. "Headspace sampling and gas chromatography of plants: A successful combination to study the composition of a plant volatile fraction." *Encyclopedia of analytical chemistry: Applications, theory and instrumentation*. John Wiley & Sons, Ltd. 1–31. DOI: 10.1002/9780470027318.a9910

Šilha, David, Karolína Švarcová, Tomáš Bajer, Karel Královec, Eliška Tesařová, Kristýna Moučková, Marcela Pejchalová, and Petra Bajerová. 2020. "Chemical composition of natural hydrolates and their antimicrobial activity on Arcobacter-like cells in comparison with other microorganisms." *Molecules* 25 (23):5654.

Smelcerovic, Andrija, Aleksandra Djordjevic, Jelena Lazarevic, and Gordana Stojanovic. 2013. "Recent advances in analysis of essential oils." *Current Analytical Chemistry* 9 (1):61–70.

Stein, Stephen. 2012. *Mass spectral reference libraries: An ever-expanding resource for chemical identification*. ACS Publications.

Tholl, Dorothea, Wilhelm Boland, Armin Hansel, Francesco Loreto, Ursula SR Röse, and Jörg-Peter Schnitzler. 2006. "Practical approaches to plant volatile analysis." *The Plant Journal* 45 (4):540–560.

Tranchida, Peter Quinto, Rosaria Costa, Paola Dugo, Giovanni Dugo, and Luigi Mondello. 2008. "Micro-bore column fast gas chromatography-mass spectrometry in essential oil analysis." *Natural Product Communications* 3 (7):1934578X0800300724.

Ušjak, Ljuboš J, Milica M Drobac, Marjan S Niketić, and Silvana D Petrović. 2018. "Chemosystematic significance of essential oil constituents and furanocoumarins of underground parts and fruits of nine Heracleum L. taxa from Southeastern Europe." *Chemistry & Biodiversity* 15 (12):e1800412.

Wangchuk, Phurpa, Paul A Keller, Stephen G Pyne, Malai Taweechotipatr, and Sumalee Kamchonwongpaisan. 2013. "GC/GC-MS analysis, isolation and identification of bioactive essential oil components from the Bhutanese medicinal plant, Pleurospermum amabile." *Natural Product Communications* 8 (9):1934578X1300800930.

Wardencki, Waldemar, Tomasz Chmiel, and Tomasz Dymerski. 2013. "Gas chromatography-olfactometry (GC-O), electronic noses (e-noses) and electronic tongues (e-tongues) for in vivo food flavour measurement." *Instrumental Assessment of Food Sensory Quality*:195–229.

Zoccali, Mariosimone, Barbara Giocastro, Ivana L Bonaccorsi, Alessandra Trozzi, Peter Q Tranchida, and Luigi Mondello. 2019. "In-depth qualitative analysis of lime essential oils using the off-line combination of normal phase high performance liquid chromatography and comprehensive two-dimensional gas chromatography-quadrupole mass spectrometry." *Foods* 8 (11):580.

Zoccali, Mariosimone, Peter Q Tranchida, Ivana L Bonaccorsi, Paola Dugo, Luigi Mondello, and Giovanni Dugo. 2017. "Detailed profiling of the volatile oxygenated fraction of mandarin essential oils by using the off-line combination of high-performance liquid chromatography and comprehensive two-dimensional gas chromatography-mass spectrometry." *Food Analytical Methods* 10:1106–1116.

Zwenger, Sam, and Chhandak Basu. 2008. "Plant terpenoids: Applications and future potentials." *Biotechnology and Molecular Biology Reviews* 3 (1):1.

# 3 Sophisticated Development of Various Advanced Techniques Employed in the Characterization of Essential Oils and Their Pharmaceutical Preparation

*Kiran Dobhal, Jyotsana Suyal,
Naveen Chandra Joshi, and
Vikash Jakhmola*

## 3.1 INTRODUCTION

In recent years, more and more focus has been placed on the advantages of essential oils' (EO) unique properties, including their antimicrobial, antifungal, and antioxidant activities, on human well-being (Sangwan et al. 2001; Bakkali et al. 2008; Guenther 1948). Public health depends on the small aromatic as well as aliphatic components found in terpenes and terpenoids, which are the fundamental building block of many EO. Terpenes are composed of plenty of isoprene ($C_5H_8$) units (Hanif et al. 2019). Terpenes with oxygen are referred to be terpenoids; 90% of EOs are composed of terpenes (Djilani, Abdelouaheb and Dicko 2012). Ocimene, myrcene, citronellol, linalool, and menthofuran are examples of acyclic monoterpenes (Förster-Fromme and Jendrossek 2010) whereas p-cymene, thymol, carvacrol, menthol, carvone, and pulegone come under the monocyclic terpenoid (Nesterkina and Iryna 2016; Camps 1967). Camphene, pinene, sabinene, fenchol, borneol, and isoborneol acetate are examples of bicyclic terpenes (OTMS 2022; Ipatieff 1947). Longifolene, elemene, cadinene, curcumins, α-caryophyllene, α-bisabolene, turmerone, and humulene are numerous sesquiterpenes found in EO (Parker, Roberts and Ramage 1967; Duhl, Helmig and Guenther 2008) (Figure 3.1).

DOI: 10.1201/9781003389774-3

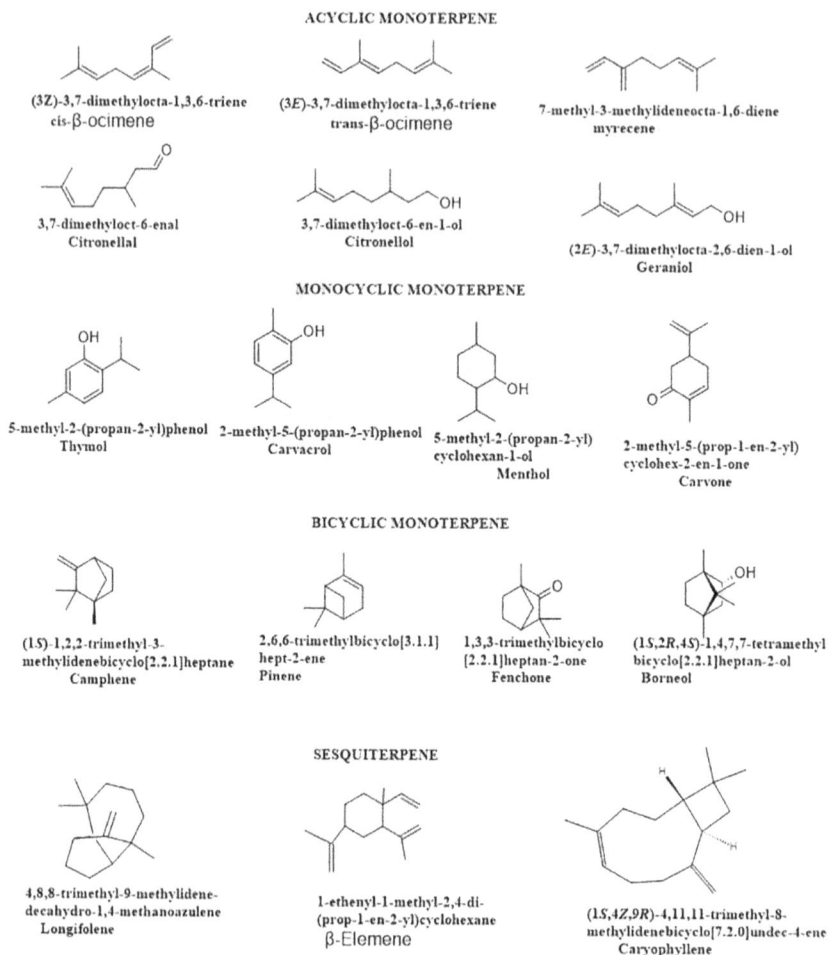

ACYCLIC MONOTERPENE

(3Z)-3,7-dimethylocta-1,3,6-triene
cis-β-ocimene

(3E)-3,7-dimethylocta-1,3,6-triene
trans-β-ocimene

7-methyl-3-methylideneocta-1,6-diene
myrecene

3,7-dimethyloct-6-enal
Citronellal

3,7-dimethyloct-6-en-1-ol
Citronellol

(2E)-3,7-dimethylocta-2,6-dien-1-ol
Geraniol

MONOCYCLIC MONOTERPENE

5-methyl-2-(propan-2-yl)phenol
Thymol

2-methyl-5-(propan-2-yl)phenol
Carvacrol

5-methyl-2-(propan-2-yl)
cyclohexan-1-ol
Menthol

2-methyl-5-(prop-1-en-2-yl)
cyclohex-2-en-1-one
Carvone

BICYCLIC MONOTERPENE

(1S)-1,2,2-trimethyl-3-
methylidenebicyclo[2.2.1]heptane
Camphene

2,6,6-trimethylbicyclo[3.1.1]
hept-2-ene
Pinene

1,3,3-trimethylbicyclo
[2.2.1]heptan-2-one
Fenchone

(1S,2R,4S)-1,4,7,7-tetramethyl
bicyclo[2.2.1]heptan-2-ol
Borneol

SESQUITERPENE

4,8,8-trimethyl-9-methylidene-
decahydro-1,4-methanoazulene
Longifolene

1-ethenyl-1-methyl-2,4-di-
(prop-1-en-2-yl)cyclohexane
β-Elemene

(1S,4Z,9R)-4,11,11-trimethyl-8-
methylidenebicyclo[7.2.0]undec-4-ene
Caryophyllene

**FIGURE 3.1** Chemical diversities in the constituent of EO (ChemDraw).

Sophisticated sample taster and ionization technologies have been introduced, and new approaches are now being developed to analyze complicated materials rapidly and accurately (Tongnuanchan and Benjakul 2014; Simon and Quinn 1988). Using specific computer software, each spectrum will be carefully examined of the famous Turkish rose EO by taking note of individual ion peaks and removing interferences, solvent peaks, and background noise from the spectrum. This sorted data will enable the separation of individual ion peaks, allowing for the simple analysis of samples' metabolites (Dhifi et al. 2016; Cebi, Arici and Sagdic 2021). An impressive range of EO applications and possible health claims are viewed favorably by a growing body of pharmacological and clinical investigations. Global regulation of EOs was aggressively pursued by several international organizations, such as the World Health Organization, Geneva (Switzerland); the Food and Drug Administration, Maryland (United State); the FAO/WHO Codex Alimentarius Commission, Rome (Italy); the International Organization for Standardization, Geneva (Switzerland); and the International Federation of EO and Aroma Trades, London (United Kingdom). Component levels for several essential oils were established by ISO and the Organisation Française de Normalisation (AFNOR). Citrus fruits like orange (*Citrus sinensis*), lemon (*Citrus limon*), lime (*Citrus aurantiifolia*), corn mint (*Mentha arvensis*), peppermint (*Mentha x piperita*), spearmint (*Mentha spicata*), eucalyptus (*Eucalyptus globulus, E. polybractea*), clove (*Syzygium aromaticum*), and others are a reliable source of EO with a significant global market projection value (Es, Khaneghah and Akbariirad 2017; Van Boeckel 2017; Kuttan and Liju 2017; Falleh et al. 2020).

## 3.2   METHOD FOR EO ANALYSIS

Around 3000 volatile oils are already recognized, of which 300 are commercially useful, mainly in the sanitary, agronomic, perfumery, pharmaceutical, and food industries. The chemical composition of essential oils can be determined using analytical techniques such as gas chromatography with mass spectrometry (GC-MS) (Hashemi et al. 2017; Dima and Dima 2015), high-performance liquid chromatography (HPLC) (Turek and Stintzing 2013), gas chromatography-olfactometry (GC-O) (Delahunty, Eyres and Dufour 2006), enantio-selective gas chromatography, LC-APCIMS (liquid chromatography-atmospheric ionization mass spectrometry) (Kostiainen et al. 2003), [13]C-NMR spectroscopy (Tomi and Casanova 2006), capillary gas chromatography, multidimensional gas chromatography (MDGC) (Kubeczka and Formáček 2002; Sandra and Bicchi 1987), GC connected with flame ionization detect (FID), headspace GC (HSGC) (Belhachemi, Maatoug and Canela-Garayoa 2022; Ordoudi et al. 2020), etc., which are extensively employed for EO analysis. The most crucial method for characterizing the components in an EOs analysis is GC-MS (Figure 3.2).

The distinctive flavor and biological activity of Basil (*Ocimum* L.) are attributed to its essential oils. Based on the composition of the EO, Lawrence distinguished four main chemotypes of basil which were rich in methyl chavicol (estragole), linalool, methyl eugenol, and methyl cinnamate (Abdulkarem, Hussein and Ibrahim Lebnane 2017). Lettuce leaf, purple, Ohre, dark green, mammolo Genovese, manes, and red rubin were the different species of basil that were investigated. Manes was outlined for the first time. GC pattern was recorded through trace GC from Thermo Finnigan (Waltham, MA, USA) coupled with trace DSQ from Thermo Finnigan, Waltham, Massachusetts, USA. Sampling was done by AS 2000. Thermo Finnigan's Xcalibur 1.3 software was employed to execute the GC-MS data. GC-MS pattern illustrates that Ohre, lettuce leaf, purple opal, and dark green showed linalool content whereas mammolo Genovese, manes, and red rubin showed eucalyptol abundantly. Except for lettuce leaf, the content of eugenol varies with climate, specifically sunlight, humidity, and temperature. All the chemical constituents were compared with NIST (National Institute of Standards and Technologies) 02 Library software (Thermo Finnigan, Waltham, MA, USA) (Muráriková et al. 2017).

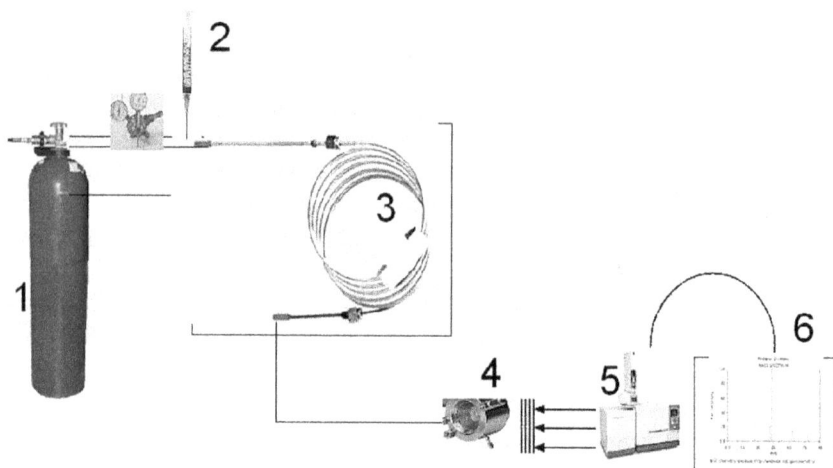

**FIGURE 3.2** Graphical representation of GC-MS 1) Helium cylinder 2) Injector 3) GC column along with oven 4) Ionization source 5) Focusing lens 6) MS detector (Drawn by Microsoft Visio Professional 2002 SR-1).

Coriander, cumin, fennel, and Indian mustard seed were investigated for EO composition by GC-MS. Shimadzu mass spectrometer (MS), model GC/MS – QP2020 NX SHIMADZU, was used to analyze the EO along with a Rxi-5 Sil MS fused silica capillary column (20 m*0.18 mm, 0.18 μm). The helium gas flow rate was done at 1 ml/min. Temperatures for the injector and detector were set at 290°C and 260°C, respectively. In accordance with the GC-MS pattern, coriander, cumin, fennel, and Indian mustard EO, respectively, have 11, 14, 09, and 13 components. Linalool had a computed level of 54.23% in coriander, followed by 17.01% cinnamaldehyde and 6.12% α-pinene. 1,4-p-menhaden-7-al, p-cumin aldehyde, γ-terpinene, and β-pinene were additional chemical components. The fennel EO contained the most anethole, at 69.01%, followed by estragole, fenchone, and limonene. The mustard seed EO contained 84.36% of 3-butenyl isothiocyanate and 8.52% of allyl-isothiocyanate. Monoterpenes, such as 31.48% of 1,4-p-menthadien-7-al, 26.65% of p-cumic aldehyde, 14.46% of α-pinene, 11.79% of γ-terpinene, and 3.81% of 2-caren-10-al, are the important ingredients of cumin EO (Ashokkumar et al. 2021).

Leaves of *Tagetes minuta* (Mexican marigold) and *Lantana camara* (tick berry leaf), *Zingiber officinale* (ginger) rhizome, and *Allium sativum* (garlic) bulb in Kenya were investigated for the chemical makeup of the EO. Steam distillation was the method to get essential oils; followed by GC-MS. It was performed using an Agilent 7890B GC and an Agilent 5977 mass detector; MS ChemStation was used to compute the data. GC has an extremely polar DB-wax capillary column with a stationary phase made entirely of polyethylene glycol (30.0 mx*0.25 mmx, 0.25 m). The GC condition, a 40°C starting oven temperature was maintained for 3 minutes. GC study revealed that Mexican marigold essential oils have the major chemical composition (71.2%), followed by ginger (55.8%), tick berries, and garlic

(53.8%). Mexican marigolds detected the presence of chrysantenyl 2- methyl butanoate, papaveroline, t-butyl hydroquinone, and dodecanoic acid while zingiberene, corymbolone, and bicyclo germacrene are the subsequent most abundant compounds in ginger EO. The main component of garlic was allyl(Z)-prop-1-enyl trisulfide; followed by 2-((2R,4aR,8aS)-4a-methyl-8-methylenedecahydronaphthalen-2-yl)-prop-2-en-1-ol, and longifolenaldehyde. The main composition in tick berries were bicyclogermacrene and 3-carene, cholesterol, 1R, 7S, E-7-isopropyl-4, 10-dimethyl-enecyclodec-5-enol, and bicyclo[5.2.0]nonane,2-methylene-4,8,8-trimethyl-4-vinyl (Mugao et al. 2020; Topi 2020).

With GC connected with an Agilent Technologies 7890A coupled mass selective detector, a VLMSD, and an Agilent 5975C equipped with a non-polar Agilent HP-5MS, researchers were able to characterize extracted from fresh *Pandanus candalabrum* (screw pine) leaves in Nigeria. GC-MS pattern revealed the presence of camphene, cembrene, phytol, kaur-16-ene, and phenanthrene. Kaur-16-ene was confirmed for analgesic and anti-inflammatory effects. FT-IR spectra showed fingerprint region at $2958.08 cm^{-1}$, $1598.10 cm^{-1}$, and $1457.86 cm^{-1}$ for carboxylic (-COOH), alkenes ($-CH_2=CH_2-$), and arenes ($-C_6H_5$) respectively (Ogwuche and Edema 2020).

GC-MS analysis of caraway EO identified the thirteen compounds, i.e., p-cymene, sylvestrene, cis-dihydrocarveol, trans-dihydrocarveol, carvcol, carvone, perilla aldehyde, nonacosane, triacontane, unitriacontane, triacontene, tetratriacontene, and pentatriacontane. Meanwhile, carvone (63.7%) and sylvestrene (14.8%) were confirmed in the caraway EO. Shimadzu GC/MS-QP2020, Kyoto (Japan) connected with Rtx-1MS fused bonded column (30 m*0.25 mm, 0.25 m). Restek, USA was employed to analyze the EO. Helium was utilized as the carrier gas with a flow rate of 1.37 mL/min, and the injector temperature was set to 280°C (Fekry et al. 2022). EO obtained from *Cinnamomum camphora* leaves; in the Qassim region of Saudi Arabia was scrutinized against different bacteria received from hospitals, i.e., *Pseudomonas aeruginosa* 89WS (wound swab), *Acinetobacter baumannii* 28TA (trachea aspiration), *Acinetobacter baumannii* 21SP (sputum), *Klebsiella pneumonia* 192U (urine), *Klebsiella pneumonia* 81TA (trachea aspiration), *Escherichia coli* 324U (urine), *Staphylococcus aureus* 24ABS (abscess), and *Staphylococcus aureus* 418BLD (blood). EO was subjected to GC-MS analysis of Shimadzu's 2010 QP Ultra Plus mass detector coupled with Thermo (TR5MS) column (25 m*250 mm). By comparing their MS with reference compounds from the NIST library, there were many different chemical components in the essential oil, including eucalyptol, 2,6,6-trimethyl bicyclo(3,1,1)hept-2-ene, D-limonene, bicyclo[3.1.1]heptane-3-ol, 6,6-dimethyl-2-methylene, α-terpineol, and 3-cyclohexene-1-ol (Mujawah et al. 2022).

EO was screened against gram-positive strains of *Staphylococcus aureus*, *Bacillus licheniformis*, and gram-negative strains of *Escherichia coli* and *Klebsiella pneumonia* using *Xylopia aethiopica* (Dunal) fruits from Ghana and Nigeria. A gas chromatograph from the Agilent 7890B series that was connected to a mass spectrometer (5977A) and a fused capillary column (HP-5MS) were used characterize the EO. 1R-pinene, 1-methyl-1-(1-methylethenyl)-cyclohexene, 2-carene, 5-methyl-3-(1-methylethenyl)-cyclohexene, trans-(-)-cyclohexene, 6-isopropylidene-1-methyl, eucalyptol, ethyl 2-(5-methyl-5-vinyltetrahydrofuran-2-yl) propan-2-carbonate were the identified compound in the EO of *Xylopia aethiopica*. The dominant metabolite detected in the fruits was isogeraniol, together with campholenal, L-trans-pinocarveol, pinocarvone, myrtenal, and myrtenol (-)-spathulenol (Alolga et al. 2019).

Design the simplest formulation, consider the impact of ingredients on preparation textural characteristics, and formulate oleogel using thyme EO that may have antibacterial activity. The concentrations of thymol and carvacrol in the thyme essential oil were measured using gas chromatography with fame ionization detection. GC-2010 Plus connected with a capillary column made of Crossbond 5% diphenyl/95% dimethyl polysiloxane Rxi-5 (Restek, USA) was used to separate the compound. *Candida albicans* were successfully eradicated by oleogel containing thyme EO (Kasparaviciene et al. 2018).

Using GS-MS analysis, the EO content of methanolic extract from *Elettaria cardamom* leaves was determined. A GCMS-QP2010 Plus analyzer was used. As a carrier gas, helium was used at a constant flow rate. The FT-IR examination using a Perkin Elmer spectrophotometer system revealed the characteristic peaks, the attenuated total reflectance component, and their functional groups. The wave number range for the IR fingerprint region was 4000–550 cm$^{-1}$. The findings showed that one of the main components in the methanol extract has antioxidant, anticancer, antitumor, anti-bronchitic, and anti-inflammatory properties. Other components include vitamin E, pentadecanoic acid, eucalyptol, octadecanoic acid, squalene, 4-phenyl-2-butanone, 3-heptanone, 5-hydroxy-1, 7-diphenyl, and 1-penten-3-one. The presence of alcohols, phenols, alkanes, aromatic rings, alkyl halides, ether linkage, and alkynes was verified by FT-IR analysis (Khatri et al. 2017).

The polymeric nanocapsules containing the essential oils (EO) of *R. officinalis* and *L. dentata* were detected by employing GC-MS and GC-FID analyses. The nanoprecipitation method was utilized to collect EO, and the GC-FID method was employed to analyze them for direct quantification. A GC model 6890N (Agilent Technologies, USA) connected 5973 INERT (ionisation energy 70 eV) mass detector and an HP 5MS column (30 m*0.25 mm, 0.25 m). The carrier gas was helium (99.99%) and the flow rate was 0.5 mL per minute. An Elite-5 capillary column and a flame ionization detector were utilized in conjunction with a gas chromatograph named the Clarus 480 (Perkin Elmer, USA) to analyze the EO (30 m*0.25 mm, 0.25 m, PerkinElmer, USA). While 1,8-cineole and -pinene were detected in EO of *L. dentata*; and camphor and 1,8-cineole were detected in *R. officinalis*, correspondingly (Silva-Flores et al. 2019).

HPLC-UV is a promising technology to authenticate the EO by using a very small concentration due to its adaptability, selectivity, and sensitivity phenomenon (Waseem and Kah Hin Low 2015; Reang, Mishra and Prasad 2020). See Figure 3.3.

Thymol and carvacrol were widely present in several pharmaceutical dose forms, abundant in thyme (*Thymus vulgaris*) EO. The HPLC method was established for the analysis of these two components in thyme EO. An HPLC experiment was carried out with the use of a Waters Alliance system that included a vacuum degasser, quaternary solvent mixing, auto-sampler, and a Waters 2996 diode array detector. UV data were gathered between 200–900 nm. For instrument control, data gathering, and data processing, Empower software was used. A 4.6 x 250 mm, 5 m, ACE C18 column was employed. Acetonitrile (ACN): H$_2$O (50:50) was the

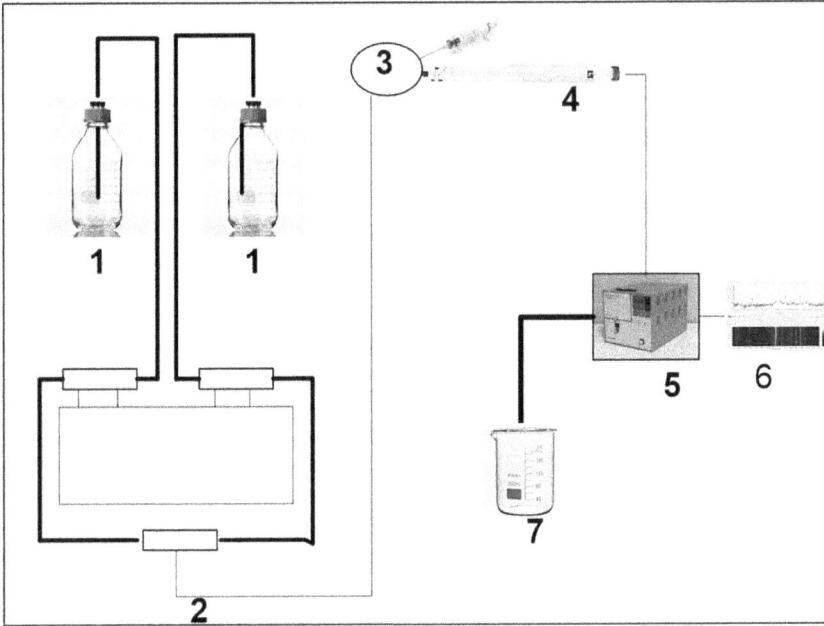

**FIGURE 3.3** Graphical representation of HPLC 1) Solvent reservoir 2) Solvent delivery system 3) Sample delivery system 4) Chromatographic column 5) Detector 6) Integrator 7) Effluent (Drawn by Microsoft Visio Professional 2002 SR-1).

isocratic mobile phase, flowing at a rate of 1 ml/min. It was established that the HPLC approach for measuring thymol and carvacrol was linear, selective, precise, and recoverable. Thymol and carvacrol are included in thymus prescription dose forms, although GC analysis was not feasible. For analyzing these compounds in plants, this method is a suitable replacement for the methods now in use. As a result, it can be said that this technique is not only beneficial for measuring these components in thyme EO, but also a reliable quality control approach for measuring thymol and carvacrol in thyme pharmaceutical dosage forms that cannot be measured by GC (Hajimehdipoor et al. 2010).

Chavibetol and methyl eugenol were simultaneously separated from the crude EO of screw pine (*P. pseudocaryophyllus*) leaves using the HPLC technique by using hexane and ethanol mobile phase. Shimadzu HPLC (Kyoto, Japan) with an analytical flow cell was utilized for the HPLC analysis and isolation. This Shimadzu HPLC connected LC-6AD pump, UV-Vis detector (SPD-10AV VP), and a SCL-10 VP system controller, Phenomenex Luna amino column (4.6 mm*150 mm, 10 m) with flow rate 1 mL/min, 10 L of injection; detected at 230 nm (Niculau et al. 2018).

*Plectranthus arabicus*, *P. asirensis*, *P. pseudomarrubioides*, *P. barbatus*, *P. hijazensis*, and *P. aegyptiacus*, cultivated in Saudi Arabia, were investigated for antioxidant capacity and the HPLC-PDA (photodiode array detector) profile of phenolic components. Waters Alliance HPLC (Waters Corp, Milford, MA, USA) connected with Waters e2995 separation module, Waters 2998 PDA, and Empower 2 software. Distinctive phenolic acids and flavonoids in the were qualitatively and quantitatively determined. The extracts were treated to solid phase extraction with a water:methanol ratio of 75:25 using an RP-C18 silica gel finger column. Ten different compounds, including gallic acid, caffeic acid, ferulic acid, rutin, rosmarinic acid, cinnamic acid, scutellarein, acacetin 7-o-methyltaxifolin, and 7,3'-di-o-methyltaxifolin, showed distinctive separation (Shaheen et al. 2017).

A total of thirteen cannabinoids, cannabinol (CBN), cannabigerol (CBG), cannabinolic acid (CBNA), cannabigerolic acid (CBGA), cannabidivarin (CBDV), tetrahydrocannabivarin (THCV), cannabidavarinic acid (CBDVA), tetrahydrocannabivarinic acid (THCVA), cannabichromenic acid (CBCA), cannabicyclolic acid (CBLA), tetrahydrocannabinolic acid (THC), cannabidiolic acid, $\delta$-8-tetrahydrocannabinol ($\delta$-8 THC), $\delta$-9 THC, cannabicyclol (CBL), cannabichromene (CBC), and tetrahydrocannabinolic acid (THCA) were characterized by using HPLC. The LabSolutions software-controlled CTO-20A column oven, LC20AB pump, DGU-20A5R degasser, SIL-20AHT autosampler, and SPD-20A UV detector were all components of the Shimadzu HPLC system. The separation process was conducted using a Restek Raptor ARC-18. Using an isocratic technique with 5 mM ammonium formate and 0.1% formic acid (for 25%), and 0.1% formic acid in acetonitrile (for 75%), chromatographic separation was accomplished in 11 min. The 228 nm setting on the UV detector (Galettis et al. 2021).

## 3.3   CONCLUSION

Consumers are learning about the advantages and possible uses of medicinal and aromatic plants, as well as their metabolites, as they become more knowledgeable about concerns relating to food, health, and nutrition. Essential oils are among the many secondary metabolites that these plants generate. To monitoring the quality of herbal medicines, several chromatographic and electrophoretic methods have been successfully used to date. The major chemical components could be detected by GC; however, it was challenging to identify the extracts' smaller components due to their low levels of presence. Mass spectrometry has other drawbacks as well, such as the inability to distinguish between closely related isomers due to extremely similar mass spectra, the absence of the compounds under investigation from the library of spectroscopy, and the computer's incorrect selection of a chemical based on similar mass. The assessment of medicinal herbs does not accurately reflect the quality of herbal medicines since a single analytical approach only provides limited information. Because of its excellent separation effectiveness and sensitive detection, GC-MS has established itself as a potent and useful technique for the determination of volatile chemicals. GC-MS has been a top tool for analyzing and characterizing EO extracts for the past 20 years and continues to be so in new studies. There will consequently be a need for a superior chemical summary based on the characterization of natural EO resources for forthcoming consequences. Specific secondary metabolites that need particularly precise sample preparation and analytical techniques to be investigated are flavonoids, terpenoids, and alkaloids. Just certain EOs were regulated, and standardization and regulation of EOs were still in their infancy. See Table 3.1.

## TABLE 3.1
## Characterization of EO by GC, GC-MS, GC-FID

| Source | GC Features | Outcomes |
|---|---|---|
| Aerial part Plan of *Ocimum* species, i.e., Ohre, lettuce leaf, purple opal, dark green, mammolo Genovese, manes, and red rubin | Trace GC, Thermo Finnigan (Waltham, MA, USA) with autosampler AS 2000 (Thermo Finnigan, Waltham, MA, USA) along with mass spectrometry detector Trace DSQ (Thermo Finnigan, Waltham, MA, USA). Data execution by Thermo Finnigan Xcalibur 1.3 software (Thermo Finnigan, Waltham, MA, USA) | Revealed the confirmation that lettuce leaf contains linalool and estragole in 1:0.9, dark green reveals linalool and eucalyptol in 1:0.7, mammolo Genovese showed eucalyptol and eugenol in 1:0.9, manes contains eucalyptol, linalool and eugenol in 1:0.6:0.4, red rubin contains eucalyptol, linalool, and eugenol in 1:0.6:0.7 |
| Coriander, cumin, fennel, and Indian mustard seed | GC QP2020 NX SHIMADZU, Shimadzu Corp., Tokyo, Japan coupled with Shimadzu mass spectrometer (MS) along with a Rxi-5 Sil MS fused silica capillary column | Revealed the confirmation of linalool, cinnamaldehyde, $\alpha$-pinene, 1,4-p-menhaden-7-al, p-cumin aldehyde, $\delta$-terpinene, $\beta$-pinene, anethole, estragole, fenchone, limonene |
| Leaves of Mexican marigold and tick berry leaf, ginger rhizome, and garlic bulb (*Allium sativum*) in Kenya | GC Agilent 7890B coupled Agilent 5977A mass detector and pattern was executed by GC-MS ChemStation software. DB-wax capillary column was installed | Revealed the confirmation of chrysantenyl 2-methylbutanoate, papaveroline, 1,2,3,4-tetrahydro-3-O-methyl-, 3,5-dimethylanisole, t-butylhydroquinone, dodecanoic acid, Zingiberene, corymbolone, bicyclogermacrene, allyl(Z)-prop-1-enyl trisulfide, 2-((2R,4ar,8as)-4a-methyl-8-methylenedecahydronaphthalen-2-yl)-prop-2-en-1-ol, Bicyclogermacrene and 3-carene, cholesterol, 1R, 7S, E -7-Isopropyl-4, 10-dimethylenecyclodec-5-enol, bicyclo [5.2.0] nonane,2-methylene-4,8,8-trimethyl-4-vinyl |
| Fresh leaves of screw pine | GC (Agilent Technologies 7890A) connected with a mass selective detector (VLMSD, Agilent 5975C) equipped with a nonpolar Agilent HP-5MS (5 %-phenyl methyl polysiloxane). | Revealed the confirmation of camphene, cembrene, phytol, kaur-16-ene, and phenanthrene |

*(Continued)*

**TABLE 3.1** (*Continued*)
## Characterization of EO by GC, GC-MS, GC-FID

| Source | GC Features | Outcomes |
|---|---|---|
| Caraway fruit essential oil | Shimadzu GC/MS-QP2020 (Kyoto, Japan) connected with Rtx-1MS fused bonded column (Restek, USA) | Revealed the confirmation of p-cymene, sylvestrene, cis dihydrocarveol, trans-dihydrocarveol, carveol, carvone, perilla aldehyde, nonerosive, triacontane, unitriacontane, triacontene, tetratriacontene, pentatriacontene |
| Cinnamomum leaves | Shimadzu QP ultra plus 2010 mass detector coupled with Thermo (TR5MS) column | eucalyptol, (62.13 2,6,6-trimethylbicyclo (3,1,1) hept-2-ene (12.20%), D-limonene (6.42%), bicyclo [3.1.1], heptane-3-ol, 6,6-dimethyl-2-methylene, α-terpineol, 3-cyclohexene-1-ol |
| Dunal fruits from Ghana and Nigeria | mzData format using DA reprocessor (Agilent) which further analyzed using SIMCA 14.1 (Umetrics, Umea, Sweden) | Revealed the confirmation of 1R-α-pinene, β-pinene, 2-carene, cyclohexene, 6-isopropylidene-1-methyl, eucalyptol, ethyl 2-(5-methyl-5-vinyl tetrahydrofuran-2-yl) propan-2-yl carbonate, isogeraniol, l-trans-pinocarveol, pinocarvone, myrtenal. |
| Oleogel using thyme essential oil | GC-2010 Plus (Shimadzu Corporation, USA) coupled with Restek, USA capillary column. | Oleogel prepared by thyme EO showed antibacterial activity against *Candida albicans* |
| Leaves of cardamom | GCMS-QP2010 Plus analyzer | Revealed the confirmation of vitamin E, squalene, eucalyptol, stigmast-5-en-3-ol, 4h-1-benjopyran-4-one, 2,3-dihydro5, 7-dihydroxy-2-pheny, octadecanoic acid, phytol, hexadecanoic acid |
| Thyme | GC model 6890N (Agilent Technologies, USA) coupled with 5973 INERT mass selective detector and an HP 5MS column | GC-FID spectra of thyme oil revealed the reduction of thymol and carvacrol content in the thyme oil |
| Nanoencapsulation of fresh essential oil from aerial parts of *R. officinalis* and *L. dentata* | 6890N (Agilent Technologies, USA) connected with a 5973 INERT mass selective spectrometer and HP 5MS column | Revealed the confirmation of camphor, 1,8-cineole, β-pinene |

Argentina is a significant supplier of essential oils since its agroclimatic conditions are ideal for the growth of aromatic plants, both domestic and foreign. In this sense, GC is the procedure that ensures conformity with the requirements agreed between the parties because the primary market for these items is European nations, which have high standards for quality (Kalita et al. 2011; Singh et al. 2022). Excellent information on the content and nature of complicated matrix components is provided by the application of HPLC-MS. With their advantages and some unwanted characteristics, innovative analytical practices for the extraction of EOs are more dependable than traditional approaches. According to several research studies, coupling extraction techniques can be used to separate the challenging EO matrices for plants' primary and secondary metabolites.

## ACKNOWLEDGMENT

Authors conveyed special thanks to Mr. Jitender Joshi, Chancellor, and Dr. Dharam Buddhi, Vice Chancellor of Uttaranchal University for encouragement for writing this communication.

## CONFLICT OF INTEREST

The authors declare that there is no conflict of interest.

## REFERENCES

Abdulkarem, Ahlam H., Ahmed Khaled Hussein, and H. Alsyari Hassan M. Ibrahim Lebnane. "Chemotaxonomy and spectral analysis (GC/MS and FT-IR) of essential oil composition of two Ocimum basilicum L. varieties and their morphological characterization." *Jordan Journal of Chemistry (JJC)* 12, no. 3 (2017): 147–160.

Alolga, Raphael N., María ASC Chávez León, George Osei-Adjei, and Vitus Onoja. "GC-MS-based metabolomics, antibacterial and anti-inflammatory investigations to characterize the quality of essential oil obtained from dried Xylopia aethiopica fruits from Ghana and Nigeria." *Journal of Pharmacy and Pharmacology* 71, no. 10 (2019): 1544–1552.

Ashokkumar, K., S. Vellaikumar, M. Murugan, M. K. Dhanya, A. Karthikeyan, G. Ariharasutharsan, P. Arjun, P. Sivakumar, and S. Aiswarya. "GC/MS analysis of essential oil composition from selected seed spices." *National Academy Science Letters* 44 (2021): 503–506.

Bakkali, Fadil, Simone Averbeck, Dietrich Averbeck, and Mouhamed Idaomar. "Biological effects of essential oils: A review." *Food and Chemical Toxicology* 46, no. 2 (2008): 446–475.

Belhachemi, Asma, M'hamed Maatoug, and Ramon Canela-Garayoa. "GC-MS and GC-FID analyses of the essential oil of Eucalyptus camaldulensis grown under greenhouses differentiated by the LDPE cover-films." *Industrial Crops and Products* 178 (2022): 114606.

Camps, Francisco, Jose Coll, and Jose Pascual. "Monocyclic terpene alcohols. IV. Birch reduction of p-isopropylbenzoic acid (cumic acid)." *The Journal of Organic Chemistry* 32, no. 8 (1967): 2563–2566.

Cebi, Nur, Muhammet Arici, and Osman Sagdic. "The famous Turkish rose essential oil: Characterization and authenticity monitoring by FTIR, Raman and GC-MS techniques combined with chemometrics." *Food Chemistry* 354 (2021): 129495.

Delahunty, Conor M., Graham Eyres, and Jean-Pierre Dufour. "Gas chromatography-olfactometry." *Journal of Separation Science* 29, no. 14 (2006): 2107–2125.

Dhifi, Wissal, Sana Bellili, Sabrine Jazi, Nada Bahloul, and Wissem Mnif. "Essential oils' chemical characterization and investigation of some biological activities: A critical review." *Medicines* 3, no. 4 (2016): 25.

Dima, Cristian, and Stefan Dima. "Essential oils in foods: Extraction, stabilization, and toxicity." *Current Opinion in Food Science* 5 (2015): 29–35.

Djilani, Abdelouaheb, and Amadou Dicko. "The therapeutic benefits of essential oils." *Nutrition, Well-Being and Health* 7 (2012): 155–179.

Duhl, T. R., D. Helmig, and A. Guenther. "Sesquiterpene emissions from vegetation: A review." *Biogeosciences* 5, no. 3 (2008): 761–777.

Es, Ismail, Amin Mousavi Khaneghah, and Hamid Akbariirad. "Global regulation of essential oils." *Essential Oils in Food Processing: Chemistry, Safety and Applications* (2017): 327–338.

Falleh, Hanen, Mariem Ben Jemaa, Mariem Saada, and Riadh Ksouri. "Essential oils: A promising eco-friendly food preservative." *Food Chemistry* 330 (2020): 127268.

Fekry, Mona, Galal Yahya, Ali Osman, Mohammed W. Al-Rabia, Islam Mostafa, and Hisham A. Abbas. "GC-MS analysis and microbiological evaluation of caraway essential oil as a virulence attenuating agent against pseudomonas aeruginosa." *Molecules* 27, no. 23 (2022): 8532.

Förster-Fromme, Karin, and Dieter Jendrossek. "AtuR is a repressor of acyclic terpene utilization (Atu) gene cluster expression and specifically binds to two 13 bp inverted repeat sequences of the atuA-atuR intergenic region." *FEMS Microbiology Letters* 308, no. 2 (2010): 166–174.

Galettis, Peter, Michelle Williams, Rebecca Gordon, and Jennifer H. Martin. "A simple isocratic HPLC method for the quantitation of 17 cannabinoids." *Australian Journal of Chemistry* 74, no. 6 (2021): 453–462.

Guenther, Ernest, and Darrell Althausen. *The Essential Oils.* Vol. 1. New York: Van Nostrand, 1948.

Hajimehdipoor, H., M. Shekarchi, M. Khanavi, N. Adib, and M. Amri. "A validated high performance liquid chromatography method for the analysis of thymol and carvacrol in Thymus vulgaris L. volatile oil." *Pharmacognosy Magazine* 6, no. 23 (2010): 154.

Hanif, Muhammad Asif, Shafaq Nisar, Ghufrana Samin Khan, Zahid Mushtaq, and Muhammad Zubair. "Essential oils." *Essential Oil Research: Trends in Biosynthesis, Analytics, Industrial Applications and Biotechnological Production* (2019): 3–17.

Hashemi, Seyed Mohammed Bagher, Amin Mousavi Khaneghah, and Anderson de Souza Sant'Ana, eds. *Essential Oils in Food Processing: Chemistry, Safety and Applications.* Hoboken, NJ: John Wiley & Sons, 2017.

Ipatieff, V. N., Herman Pines, Vladimir Dvorkovitz, R. C. Olberg, and Michael Savoy. "Studies in the terpene series. VI. Cyclic isomerization of limonene (1)." *The Journal of Organic Chemistry* 12, no. 1 (1947): 34–42.

Kalita, H., A. Kumar, K. Kishore, H. Rahman, R. Helim, and B. Das. *Aromatic Plants-Production and Potential in Sikkim.* Sikkim: ICAR Research Complex for NEH Region, Sikkim Centre (2011).

Kasparaviciene, Giedre, Zenona Kalveniene, Alvydas Pavilonis, Ruta Marksiene, Jurgita Dauksiene, and Jurga Bernatoniene. "Formulation and characterization of potential antifungal oleogel with essential oil of thyme." *Evidence-Based Complementary and Alternative Medicine* 2018 (2018).

Khatri, Poonam, J. S. Rana, Pragati Jamdagni, and Anil Sindhu. "Phytochemical screening, GC-MS and FT-IR analysis of methanolic extract leaves of Elettaria cardamomum." *International Journal of Research* 5, no. 2 (2017): 213–224.

Kostiainen, R., T. Kotiaho, T. Kuuranne, and S. Auriola. "Liquid chromatography/atmospheric pressure ionization-mass spectrometry in drug metabolism studies." *Journal of Mass Spectrometry* 38, no. 4 (2003): 357–372.

Kubeczka, Karl-Heinz, and Viktor Formáček. *Essential Oils Analysis by Capillary Gas Chromatography and Carbon-13 NMR Spectroscopy*. No. Ed. 2. Hoboken, NJ: John Wiley & Sons Ltd, 2002.

Kuttan, Ramadasan, and Vijayasteltar B. Liju. "Safety evaluation of essential oils." *Essential Oils in Food Processing: Chemistry, Safety and Applications* (2017): 247–292.

Mugao, Lydia G., Bernard M. Gichimu, Phyllis W. Muturi, and Simon T. Mukono. "Characterization of the volatile components of essential oils of selected plants in Kenya." *Biochemistry Research International* 2020 (2020).

Mujawah, A. A. H., E. M. Abdallah, S. A. Alshoumar, M. I. Alfarraj, S. M. I. Alajel, A. L. Alharbi, S. A. Alsalman, and F. A. Alhumaydhi. "GC-MS and in vitro antibacterial potential of Cinnamomum camphora essential oil against some clinical antibiotic-resistant bacterial isolates." *European Review for Medical and Pharmacological Sciences* 26, no. 15 (2022): 5372–5379.

Muráriková, Andrea, Anton Ťažký, Jarmila Neugebauerová, Alexandra Planková, Josef Jampílek, Pavel Mučaji, and Peter Mikuš. "Characterization of essential oil composition in different basil species and pot cultures by a GC-MS method." *Molecules* 22, no. 7 (2017): 1221.

Nesterkina, Mariia, and Iryna Kravchenko. "Synthesis and pharmacological properties of novel esters based on monocyclic terpenes and GABA." *Pharmaceuticals* 9, no. 2 (2016): 32.

Niculau, Edenilson dos Santos, Leandro do Prado Ribeiro, Thiago Felipe Ansante, João Batista Fernandes, Moacir Rossi Forim, Paulo Cezar Vieira, José Djair Vendramim, and Maria Fátima das Graças Fernandes Da Silva. "Isolation of chavibetol and methyleugenol from essential oil of Pimenta pseudocaryophyllus by high performance liquid chromatography." *Molecules* 23, no. 11 (2018): 2909.

Ogwuche, C. E., and M. O. Edema. "GC-MS and FTIR characterization of essential oil from the fresh leaves of Pandanus candalabrum obtained from Bayelsa state, Nigeria." *Nigerian Journal of Chemical Research* 25, no. 1 (2020): 1–10.

Ordoudi, Stella A., Maria Papapostolou, Stella Kokkini, and Maria Z. Tsimidou. "Diagnostic potential of FT-IR fingerprinting in botanical origin evaluation of Laurus nobilis L. essential oil is supported by GC-FID-MS Data." *Molecules* 25, no. 3 (2020): 583.

OTMS, O. OTMS. "8.4 Bicyclic Terpene Building Blocks." In. *Chiral Building Blocks in Asymmetric Synthesis* (2022). Wiley publication.

Parker, W., J. S. Roberts, and R. Ramage. "Sesquiterpene biogenesis." *Quarterly Reviews, Chemical Society* 21, no. 3 (1967): 331–363.

Reang, Sania Pallabi, J. P. Mishra, and Rajendra Prasad. "In vitro antifungal activities of five plant essential oils against Botrytis cinerea causing gray mold of orange." *Journal of Pharmacognosy and Phytochemistry* 9, no. 3 (2020): 1046–1048.

Sandra, Pat, and Carlo Bicchi. *Capillary gas chromatography in essential oil analysis*. (1987). Huethig Publishers.

Sangwan, N. S., A. H. A. Farooqi, F. Shabih, and R. S. Sangwan. "Regulation of essential oil production in plants." *Plant Growth Regulation* 34 (2001): 3–21.

Shaheen, Usama, K. Abdel Khalik, Mohamed IS Abdelhady, Saad Howladar, Mohammed Alarjah, and Mohammed A. S Abourehab. "HPLC profile of phenolic constituents, essential oil analysis and antioxidant activity of six Plectranthus species growing in Saudi Arabia." *Journal of Chemical and Pharmaceutical Research* 9, no. 4 (2017): 345–354.

Silva-Flores, Perla Giovanna, Luis Alejandro Pérez-López, Verónica Mayela Rivas-Galindo, David Paniagua-Vega, Sergio Arturo Galindo-Rodríguez, and Rocío Álvarez-Román. "Simultaneous GC-FID quantification of main components of Rosmarinus officinalis L. and Lavandula dentata essential oils in polymeric nanocapsules for antioxidant application." *Journal of Analytical Methods in Chemistry* 2019 (2019).

Simon, James E., and James Quinn. "Characterization of essential oil of parsley." *Journal of Agricultural and Food Chemistry* 36, no. 3 (1988): 467–472.

Singh, Preet Amol, Neha Bajwa, Sampath Chinnam, Arun Chandan, and Ashish Baldi. "An overview of some important deliberations to promote medicinal plants cultivation." *Journal of Applied Research on Medicinal and Aromatic Plants* (2022): 100400.

Tomi, F., and J. Casanova. "13C NMR as a tool for identification of individual components of essential oils from labiatae: A review." In *I International Symposium on the Labiatae: Advances in Production, Biotechnology and Utilisation 723*, pp. 185–192. 2006.

Tongnuanchan, Phakawat, and Soottawat Benjakul. "Essential oils: Extraction, bioactivities, and their uses for food preservation." *Journal of Food Science* 79, no. 7 (2014): R1231-R1249.

Topi, Dritan. "Volatile and chemical compositions of freshly squeezed sweet lime (Citrus limetta) juices." *The Journal of Raw Materials to Processed Foods* 1, no. 1 (2020): 22–27.

Turek, Claudia, and Florian C. Stintzing. "Stability of essential oils: A review." *Comprehensive Reviews in Food Science and Food Safety* 12, no. 1 (2013): 40–53.

Van Boeckel, Lex. *Maps and Essential Oils from Nepal: Market Analysis and Market Entry Strategy in the Indian Market.* Deutsche Gesellschaft fur Internationale Zusammenarbeit (GIZ) GmbH, 2017.

Waseem, Rabia, and Kah Hin Low. "Advanced analytical techniques for the extraction and characterization of plant-derived essential oils by gas chromatography with mass spectrometry." *Journal of Separation Science* 38, no. 3 (2015): 483–501.

# 4 Components of Essential Oils as Building Blocks of Functional Materials for Nanomedicine
## *Metal-Phenolic Networks and Self-Assembly Approaches*

*V. C. Cajiao Checchin, A. Gonzalez,*
*D. I. Arrieta Gamarra, N. S. Fagali, and*
*M. A. Fernández Lorenzo de Mele*

## 4.1 INTRODUCTION

Phytophenols (PPs) are secondary metabolites of plants. They play essential roles related to protection against UV radiation and diverse plant pathogens such as micro-organisms and insects. PPs are exceptional health assistants as antioxidants reducing the risk of degenerative diseases with anti-inflammatory, anticancer, antimicrobial, and cardio-, kidney-, lung-, UV-, and neuro-protective abilities (Liang et al. 2019). Polymers of PPs (poly-PPs) can assemble on diverse substrata conferring mechanical/thermal stability, pH responsive disassembly, protection against bacteria, and sensitive bioactivity that have attracted interest (Liang et al. 2019). In view of their natural source, PPs have been considered suitable for substituting diverse petroleum-derived materials (Lei et al. 2011).

A great variety of phenolic-enable nanotechnologies has been developed due to PPs' exceptional physicochemical properties. The ability to establish electrostatic coordination, hydrogen and covalent bonds, $\pi$ interactions, pH sensitivity, redox potentials, and radical scavenging have made PPs a distinct class of structural motifs for the synthesis of functional materials (Rahim et al. 2019; Ejima, Richardson, and Caruso 2017; Cajiao Checchin et al. 2022; Zhong et al. 2019).

DOI: 10.1201/9781003389774-4

### 4.1.1  SELF-ASSEMBLY/POLYMERIZATION (SAP) BY PPS

PPs like tannic acid (TA), dopamine (Dop), gallic acid (GA), caffeic acid (CA), pyrogallol (PG), thymol, and carvacrol can form, by SAP, thin layers (Figure 4.1) owed to their high surface bonding affinity (Lu et al. 2020; Gonzalez et al. 2020; Cajiao Checchin et al. 2022). Several works reported methods for easy deposition of PPs on diverse surfaces either spontaneously (M. Bertuola, Grillo, and Fernández Lorenzo de Mele 2016; Gonzalez et al. 2020), under a potential field (M. Bertuola et al. 2016, 2017), or as ingredients of more complex coatings (Sileika et al. 2013). Thin adherent SAP films can be formed by simple immersion of substrata of different nature in PPs solutions (Z. Wang and Cohen 2009). Thus, PPs can form SAP multifunctional structures such as coating films, hydrogels, and SAP-coated NPs for medical treatments in cancer and infections. Particularly, the use of functional poly-PPs-NPs fabricated with epigallocatechin gallate (EGCG)-conjugated polyethylene glycol (PEG) and the photosensitizer chlorin e6 (Ce6) has a promissory future for applications in cardiovascular or neurodegenerative diseases (T. Liu, Zhang, et al. 2018). Remarkably, the high ability of TA to assemble with protein, peptides, and polymers has been emphasized due to the interesting implications of this property for materials design (T. Liu, Zhang, et al. 2018).

The interaction of PPs with metal (Me) and Me-oxide surfaces deserves a special analysis. Particularly, the amino group in Dop can interact with Au Me surface, and construction and release of SAP monolayers can be achieved by electrochemical modulation (J. Li et al. 2019). Besides, the catechol (Cat) group can be useful in improving the stability and biocompatibility of superparamagnetic iron oxide nanoparticles (SPIONs).

In the case of the SAP approach, fundamental aspects of Me/substrata interactions with PPs can be followed by electrochemical techniques, since the presence of alcohol groups derives in oxidation. This oxidation is affected by the presence of substituents in the aromatic ring and depends on the Me nature. After the irreversible phenol electro-oxidation to phenoxy radicals, the reactivity of the Me electrode is usually partially or totally blocked due to the SAP layer (Ferreira et al. 2006; Chiorcea-Paquim et al. 2020) (Figure 4.1). Different electrochemical responses were reported for Pt, Au, Mg, Cu, and Ti, according to the Me reactivity (Ferreira et al. 2006; M. Bertuola, Grillo, and Fernández Lorenzo de Mele 2016; M. Bertuola, Fagali, and Fernández Lorenzo de Mele 2020; M. Bertuola et al. 2016, 2018).

On the other hand, due to their reducing capacity, PPs have been extensively used to reduce noble Me ions such as Ag(I), Au(III), Pt(IV), as a green method to synthesize NPs (Ying et al. 2022). They are also employed with non-metallic substrata such as carbon materials (graphene, carbon nanotubes, and carbon quantum dots) as reducing or stabilizing agents (Lei et al. 2011). Also, silica NPs can be obtained by the assistance of PPs such as GA and TA (Postnova and Shchipunov 2022). Moreover, PPs films are likewise formed on organic surfaces (polymer fibres, protein, and polysaccharide NPs) (Wu and Chen 2013).

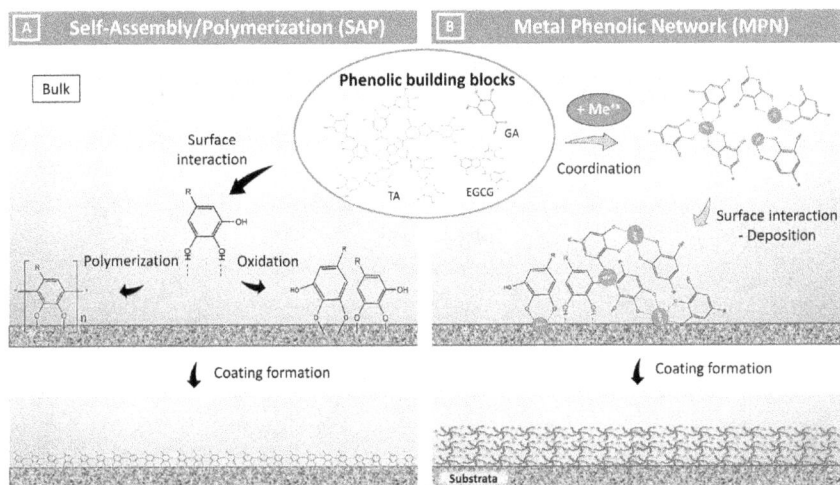

**FIGURE 4.1** Coating formation on different surfaces by A) SAP or B) MPN strategies.

## 4.1.2 METAL-PHENOLIC NETWORK (MPN) FORMATION BY PPS

The high coordination affinities of PPs allow them to function as raw materials of inorganic-organic networks for applications in diverse areas. One of the most investigated issues is the coordination between phenolics and Me ions since diverse arrangements known as Metal Phenolic Networks (MPNs) can be created (Z. Wang and Cohen 2009).

MPNs are supra-molecular structures formed from primary building assemblies consisting of central Me ions joint to phenolic molecules that contain dihydroxyphenyl (Cat) or trihydroxyphenyl (galloyl) groups (Figure 4.2). Diverse Me cations (Fe[III], Al[III], Zr[IV], Cu[II], Ce[III], Ti[IV], Zn[II], etc.) can be components of MPNs (Yaping Zhang et al. 2021) and modulate the assembly rate of PPs. In case of Dop polymerization it is greatly accelerated in presence of Cu(II) in alkaline media (C. Zhang et al. 2016) whereas formation of Fe(III)-TA healable film is improved by the oxidation of Fe(II) to Fe(III) when $O_2$ is present (H. Lee et al. 2018). The Cat or galloyl groups are the main phenolic constituents that interact with cations, Fe(III) being one of the most employed. Among PPs, TA is characterized by its five digalloyl ester groups that easily join to Me cations to build a net (Lu et al. 2020). TA is a dendritic PP (Figure 4.2) that may confer antioxidant, corrosion protection, antibacterial, antimutagenic, and anticarcinogenic properties to the surfaces (W. Xie et al. 2021). MPNs are able to form stimuli-responsive coatings and may include biomolecules (Liang et al. 2019; Guo et al. 2017).

Accordingly, MPNs exhibit unique structure and composition with outstanding properties useful for several medical applications that will be detailed in the next section. Their most important characteristics are i) *Adhesiveness*: MPN presents high bioadhesion capacity suitable for substrates of different nature and

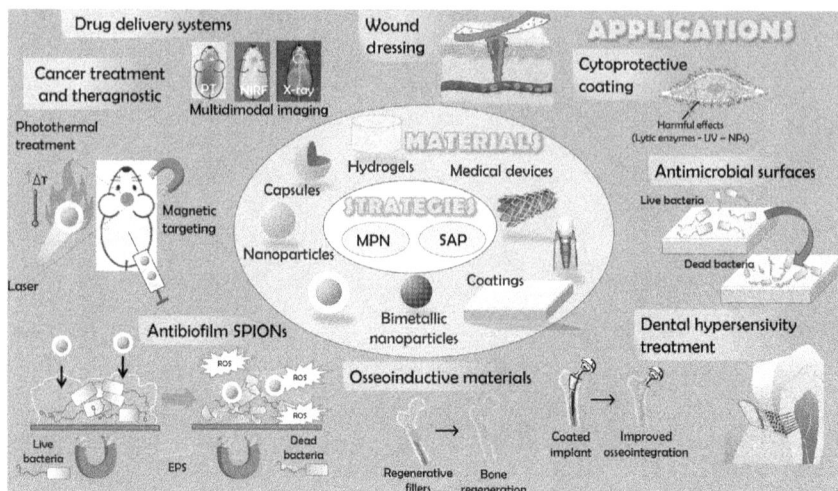

**FIGURE 4.2**   Schematic description of uses and applications of the materials obtained with the MPN and SAP strategies.

topography, providing favourable conditions for multiple drug encapsulation in nano-vehicles; ii) *Photothermal conversion*: MPNs exhibits strong absorption in the near-infrared (NIR) windows and can transduce NIR light in thermal energy, acting as photothermal nanomaterial; iii) *Fenton reaction enhancement*: PPs components of MPN convert Fe(III) into Fe(II) (of better catalytic efficacy), leading to higher levels of reactive oxygen species (ROS) production; and iv) *Quenching effect*: Useful in fluorescence techniques to localize abnormal tissues by magnetic resonance imaging (MRI).

## 4.2   USES AND APPLICATIONS OF MPNS AND SAP-COATINGS

In this section, several examples of materials/devices formed through the use of MPNs or SAP strategies are reported. They are summarized in Table 4.1, together with their main applications in medicine.

### 4.2.1   Osteoinductive Applications

One of the various applications of MPNs is improving the biocompatibility of bone implants. In this regard, Asgari et al. (2019) modified the surface of degradable Mg-based implants with a TA-Mg(II) coating. The goal of this dip coating capping is to reduce the corrosion rate of the implant, avoiding the hydrogen gas production that leads to the formation of cavities in the implant/tissue contact area, decreasing its post-implantation success. An important factor in the formation of these nanostructured coatings was the concentration of Mg(II). In the case of Mg(2.4%)-TA a reduction in degradation rate of almost three times, compared to the control, was found. In addition, a decrease in cytotoxicity and an increase in the adhesion and proliferation of the MC3T3-E1 cell line were achieved. *In vivo* tests in rats confirmed the success of the implant in reducing hydrogen production.

Other important application of MPNs are bone fillers with bioactive agents. Gao et al. (2021) worked on the development of next-generation multifunctional immunomodulatory biocomposites based on polycaprolactone, TA and Mg(II), using the electrospinning technique. The fillers showed a remarkable performance in ROS-scavenging activity, particularly against stable radical species DPPH, ABTS, and PTIO. The authors believe that the release of TA and Mg(II) would generate an anti-inflammatory microenvironment. When the new materials were employed in *in vivo* tests as scaffold for natural bone formation, they found a significant increase in osteogenesis.

In case of materials such as Ti alloys used in permanent implants, surface modifications are usually carried out to improve the osteogenic activity. S. Lee et al. (2020) developed a MPN-coating based on EGCG and Mg(II). They carried out osteogenic cell differentiation assays with adipose tissue cells and found an increase in alkaline phosphatase activity and expression of osteogenic markers. Also, an increase in mineralization compared to the control surface was found. It was also reported that the combination of EGCG and Mg(II) showed a synergistic effect in the decrease of maturation of macrophages Raw264.7 to osteoclastic form to avoid the administration of anti-osteoporotic drugs. Another example of MPN used on Ti is the coating based on Sr(II) and Cu(II) and TA developed by Xu et al. (2020). The authors reported that the deposition onto the substrates begins by the adhesion of TA-Me ion nuclei followed by the generation of homogeneous layers along the surface. They found that the cation release from the coatings, particularly anti-inflammatory and osteogenic cations, was faster in acid solutions. This is a remarkable result since a pH decrease can occur around the tissue due to surgery, repair processes, or infections (Teitelbaum 2000). Additionally, a greater area covered by better anchored mesenchymal stem cells and a lower fraction of apoptotic cells in the case of Sr-MPN and Sr/Cu-MPN were found.

### 4.2.2 Dental Hypersensitivity Treatment and Bone Tissue Regeneration

Oh et al. (2015) created an easy and rapid solution to seal the dentinal tubule entrances as a treatment for dental hypersensitivity. They used a diluted solution of TA-Fe(III) complex that quickly formed a MPN narrowing the dental tubule entrances. Additionally, this coating induced remineralization by Ca-absorption that promoted hydroxyapatite deposit. Recently, it was also demonstrated that TA lead to biomineralization by cross-linking with collagen fibres and by surface modification (Kong et al. 2022). Other authors reported an improvement in osteoconductivity and stimuli in bone formation *in vivo* thanks to TA, GA, and other PPs (Onat et al. 2018; Cajiao Checchin et al. 2022).

### 4.2.3 ANTIMICROBIAL STRATEGIES

Jiang et al. (2018) designed TA/Fe-MPN coatings using the layer-by-layer method on polymers generally used as part of materials in endoscopes or catheters. They reported that the bacteria repellence was 25% and 45% for *Staphylococcus aureus* and *Escherichia coli* respectively for TA/Fe(III). In case of TA-Ce(IV), the performance is better (93% and 85% respectively) since Ce acts as biocatalyst, accelerating the hydrolysis of DNA excreted by bacteria to form the matrix in biofilm.

TA can rapidly and spontaneously form a gel with elements of group IVB as Ti(IV) and Zr(IV). This kind of gel has been used in the pharmaceutical industry for years to induce crystallisation of active principles (Y. Li et al. 2022). Anh, Huang, and Huang (2019) showed that the gel made of TA/Ti(IV)-MPN was able to incorporate other Me ions (such as Cu[II]) that were studied by their antimicrobial and wound-healing properties. The authors discovered that acidic pH and $H_2O_2$, which are generated in infected wounds, triggered the Cu(II) release from the TA-Ti(IV) gel. Consequently, it can be employed as a smart dressing for controlled release of antimicrobial Me ions. Also, a TA-loaded gellan/gelatine binary blend hydrogel was able to stimulate wound healing (Y. Zheng et al. 2018).

Balne et al. (2018) developed antibacterial coatings with poly-PG and Ag(I) or Mg(II) to be used on catheters to prevent nosocomial infections. Coating with these cations and poly-PG(1%) eradicated methicillin-resistant *S. aureus* (MRSA). However, in the case of *E. coli*, only the inhibition of growth was attained using poly-PG(1%)-Ag. J.Y. Lee et al. (2019) created a poly-CA-based coating on Ti substrates by exposing it to $AgNO_3$ solution, with the aim of capturing Ag(I) cations and reducing them to $Ag°$ NPs in this matrix. They performed *in vitro* assays with the MC3T3 pre-osteoblastic cell line and reported an enhancement in biocompatibility compared to the control and an increase in the inhibition halo in case of *S. aureus*, *E. coli*, and *P. aeruginosa* strains.

Another way to obtain MPNs with increased antimicrobial activity is to generate bimetallic nanostructures. Y. Xie et al. (2022) developed a coating for a wound dressing that helps fight infection and at the same time promotes the microvascular network to have a speedy recovery. They relied on spontaneous co-reduction of Ag(I) + 1e è $Ag°$ and Cu(I)èCu°+Cu(II), forming Ag/Cu-TA MPN films. Assays with *E. coli* and *S. aureus* demonstrated a noteworthy decrease (almost 100%) in bacterial adhesion to the substrate coated with Ag/Cu-TA. In contrast, for the monometallic coatings lower yields were found for both strains, ~58% with Cu-TA and ~89% with Ag-TA.

Exploiting the antibacterial property of Cu, Tu et al. (2019) developed Cu(II)-based MPNs coating, with TA and cysteamine (CS) to cover polyvinyl chloride (PVC) with the aim of decreasing infections in vascular devices. They exposed the surface to *E. coli* and *S. aureus* strains and achieved ~99% antibacterial effectiveness for Cu(20 mg/ml)-TA-CS. Additionally, the decrease in platelet adhesion and its activation (anti-thrombogenic activity) were reported. X. Li et al. (2018) also used Cu(II) with Dop, norepinephrine, and TA to functionalized stainless steel and PVC. These coatings showed 95% of antibacterial effect with *S. aureus* and *E. coli* strains. Moreover, the films exhibited antioxidant, anti-inflammatory, and anticoagulant activity *ex vivo* related to the properties of their building block components.

### 4.2.4 PHOTOTHERMAL TREATMENTS

NIR light has been applied in a broad range of biomedical strategies such as photo-thermal therapy or drug delivery systems. Due to the strong absorption and the trans-duction of NIR light in thermal energy MPNs can act as photothermal nanomaterial and also in photodynamic therapy against cancer (Chang et al. 2021). ROS formation during irradiation is promoted being useful for cancer treatment or bacterial biofilm eradication.

When TA/Fe(III) mixtures were included in a polyacrylamide hydrogel, they confer excellent photothermal properties (X. Zhang et al. 2021; Y. Wang et al. 2020) with a high photothermal efficiency (near 40%), which was remarkably superior to the Au nanorods.

### 4.2.5 CYTOPROTECTIVE COATINGS

Great advances have been made in cytoprotective coatings that, inspired by biology, try to recreate the bacterial endospores generated under stress as a protective strat-egy, until the harmful effect of their surroundings disappears. These cytoprotective coatings were mostly emulated with TA and Fe(III) solutions, creating a biocompati-ble defending layer capable of being modified (H. Wang et al. 2020; Park et al. 2016). Park et al. (2014) obtained a cytoprotective and degradable coating on individual *Saccharomyces cerevisiae* that protects the yeast from multiple external aggressors such as UV-C, lytic enzymes, and silver NPs (AgNPs). In turn, Kim et al. (2017) devised nanocapsules using a biphasic system of TA in an aqueous medium, and Fe(III) as immiscible continuous phase. They obtained protective UV-C irradiation coatings with a percentage of viability of *S. cerevisiae* after irradiation of ~65.1% compared to the uncoated control of ~6.8%. Wasuwanich et al. (2022) designed a coating to supply the beneficial bacteria *Bacillus subtilis* into the gut in a viable state, protecting it from the stress of the process. They found that the degree of protection against lyophilization depends on the size of the PP molecule (GA->TA->EGCG-protection), on the stability of the Me-phenol coordination and on the cation charge/size (GA-Fe[III]<GA-Al[III]<GA-Zn[II]).

### 4.2.6 DRUG DELIVERY WITH MPNs-CAPSULES

There is also a large field for the designing of MPN-coatings or -capsules that allow the incorporation of active ingredients or drugs with anti-inflammatory, antican-cer, or antimicrobial properties, necessary to combat specific medical problems (H. Wang et al. 2020; Y. Wang et al. 2022). Among them, Guo et al. (2014) developed capsules based on TA and different Me, which can be applied in drug delivery and imaging. They studied the degradation of FITC-dextran-loaded Al(III)-capsules and confirmed a successful internalization with conserved capsule shape. At the same time, this procedure allows tracking through positron emission tomography (PET) phantom images, very useful to see *in vivo* biodistribution.

### 4.2.7 DRUG DELIVERY WITH SPIONS

Biomedical applications based on SPIONs require NPs systems with a high magnetization value, a narrow particle size distribution, and a biocompatible surface coating (Santos et al. 2016).

TA-based coating for NPs systems provides the nanocarrier with important properties, such as better water dispersibility, higher cellular internalization (Santos et al. 2016), antioxidant activity and longer circulation in the body (Shagholani and Ghoreishi 2017). In addition, the incorporation of TA and GA (Santos et al. 2016; Shagholani and Ghoreishi 2017) leads to the reduction in the NPs size.

Antimicrobial, anti-inflammatory, tissue imaging, and theragnostic properties will be summarized in this section while the applications for cancer treatments will be detailed in Section 2.8.

#### 4.2.7.1 Antimicrobial Strategies

SAP-coated SPIONs have been proposed as antibacterial and/or antifungal agents. X. Wang et al. (2017) created a magnetic nanocomposite by the deposit of TA and the anchoring of AgNPs on the surface of magnetite NPs to fulfil antibacterial functions against Gram positive and Gram negative bacteria. The pH sensitivity of TA allows the controlled release of Ag(I) ions that cause bacterial killing. Since the NPs are magnetic, the authors reported the possibility of recovering them with a magnet and recycling after disinfection. The authors also presented (X. Wang et al. 2018) a highly efficient magnetic nanoplatform for planktonic inactivation and biofilm disruption. The nanoplatform consisted of a magnetite core and a multilayer coating composed of TA, the antibiotic gentamicin, AgNPs, and an outer layer of hyaluronic acid. The nanoplatform was a potent nanocarrier for AgNPs delivery and release on demand in response to the microenvironment of bacterial infection. Moreover, the use of SPIONs contributes to overcoming bacterial resistance since the mechanical disruption of the biofilm matrix can be triggered with an external changing magnetic field.

#### 4.2.7.2 Anti-Inflammatory Treatments

SAP-coated SPIONs have been proposed as anti-inflammatory or healing agents. For example, Ardeshirzadeh et al. (2022) studied the degranulation of mast cells and the presence of inflammatory cells in wounds of mice with diabetes, and concluded that the controlled and localized release of curcumin by magnetic NPs accelerates the wound healing process. Fatemi Abhari et al. (2020) proposed the inoculation of curcumin-coated SPIONs as a treatment for polycystic ovary syndrome (PCOS). Assays in PCOS-induced mice demonstrate that ovarian lesions and cell apoptosis were efficiently suspended by curcumin released from NPs.

### 4.2.7.3  Tissue Imaging and Theragnostic

MRI is one of the most used techniques for diagnosing cancer early. SPIONs are excellent MRI contrast agents due to their large magnetic moment, which induces a high characteristic transverse relaxation and increased susceptibility effect (Richard et al. 2016). Ren et al. (2020) reported the combination of Fe(III) with EGCG to prepare nanodrugs which were combined with Gd(III) to obtain a whiter image in tumour areas and a MRI signal increasing over time. Additionally, these NPs included cisplatin that can function as a catalyst to produce high intracellular levels of ROS with excellent anticancer properties, avoiding the systemic toxicity. Bimetallic capsules can be prepared to be detected by more than one imaging technique. Thus, Cu(II) and Eu(III) were detected by energy dispersive X-ray spectroscopy (EDX), PET, and fluorescence imaging (Guo et al. 2014). SAP-coated SPIONs with curcumin also have theragnostic applications. Gholibegloo et al. (2019) proposed a nanosponge that has a core of magnetite, coated with curcumin and decorated with folic acid. Its objective is the release of PPs in cancer cells with increased negative signal of diagnostic imaging.

Another PP of interest for improving imaging is CA. This PP is also a perfect complement to SPIONs in brain tumour investigations due to its potential as an anticancer drug and regenerative properties. Richard et al. (2016) propose the inoculation of SPIONs functionalized with CA in mice. Following intravenous injection of the NPs into mice with U87 glioblastomas, negative contrast enhancement was observed on MRI in cancerous tissue.

### 4.2.8  CANCER TREATMENT

In recent years a great effort has been made in order to target the cancer treatment directly to the tumour, avoiding the cytotoxic effects in the rest of the body (P. Liu et al. 2021; Q. Li et al. 2021). MPNs are versatile platforms capable of improving and complementing traditional therapies against tumour eradication with very promising results that can change future treatments to combat cancer worldwide. Fe(II)/Fe(III) triggered Fenton reaction has been proposed to obtain cytotoxic hydroxyl radicals (•OH) for several biomedical applications. The presence of PPs in Fe-based-MPNs leads to higher levels of ROS production (Xu et al. 2020; Teitelbaum 2000). In this way, MPNs can be used in ROS-mediated ferroptosis therapies and their photothermal capacity makes MPNs interesting targets to replace current chemotherapy with less invasive treatments (Zhou et al. 2021). However, it is necessary to carry out further complementary studies on the tissues and organs surrounding the tumour location, since hyperthermia treatments and the increase in ROS may cause severe damage on them (P. Liu et al. 2021; Yanbing Wang, Liu, et al. 2019).

Different MPNs applications in cancer treatments and their principal effects, biosafety and biocompatibility are reviewed in Table 4.1. In brief, Table 4.1 reports i) the advantages of the MPN-nanovehicles that enhances the antitumor activity in relation with the pure drugs (Shen et al. 2016; Le et al. 2018; C. Wang et al. 2018; Luo et al. 2020; L. Zhang et al. 2018; Yang et al. 2020; Dong et al. 2019; Hao et al. 2020; Shan et al. 2019; Ren et al. 2020; S. Chen et al. 2020); ii) the increased efficacy of the

**TABLE 4.1**
**Summary of Principal MPN-Based Therapies for Cancer Applications**

| MPN | Based Material | Cancer Applications | Principal Effects | Biosafety and Biocompatibility of Studied System | References |
|---|---|---|---|---|---|
| TA-Fe(III) NPs | PTX | Chemotherapy (drug delivery) | Better antitumour activity than pure PTX. Good oral bioavailability. | Non-cytotoxic effect in heart, lung, liver, spleen, brain, and kidneys in mice model. Good intestinal absorption. | Shen et al. 2016; Le et al. 2018 |
| | Ce6 | Photodynamic therapy | Selective accumulation in tumour and enhanced photodynamic therapy. | Not evaluated. | Liu et al. 2017 |
| | Rapamycin/ Ce6 | Photodynamic therapy | Strong effect for photodynamic therapy under hypoxia conditions. | Not evaluated. | Liu et al. 2019 |
| | BTZ | Chemotherapy (drug delivery) and MRI | Increased apoptosis on cancer cells and suppressed tumour growth. | High biocompatibility to blood in mice model. | C. Wang et al. 2018 |
| | SRF | Photodynamic and ferroptosis therapy | Increased ferroptosis and complete tumour elimination. | Non-cytotoxic effect in heart, lung, liver, spleen, and kidneys in mice model. | Liu et al. 2018 |
| | DOX | Chemotherapy (drug delivery), MRI, photothermal, and photoacoustic therapy | ATP-depletion, enhanced effect of chemotherapy. Suitable for photoacoustic and photothermal imaging. | Non-cytotoxic effect in heart, lung, liver, spleen, brain, and kidneys in mice model. | Luo et al. 2020 |

| | | | | |
|---|---|---|---|---|
| **TA-Fe(III) coatings** | PNSs nanospheres | Photothermal and photoacoustic therapy guided by imaging | Complete elimination of tumour and enhanced photothermal and photoacoustic imaging. | Not evaluated. | Liu et al. 2018 |
| | GOx@ZIF NPs | Chemodynamic therapy | Enhanced Fenton reaction and thus increased ROS production. | Non-cytotoxic effect was found in heart, lung, liver, spleen, brain, and kidneys in mice model. | Zhang et al. 2018 |
| | PG-g-mPEG NPs | Photothermal and photoacoustic therapy | Effective NPs accumulation in tumour tissue and photothermal effect. | Not evaluated. | Wang et al. 2019 |
| | Mesoporous silica NPs | Chemotherapy (drug delivery) and photothermal therapy | Increased photothermal effect and effectiveness to kill cancer cells. | Not evaluated. | Yang et al. 2020 |
| | PEI/p53 NPs | Ferroptosis therapy | Increased ferroptosis and suppressed the tumour growth. Decreased blood, lung, and liver metastasis. | Not evaluated. | Zheng et al. 2017 |
| | DOX NPs | Chemodynamic and ferroptosis therapies | Elevated ROS and Fenton reaction, increased chemodynamic and ferroptosis effect. | Not evaluated. | Guo et al. 2019 |
| **GA-Fe(III)-coatings** | PVP NPs | MRI imaging guided photothermal therapy | Increased tumours-imaging sensitivity and MRI-guided photothermal therapy. Complete suppression of tumour growth. | No cytotoxic effect (histochemical, hematologic and blood biochemical analyses). | Liu et al. 2015 |
| | $MoS_2$-nanosheets | Imaging-guided chemodynamic therapy | Enhanced •OH radical generation. | No cytotoxic hematologic effects. | Zheng et al. 2021 |

(Continued)

**TABLE 4.1 (Continued)**
**Summary of Principal MPN-Based Therapies for Cancer Applications**

| MPN | Based Material | Cancer Applications | Principal Effects | Biosafety and Biocompatibility of Studied System | References |
|---|---|---|---|---|---|
| | UCNP-nanoprobe | Photothermal therapy and MRI | Improved ligand-free tumour targeting ability, enriched MRI performance, and enhanced therapeutic effects against tumours *in vivo*. | Not evaluated. | Zhang et al. 2021 |
| | GOx/ZIF-8/BSA | Photothermal and ferroptosis therapy | Accelerated Fenton reaction and enhanced photothermal and ferroptosis therapies. | Not evaluated. | An et al. 2019 |
| **GA-Fe(II)** | BSO liposome | Radiotherapy and Chemotherapy (drug delivery). | Amplified intracellular and intratumoural oxidative stress via increasing •OH generation and reducing GSH biosynthesis. | Not evaluated. | Dong et al. 2019 |
| | DOX-liposomes | MRI, photothermal, and ferroptosis therapies | Increased intracellular ROS levels and induced ferroptosis. Superior photothermal responsiveness and MRI capabilities. | Not evaluated. | Zhang et al. 2021 |
| | GOx-DMAA-PEGDA-nanocomplex | Chemodynamic therapy | •OH generation with glucose depletion, effective destruction of breast cancer tumours by chemodynamic-starvation therapy. | Not evaluated. | Hao et al. 2020 |

| | Material | Therapy | Outcome | Toxicity | Reference |
|---|---|---|---|---|---|
| **EGCG-Fe(III)-coating** | DOX and PEG NPs | Chemotherapy | Better antitumor effect than free drugs (DOX). | Reduced cardiac toxicity in mice model. | Shan et al. 2019 |
| | PEG-polymer NPs | Chemotherapy (drug delivery) and chemodynamic therapy | Increased intracellular $H_2O_2$ level and ROS. Improved anticancer efficacy. | Not evaluated. | Ren et al. 2020 |
| | DOX NPs | Chemotherapy and photothermal therapy | Elimination of tumour was achieved. | Non-cytotoxic effect was found in heart, lung, liver, spleen, and kidneys in mice model. | Chen et al. 2019 |
| | DOX NPs | Chemotherapy (drug delivery) | Accumulation in tumour tissue, prevention of the occurrence of tumour metastasis. | Non-cytotoxic effect was found in heart, liver, spleen, and kidneys in mice model. | Chen et al. 2020 |
| | DOX NPs | Ferroptosis therapy | Increased Fenton reaction and generation of ROS inducing lethal ferroptosis. | Not evaluated. | Mu et al. 2020 |
| | Ce6-NPs | Photodynamic therapy | Better performance in intracellular uptake, ROS generation, penetrability into multicellular tumour spheres than pure drugs, and feasibility to function as photodynamic agents. | Not evaluated. | Chen et al. 2020 |

*Abbreviations*: PTX: paclitaxel; BTZ: bortezomib; SRF: sorafenib; DOX: doxorubicin; PNSs: Poly(lactic-*co*-glycolic acid)-based polymeric nanospheres; PEI: polyethylenimine; PLG-g-mPEG: poly glutamic acid-graft-methoxy PEG; GOx: glucose oxidase; ZIF: zeolitic imidazolate framework; PVP: polyvinylpyrrolidone; UCNP: upconversion NP; BSA: bull serum albumin; BSO: L-buthionine sulfoximine; DMAA: N,N-dimethylacrylamide.

MPN-vehicles in comparison with single-photosensitizers in photothermal therapies (Y. Liu et al. 2017; P. Liu et al. 2019; T. Liu, Liu, et al. 2018; T. Liu, Zhang, et al. 2018; Yanbing Wang, Wang, et al. 2019; F. Liu et al. 2015; P. Zhang et al. 2019; An et al. 2019; Yulin Zhang et al. 2021; X. Chen et al. 2019, 2020); iii) the enriched ROS production of MPN-based developments (T. Liu, Liu, et al. 2018; An et al. 2019; Yulin Zhang et al. 2021; D. W. Zheng et al. 2017; Kang et al. 2019; H. Zheng et al. 2021; Mu et al. 2020); and iv) the excellent capacity of MPN-systems to localize cancer tissues by MRI either for diagnosis or for guided-imaging therapies (theragnosis) (T. Liu, Zhang, et al. 2018; C. Wang et al. 2018; Luo et al. 2020; F. Liu et al. 2015; P. Zhang et al. 2019; Yulin Zhang et al. 2021; H. Zheng et al. 2021).

According to these results most *in vivo* studies have been conducted with drug delivery agents, contain Fe(II)/Fe(III) ions and do not have cytotoxic effects in blood or in vital organs. Accordingly, the use of these systems in medical treatments is promissory. However, *in vivo* studies are still not frequent in those systems proposed for photothermal and ferroptosis therapies.

## 4.3   CONCLUSIONS

All things considered, the interesting physical-chemical properties of PPs allow them to interact with surfaces, ions, and biomolecules of different natures and to form multifunctional coatings and nanostructures with applications in diverse areas, with special emphasis in medicine. Many of them are related to delivery vehicles, mainly in cancer theragnostics, and other new applications are focused on bacterial infection, cell therapy, anti-inflammatory therapies, and wound healing and bone regeneration. Among PPs-derived future applications a precise on-demand drug delivery could be developed since PPs can strongly interact with the proteins of tissues and consequently, the target delivery to specific organs may be achieved. After solving some remaining challenges such as stability, biosafety, and scaling-up, new developments will emerge as the next generation drug delivery systems and tissue treatments with the consequent public health benefits in the near future.

## REFERENCES

An, Peijing, Dihai Gu, Zhiguo Gao, Fengying Fan, Yong Jiang, and Baiwang Sun. 2019. "Hypoxia-Augmented and Photothermally-Enhanced Ferroptotic Therapy with High Specificity and Efficiency." *Journal of Materials Chemistry B* 8 (1). Royal Society of Chemistry: 78–87. doi:10.1039/c9tb02268f.

Anh, Ha Thi Phuong, Chun Ming Huang, and Chun Jen Huang. 2019. "Intelligent Metal-Phenolic Metallogels as Dressings for Infected Wounds." *Scientific Reports* 9 (1). Springer US: 1–10. doi:10.1038/s41598-019-47978-9.

Ardeshirzadeh, Ahmadreza, Houssein Ahmadi, Mansooreh Mirzaei, Hamidreza Omidi, Atarodalsadat Mostafavinia, Abdollah Amini, Sahar Bayat, Mohammadjavad Fridoni, Sufan Chien, and Mohammad Bayat. 2022. "The Combined Use of Photobiomodulation and Curcumin-Loaded Iron Oxide Nanoparticles Significantly Improved Wound Healing in Diabetic Rats Compared to Either Treatment Alone." *Lasers in Medical Science*, (December). Springer Science and Business Media Deutschland GmbH. doi:10.1007/s10103-022-03639-4.

Asgari, Mohammad, Ying Yang, Shuang Yang, Zhentao Yu, Prasad K.D.V. Yarlagadda, Yin Xiao, and Zhiyong Li. 2019. "Mg-Phenolic Network Strategy for Enhancing Corrosion Resistance and Osteocompatibility of Degradable Magnesium Alloys." *ACS Omega* 4 (26): 21931–21944. doi:10.1021/acsomega.9b02976.

Balne, Praveen Kumar, Sriram Harini, Chetna Dhand, Neeraj Dwivedi, Madhavi Latha Somaraju Chalasani, Navin Kumar Verma, Veluchamy Amutha Barathi, Roger Beuerman, Rupesh Agrawal, and Rajamani Lakshminarayanan. 2018. "Surface Characteristics and Antimicrobial Properties of Modified Catheter Surfaces by Polypyrogallol and Metal Ions." *Materials Science & Engineering C, Materials for Biological Applications* 90 (May). Elsevier Ltd: 673–684. doi:10.1016/J. MSEC.2018.04.095.

Bertuola, M., N. Fagali, and M. Fernández Lorenzo de Mele. 2020. "Detection of Carvacrol in Essential Oils by Electrochemical Polymerization." *Heliyon* 6 (4). doi:10.1016/j.heliyon.2020.e03714.

Bertuola, M., C.A. Grillo, and M. Fernández Lorenzo de Mele. 2016. "Reduction of Copper Ions Release by a Novel Ecofriendly Electropolymerized Nanolayer Obtained from a Natural Compound (Carvacrol)." *Journal of Hazardous Materials* 313: 262–271. doi:10.1016/j.jhazmat.2016.03.086.

Bertuola, M., C.A. Grillo, D.E. Pissinis, E.D. Prieto, and M. Fernández Lorenzo de Mele. 2017. "Is the Biocompatibility of Copper with Polymerized Natural Coating Dependent on the Potential Selected for the Electropolymerization Process?" *Colloids and Surfaces B: Biointerfaces* 159. doi:10.1016/j.colsurfb.2017.08.029.

Bertuola, M., A. Miñán, C.A. Grillo, M.C. Cortizo, and M.A. Fernández Lorenzo de Mele. 2018. "Corrosion Protection of AZ31 Alloy and Constrained Bacterial Adhesion Mediated by a Polymeric Coating Obtained from a Phytocompound." *Colloids and Surfaces B: Biointerfaces* 172 (August). Elsevier: 187–196. doi:10.1016/j.colsurfb.2018.08.025.

Bertuola, Marcos, Diego E. Pissinis, Aldo A. Rubert, Eduardo D. Prieto, and Mónica A. Fernández Lorenzo de Mele. 2016. "Impact of Molecular Structure of Two Natural Phenolic Isomers on the Protective Characteristics of Electropolymerized Nanolayers Formed on Copper." *Electrochimica Acta* 215 (October). Pergamon: 289–297. doi:10.1016/J.ELECTACTA.2016.08.100.

Cajiao, Checchin, Valentina Chiara, Ariel Gonzalez, Marcos Bertuola, and Mónica Alicia Fernández Lorenzo de Mele. 2022. "Multifunctional Coatings of Phenolic Phytocompounds of Medical Interest: Assembly Methods and Applications." *Progress in Organic Coatings* 172 (August). doi:10.1016/j.porgcoat.2022.107068.

Chang, Mengyu, Zhiyao Hou, Man Wang, Chunxia Li, and Jun Lin. 2021. "Recent Advances in Hyperthermia Therapy-Based Synergistic Immunotherapy." *Advanced Materials* 33 (4): 1–29. doi:10.1002/adma.202004788.

Chen, Si, Jin Xuan Fan, Di Wei Zheng, Fan Liu, Xuan Zeng, Guo Ping Yan, and Xian Zheng Zhang. 2020. "A Multi-Functional Drug Delivery System Based on Polyphenols for Efficient Tumor Inhibition and Metastasis Prevention." *Biomaterials Science* 8 (2). Royal Society of Chemistry: 702–711. doi:10.1039/c9bm01646e.

Chen, Xiangyu, Zeng Yi, Guangcan Chen, Xiaomin Ma, Wen Su, Xinxing Cui, and Xudong Li. 2019. "DOX-Assisted Functionalization of Green Tea Polyphenol Nanoparticles for Effective Chemo-Photothermal Cancer Therapy." *Journal of Materials Chemistry B* 7 (25). Royal Society of Chemistry: 4066–4078. doi:10.1039/c9tb00751b.

Chen, Xiangyu, Zeng Yi, Guangcan Chen, Xiaomin Ma, Wen Su, Zhiwen Deng, Lei Ma, Qiulan Tong, Yaqin Ran, and Xudong Li. 2020. "Carrier-Enhanced Photodynamic Cancer Therapy of Self-Assembled Green Tea Polyphenol-Based Nanoformulations." *ACS Sustainable Chemistry and Engineering* 8 (43): 16372–16384. doi:10.1021/ acssuschemeng.0c06645.

Chiorcea-Paquim, Ana Maria, Teodor Adrian Enache, Eric De Souza Gil, and Ana Maria Oliveira-Brett. 2020. "Natural Phenolic Antioxidants Electrochemistry: Towards a New Food Science Methodology." *Comprehensive Reviews in Food Science and Food Safety* 19 (4): 1680–1726. doi:10.1111/1541-4337.12566.

Dong, Ziliang, Liangzhu Feng, Yu Chao, Yu Hao, Muchao Chen, Fei Gong, Xiao Han, Rui Zhang, Liang Cheng, and Zhuang Liu. 2019. "Amplification of Tumor Oxidative Stresses with Liposomal Fenton Catalyst and Glutathione Inhibitor for Enhanced Cancer Chemotherapy and Radiotherapy." *Nano Letters* 19 (2): 805–815. doi:10.1021/acs.nanolett.8b03905.

Ejima, Hirotaka, Joseph J. Richardson, and Frank Caruso. 2017. "Metal-Phenolic Networks as a Versatile Platform to Engineer Nanomaterials and Biointerfaces." *Nano Today* 12 (February). Elsevier: 136–148. doi:10.1016/J.NANTOD.2016.12.012.

Fatemi Abhari, Seyedeh Maedeh, Ramzan Khanbabaei, Nasim Hayati Roodbari, Kazem Parivar, and Parichehreh Yaghmaei. 2020. "Curcumin-Loaded Super-Paramagnetic Iron Oxide Nanoparticle Affects on Apoptotic Factors Expression and Histological Changes in a Prepubertal Mouse Model of Polycystic Ovary Syndrome-Induced by Dehydroepiandrosterone-A Molecular and Stereological Study." *Life Sciences* 249 (May). Elsevier Inc. doi:10.1016/j.lfs.2020.117515.

Ferreira, Marystela, Hamilton Varela, Roberto M. Torresi, and Germano Tremiliosi-Filho. 2006. "Electrode Passivation Caused by Polymerization of Different Phenolic Compounds." *Electrochimica Acta* 52 (2): 434–442. doi:10.1016/j.electacta.2006.05.025.

Gao, Xinghui, Qian Wang, Lulu Ren, Pei Gong, Min He, Weidong Tian, and Weifeng Zhao. 2021. "Metal-Phenolic Networks as a Novel Filler to Advance Multi-Functional Immunomodulatory Biocomposites." *Chemical Engineering Journal* 426 (December). Elsevier: 131825. doi:10.1016/J.CEJ.2021.131825.

Gholibegloo, Elham, Tohid Mortezazadeh, Fatemeh Salehian, Hamid Forootanfar, Loghman Firoozpour, Alireza Foroumadi, Ali Ramazani, and Mehdi Khoobi. 2019. "Folic Acid Decorated Magnetic Nanosponge: An Efficient Nanosystem for Targeted Curcumin Delivery and Magnetic Resonance Imaging." *Journal of Colloid and Interface Science* 556 (November). Academic Press Inc.: 128–139. doi:10.1016/j.jcis.2019.08.046.

Gonzalez, Ariel, Alejandro Guillermo Miñán, Claudia Alejandra Grillo, Eduardo Daniel Prieto, Patricia Laura Schilardi, and Mónica Alicia Fernández Lorenzo de Mele. 2020. "Characterization and Antimicrobial Effect of a Bioinspired Thymol Coating Formed on Titanium Surface by One-Step Immersion Treatment." *Dental Materials* 36 (12): 1495–1507. doi:10.1016/j.dental.2020.09.006.

Guo, Junling, Yuan Ping, Hirotaka Ejima, Karen Alt, Mirko Meissner, Joseph J. Richardson, Yan Yan, et al. 2014. "Engineering Multifunctional Capsules through the Assembly of Metal-Phenolic Networks." *Angewandte Chemie: International Edition* 53 (22): 5546–5551. doi:10.1002/anie.201311136.

Guo, Junling, Joseph J. Richardson, Quinn A. Besford, Andrew J. Christofferson, Yunlu Dai, Chien W. Ong, Blaise L. Tardy, et al. 2017. "Influence of Ionic Strength on the Deposition of Metal-Phenolic Networks." *Langmuir* 33 (40): 10616–10622. doi:10.1021/acs.langmuir.7b02692.

Guo Y, Zhang X, Sun W, Jia HR, Zhu YX, Zhang X, et al. Metal-Phenolic Network-Based Nanocomplexes that Evoke Ferroptosis by Apoptosis: Promoted Nuclear Drug Influx and Reversed Drug Resistance of Cancer. Chem Mater 2019;31:10071–84. doi:10.1021/acs.chemmater.9b03042.

Hao, Yu, Ziliang Dong, Muchao Chen, Yu Chao, Zhuang Liu, Liangzhu Feng, Y. Hao, et al. 2020. "Near-Infrared Light and Glucose Dual-Responsive Cascading Hydroxyl Radical

Generation for in Situ Gelation and Effective Breast Cancer Treatment." *Biomaterials* 228 (October 2019). Elsevier: 119568. doi:10.1016/j.biomaterials.2019.119568.

Jiang, Ru Jian, Shun Jie Yan, Li Mei Tian, Shi Ai Xu, Zhi Rong Xin, Shi Fang Luan, Jing Hua Yin, Lu Quan Ren, and Jie Zhao. 2018. "A Biomimetic Surface for Infection-Resistance through Assembly of Metal-Phenolic Networks." *Chinese Journal of Polymer Science (English Edition)* 36 (5). Springer Verlag: 576–583. doi:10.1007/S10118–018–2032-Z.

Kang, Junjie, Guoqiang Bai, Shuanhong Ma, Xinghuan Liu, Zhiyuan Ma, Xuhong Guo, Xiaolong Wang, Bin Dai, Feng Zhou, and Xin Jia. 2019. "Metal-Phenolic Networks Films: On-Site Surface Coordination Complexation via Mechanochemistry for Versatile Metal-Phenolic Networks Films (Adv. Mater. Interfaces 5/2019)." *Advanced Materials Interfaces* 6 (5): 1970031. doi:10.1002/admi.201970031.

Kim, Beom Jin, Sol Han, Kyung Bok Lee, and Insung S. Choi. 2017. "Biphasic Supramolecular Self-Assembly of Ferric Ions and Tannic Acid across Interfaces for Nanofilm Formation." *Advanced Materials* 29 (28): 1–7. doi:10.1002/adma.201700784.

Kong, Weijing, Qiaolin Du, Yinan Qu, Changyu Shao, Chaoqun Chen, Jian Sun, Caiyun Mao, Ruikang Tang, and Xinhua Gu. 2022. "Tannic Acid Induces Dentin Biomineralization by Crosslinking and Surface Modification." *RSC Advances* 12 (6). Royal Society of Chemistry: 3454–3464. doi:10.1039/d1ra07887a.

Le, Zhicheng, Yantao Chen, Honghua Han, Houkuan Tian, Pengfei Zhao, Chengbiao Yang, Zhiyu He, et al. 2018. "Hydrogen-Bonded Tannic Acid-Based Anticancer Nanoparticle for Enhancement of Oral Chemotherapy." *ACS Applied Materials and Interfaces* 10 (49): 42186–42197. doi:10.1021/acsami.8b18979.

Lee, Hojae, Won Il Kim, Wongu Youn, Taegyun Park, Sangmin Lee, Taek Soo Kim, João F. Mano, and Insung S. Choi. 2018. "Iron Gall Ink Revisited: In Situ Oxidation of Fe(II)-Tannin Complex for Fluidic-Interface Engineering." *Advanced Materials* 30 (49): 1–8. doi:10.1002/adma.201805091.

Lee, Ji Yeon, Ludwig Erik Aguilar, Chan Hee Park, and Cheol Sang Kim. 2019. "UV Light Assisted Coating Method of Polyphenol Caffeic Acid and Mediated Immobilization of Metallic Silver Particles for Antibacterial Implant Surface Modification." *Polymers* 11 (7). Multidisciplinary Digital Publishing Institute (MDPI). doi:10.3390/POLYM11071200.

Lee, Sangmin, Yun Young Chang, Jinkyu Lee, Sajeesh Kumar Madhurakkat Perikamana, Eun Mi Kim, Yang Hun Jung, Jeong Ho Yun, and Heungsoo Shin. 2020. "Surface Engineering of Titanium Alloy Using Metal-Polyphenol Network Coating with Magnesium Ions for Improved Osseointegration." *Biomaterials Science* 8 (12). The Royal Society of Chemistry: 3404–3417. doi:10.1039/D0BM00566E.

Lei, Yanda, Zhenghai Tang, Ruijuan Liao, and Baochun Guo. 2011. "Hydrolysable Tannin as Environmentally Friendly Reducer and Stabilizer for Graphene Oxide." *Green Chemistry* 13 (7): 1655–1658. doi:10.1039/c1gc15081b.

Li, Jun, Chun Lin Sun, Pengrong An, Xiaoyan Liu, Ruihua Dong, Jinghong Sun, Xingyu Zhang, et al. 2019. "Construction of Dopamine-Releasing Gold Surfaces Mimicking Presynaptic Membrane by On-Chip Electrochemistry." *Journal of the American Chemical Society* 141 (22): 8816–8824. doi:10.1021/jacs.9b01003.

Li, Quguang, Ziliang Dong, Meiwan Chen, and Liangzhu Feng. 2021. "Phenolic Molecules Constructed Nanomedicine for Innovative Cancer Treatment." *Coordination Chemistry Reviews* 439. doi:10.1016/j.ccr.2021.213912.

Li, Xiangyang, Peng Gao, Jianying Tan, Kaiqin Xiong, Manfred F. Maitz, Changjiang Pan, Hongkai Wu, Yin Chen, Zhilu Yang, and Nan Huang. 2018. "Assembly of Metal-Phenolic/Catecholamine Networks for Synergistically Anti-Inflammatory, Antimicrobial, and Anticoagulant Coatings." *ACS Applied Materials and Interfaces* 10 (47): 40844–40853. doi:10.1021/acsami.8b14409.

Li, Yue, Yong Miao, Lunan Yang, Yitao Zhao, Keke Wu, Zhihui Lu, Zhiqi Hu, and Jinshan Guo. 2022. "Recent Advances in the Development and Antimicrobial Applications of Metal: Phenolic Networks." *Advanced Science* 9 (27): 1–22. doi:10.1002/advs.202202684.

Liang, Hongshan, Bin Zhou, Di Wu, Jing Li, and Bin Li. 2019. "Supramolecular Design and Applications of Polyphenol-Based Architecture: A Review." *Advances in Colloid and Interface Science* 272: 1–13. doi:10.1016/j.cis.2019.102019.

Liu, Fuyao, Xiuxia He, Hongda Chen, Junping Zhang, Huimao Zhang, and Zhenxin Wang. 2015. "Gram-Scale Synthesis of Coordination Polymer Nanodots with Renal Clearance Properties for Cancer Theranostic Applications." *Nature Communications* 6. Nature Publishing Group: 1–9. doi:10.1038/ncomms9003.

Liu, Peng, Xinyi Shi, Shenghui Zhong, Ying Peng, Yan Qi, Jinsong Ding, and Wenhu Zhou. 2021. "Metal-Phenolic Networks for Cancer Theranostics." *Biomaterials Science* 9 (8): 2825–2849. doi:10.1039/d0bm02064h.

Liu, Peng, Xin Xie, Xinyi Shi, Ying Peng, Jinsong Ding, and Wenhu Zhou. 2019. "Oxygen-Self-Supplying and HIF-1α-Inhibiting Core-Shell Nanosystem for Hypoxia-Resistant Photodynamic Therapy." *ACS Applied Materials and Interfaces* 11 (51): 48261–48270. doi:10.1021/acsami.9b18112.

Liu, Tao, Wenlong Liu, Mingkang Zhang, Wuyang Yu, Fan Gao, Chuxin Li, Shi Bo Wang, Jun Feng, and Xian Zheng Zhang. 2018. "Ferrous-Supply-Regeneration Nanoengineering for Cancer-Cell-Specific Ferroptosis in Combination with Imaging-Guided Photodynamic Therapy." *ACS Nano* 12 (12): 12181–12192. doi:10.1021/acsnano.8b05860.

Liu, Tao, Mingkang Zhang, Wenlong Liu, Xuan Zeng, Xianlin Song, Xiaoquan Yang, Xianzheng Zhang, and Jun Feng. 2018. "Metal Ion/Tannic Acid Assembly as a Versatile Photothermal Platform in Engineering Multimodal Nanotheranostics for Advanced Applications." *ACS Nano* 12 (4): 3917–3927. doi:10.1021/acsnano.8b01456.

Liu, Yamei, Kai Ma, Tifeng Jiao, Ruirui Xing, Guizhi Shen, and Xuehai Yan. 2017. "Water-Insoluble Photosensitizer Nanocolloids Stabilized by Supramolecular Interfacial Assembly towards Photodynamic Therapy." *Scientific Reports* 7 (January). Nature Publishing Group: 1–8. doi:10.1038/srep42978.

Lu, Ruofei, Xiaoqiang Zhang, Xinxiu Cheng, Yagang Zhang, Xingjie Zan, and Letao Zhang. 2020. "Medical Applications Based on Supramolecular Self-Assembled Materials From Tannic Acid." *Frontiers in Chemistry* 8 (October). doi:10.3389/fchem.2020.583484.

Luo, Yuanli, Bin Qiao, Ping Zhang, Chao Yang, Jin Cao, Xun Yuan, Haitao Ran, et al. 2020. "TME-Activatable Theranostic Nanoplatform with ATP Burning Capability for Tumor Sensitization and Synergistic Therapy." *Theranostics* 10 (15): 6987–7001. doi:10.7150/thno.44569.

Mu, Min, Yuelong Wang, Shasha Zhao, Xiaoling Li, Rangrang Fan, Lan Mei, Min Wu, et al. 2020. "Engineering a PH/Glutathione-Responsive Tea Polyphenol Nanodevice as an Apoptosis/Ferroptosis-Inducing Agent." *ACS Applied Bio Materials* 3 (7): 4128–4138. doi:10.1021/acsabm.0c00225.

Oh, Dongyeop X., Ekavianty Prajatelistia, Sung Won Ju, Hyo Jeong Kim, Soo Jin Baek, Hyung Joon Cha, Sang Ho Jun, Jin Soo Ahn, and Dong Soo Hwang. 2015. "A Rapid, Efficient, and Facile Solution for Dental Hypersensitivity: The Tannin-Iron Complex." *Scientific Reports* 5 (June). Nature Publishing Group: 1–8. doi:10.1038/srep10884.

Onat, Bora, Salih Ozcubukcu, Sreeparna Banerjee, and Irem Erel-Goktepe. 2018. "Osteoconductive Layer-by-Layer Films of Poly(4-Hydroxy-L-Proline Ester) (PHPE) and Tannic Acid." *European Polymer Journal* 103 (June). Pergamon: 101–115. doi:10.1016/J.EURPOLYMJ.2018.03.034.

Park, Ji Hun, Daewha Hong, Juno Lee, and Insung S. Choi. 2016. "Cell-in-Shell Hybrids: Chemical Nanoencapsulation of Individual Cells." *Accounts of Chemical Research* 49 (5). American Chemical Society: 792–800. doi:10.1021/ACS.ACCOUNTS.6B00087/ASSET/IMAGES/MEDIUM/AR-2016–00087B_0009.GIF.

Park, Ji Hun, Kyunghwan Kim, Juno Lee, Ji Yu Choi, Daewha Hong, Sung Ho Yang, Frank Caruso, Younghoon Lee, and Insung S. Choi. 2014. "A Cytoprotective and Degradable Metal: Polyphenol Nanoshell for Single-Cell Encapsulation." *Angewandte Chemie International Edition* 53 (46). John Wiley & Sons, Ltd: 12420–12425. doi:10.1002/ANIE.201405905.

Postnova, Irina, and Yury Shchipunov. 2022. "Tannic Acid as a Versatile Template for Silica Monoliths Engineering with Catalytic Gold and Silver Nanoparticles." *Nanomaterials* 12 (23). Multidisciplinary Digital Publishing Institute: 4320. doi:10.3390/NANO12234320.

Rahim, Md Arifur, S.L. Kristufek, S Pan, J Richardson, F Caruso. 2019. "Phenolic Building Blocks for the Assembly of Functional Materials." *Angewandte Chemie: International Edition* 58 (7): 1904–1927.

Ren, Zhigang, Shichao Sun, Ranran Sun, Guangying Cui, Liangjie Hong, Benchen Rao, Ang Li, Zujiang Yu, Quancheng Kan, and Zhengwei Mao. 2020. "A Metal: Polyphenol-Coordinated Nanomedicine for Synergistic Cascade Cancer Chemotherapy and Chemodynamic Therapy." *Advanced Materials* 32 (6): 1–10. doi:10.1002/adma.201906024.

Richard, Sophie, Ana Saric, Marianne Boucher, Christian Slomianny, Françoise Geffroy, Sébastien Mériaux, Yoann Lalatonne, Patrice X. Petit, and Laurence Motte. 2016. "Antioxidative Theranostic Iron Oxide Nanoparticles toward Brain Tumors Imaging and ROS Production." *ACS Chemical Biology* 11 (10). American Chemical Society: 2812–28119. doi:10.1021/acschembio.6b00558.

Santos, Anderson F.M., Lucyano J.A. Macedo, Mariana H. Chaves, Marisol Espinoza-Castañeda, Arben Merkoçi, Francisco Das Chagas A. Limac, and Welter Cantanhêde. 2016. "Hybrid Self-Assembled Materials Constituted by Ferromagnetic Nanoparticles and Tannic Acid: A Theoretical and Experimental Investigation." *Journal of the Brazilian Chemical Society* 27 (4). Sociedade Brasileira de Quimica: 727–734. doi:10.5935/0103–5053.20150322.

Shagholani, Hamidreza, and Sayed Mehdi Ghoreishi. 2017. "Investigation of Tannic Acid Cross-Linked onto Magnetite Nanoparticles for Applying in Drug Delivery Systems." *Journal of Drug Delivery Science and Technology* 39: 88–94.

Shan, Lingling, Guizhen Gao, Weiwei Wang, Wei Tang, Zhantong Wang, Zhen Yang, Wenpei Fan, et al. 2019. "Self-Assembled Green Tea Polyphenol-Based Coordination Nanomaterials to Improve Chemotherapy Efficacy by Inhibition of Carbonyl Reductase 1." *Biomaterials* 210 (April). Elsevier: 62–69. doi:10.1016/j.biomaterials.2019.04.032.

Shen, Guizhi, Ruirui Xing, Ning Zhang, Chengjun Chen, Guanghui Ma, and Xuehai Yan. 2016. "Interfacial Cohesion and Assembly of Bioadhesive Molecules for Design of Long-Term Stable Hydrophobic Nanodrugs toward Effective Anticancer Therapy." *ACS Nano* 10 (6): 5720–5729. doi:10.1021/acsnano.5b07276.

Sileika, Tadas S., Devin G. Barrett, Ran Zhang, King Hang Aaron Lau, and Phillip B. Messersmith. 2013. "Colorless Multifunctional Coatings Inspired by Polyphenols Found in Tea, Chocolate, and Wine." *Angewandte Chemie International Edition* 52 (41). John Wiley & Sons, Ltd: 10766–10770. doi:10.1002/ANIE.201304922.

Teitelbaum, S.L. 2000. "Bone Resorption by Osteoclasts." *Science (New York, N.Y.)* 289 (5484). Science: 1504–1508. doi:10.1126/SCIENCE.289.5484.1504.

Tu, Qiufen, Xuehong Shen, Yaowen Liu, Qiang Zhang, Xin Zhao, Manfred F. Maitz, Tao Liu, et al. 2019. "A Facile Metal: Phenolic: Amine Strategy for Dual-Functionalization of Blood-Contacting Devices with Antibacterial and Anticoagulant Properties." *Materials Chemistry Frontiers* 3 (2). The Royal Society of Chemistry: 265–275. doi:10.1039/C8QM00458G.

Wang, Changping, Huajun Sang, Yitong Wang, Fang Zhu, Xinhao Hu, Xinyu Wang, Xing Wang, Yiwen Li, and Yiyun Cheng. 2018. "Foe to Friend: Supramolecular Nanomedicines Consisting of Natural Polyphenols and Bortezomib." *Nano Letters* 18 (11): 7045–7051. doi:10.1021/acs.nanolett.8b03015.

Wang, Hui, Changping Wang, Yuan Zou, Jingjing Hu, Yiwen Li, and Yiyun Cheng. 2020. "A Natural Polyphenols in Drug Delivery Systems: Current Status and Future Challenges." *Giant* 3 (August). Elsevier B. V. doi:10.1016/j.giant.2020.100022.

Wang, Xi, Weiwei Cao, Qian Xiang, Feng Jin, Xuefeng Peng, Qiang Li, Min Jiang, Bingcheng Hu, and Xiaodong Xing. 2017. "Silver Nanoparticle and Lysozyme/Tannic Acid Layer-by-Layer Assembly Antimicrobial Multilayer on Magnetic Nanoparticle by an Eco-Friendly Route." *Materials Science and Engineering C* 76 (July). Elsevier Ltd: 886–896. doi:10.1016/j.msec.2017.03.192.

Wang, Xi, Juan Wu, Peili Li, Lina Wang, Jie Zhou, Gaoke Zhang, Xin Li, Bingcheng Hu, and Xiaodong Xing. 2018. "Microenvironment-Responsive Magnetic Nanocomposites Based on Silver Nanoparticles/Gentamicin for Enhanced Biofilm Disruption by Magnetic Field." *ACS Applied Materials and Interfaces* 10 (41). American Chemical Society: 34905–34915. doi:10.1021/acsami.8b10972.

Wang Y, Wang Z, Xu C, Tian H, Chen X. A disassembling strategy overcomes the EPR effect and renal clearance dilemma of the multifunctional theranostic nanoparticles for cancer therapy. *Biomaterials* 2019;197:284–93. doi:10.1016/j.biomaterials.2019.01.025.

Wang, Yanan, Jingwen Zhang, Yi Zhao, Minju Pu, Xinyu Song, Liangmin Yu, Xuefeng Yan, et al. 2022. "Innovations and Challenges of Polyphenol-Based Smart Drug Delivery Systems." *NaRes* 15 (9). Tsinghua University: 8156–8184. doi:10.1007/S12274-022-4430-3.

Wang, Yanbing, Feng Liu, Nan Yan, Shu Sheng, Caina Xu, Huayu Tian, and Xuesi Chen. 2019. "Exploration of FeIII-Phenol Complexes for Photothermal Therapy and Photoacoustic Imaging." *ACS Biomaterials Science and Engineering* 5 (9): 4700–4707. doi:10.1021/acsbiomaterials.9b00711.

Wang, Yanbing, Zhuo Wang, Caina Xu, Huayu Tian, and Xuesi Chen. 2019. "A Disassembling Strategy Overcomes the EPR Effect and Renal Clearance Dilemma of the Multifunctional Theranostic Nanoparticles for Cancer Therapy." *Biomaterials* 197 (December 2018). Elsevier: 284–293. doi:10.1016/j.biomaterials.2019.01.025.

Wang, Yaran, Ting Wei, Yangcui Qu, Yang Zhou, Yanjun Zheng, Chaobo Huang, Yanxia Zhang, Qian Yu, and Hong Chen. 2020. "Smart, Photothermally Activated, Antibacterial Surfaces with Thermally Triggered Bacteria-Releasing Properties." *ACS Applied Materials and Interfaces* 12 (19): 21283–21291. doi:10.1021/acsami.9b17581.

Wang, Zhenqiang, and Seth M. Cohen. 2009. "Postsynthetic Modification of Metal: Organic Frameworks." *Chemical Society Reviews* 38 (5). The Royal Society of Chemistry: 1315–1329. doi:10.1039/B802258P.

Wasuwanich, Pris, Gang Fan, Benjamin Burke, and Ariel L. Furst. 2022. "Metal-Phenolic Networks as Tuneable Spore Coat Mimetics." *Journal of Materials Chemistry B* 10 (37). The Royal Society of Chemistry: 7600–7606. doi:10.1039/D2TB00717G.

Wu, Jie, and Jing Chen. 2013. "Adsorption Characteristics of Tannic Acid onto the Novel Protonated Palygorskite/Chitosan Resin Microspheres." *Journal of Applied Polymer Science* 127 (3): 1765–1771. doi:10.1002/app.37787.

Xie, Wensheng, Zhenhu Guo, Lingyun Zhao, and Yen Wei. 2021. "Metal-Phenolic Networks: Facile Assembled Complexes for Cancer Theranostics." *Theranostics* 11 (13). Ivyspring International Publisher: 6407–6426. doi:10.7150/THNO.58711.

Xie, Yi, Shengqiu Chen, Xu Peng, Xiaoling Wang, Zhiwei Wei, Joseph J. Richardson, Kang Liang, Hirotaka Ejima, Junling Guo, and Changsheng Zhao. 2022. "Alloyed Nanostructures Integrated Metal-Phenolic Nanoplatform for Synergistic Wound Disinfection and Revascularization." *Bioactive Materials* 16 (October). Elsevier: 95–106. doi:10.1016/J.BIOACTMAT.2022.03.004.

Xu, Kui, Mi Zhou, Ming Li, Weizhen Chen, Yabin Zhu, and Kaiyong Cai. 2020. "Metal-Phenolic Networks as a Promising Platform for PH-Controlled Release of Bioactive Divalent Metal Ions." *Applied Surface Science* 511 (May). North-Holland: 145569. doi:10.1016/J.APSUSC.2020.145569.

Yang, Bo, Shan Zhou, Jie Zeng, Liping Zhang, Runhao Zhang, Kang Liang, Lei Xie, et al. 2020. "Super-Assembled Core-Shell Mesoporous Silica-Metal-Phenolic Network Nanoparticles for Combinatorial Photothermal Therapy and Chemotherapy." *Nano Research* 13 (4): 1013–1019. doi:10.1007/s12274-020-2736-6.

Ying, Shuaixuan, Zhenru Guan, Polycarp C. Ofoegbu, Preston Clubb, Cyren Rico, Feng He, and Jie Hong. 2022. "Green Synthesis of Nanoparticles: Current Developments and Limitations." *Environmental Technology and Innovation* 26 (May). Elsevier B.V. doi:10.1016/J.ETI.2022.102336.

Zhang, Chao, Yang Ou, Wen Xi Lei, Ling Shu Wan, Jian Ji, and Zhi Kang Xu. 2016. "CuSO4/H2O2-Induced Rapid Deposition of Polydopamine Coatings with High Uniformity and Enhanced Stability." *Angewandte Chemie: International Edition* 55 (9): 3054–3057. doi:10.1002/anie.201510724.

Zhang, Lu, Shuang Shuang Wan, Chu Xin Li, Lu Xu, Han Cheng, and Xian Zheng Zhang. 2018. "An Adenosine Triphosphate-Responsive Autocatalytic Fenton Nanoparticle for Tumor Ablation with Self-Supplied H 2 O 2 and Acceleration of Fe(III)/Fe(II) Conversion." *Nano Letters* 18 (12): 7609–7618. doi:10.1021/acs.nanolett.8b03178.

Zhang, Peisen, Yi Hou, Jianfeng Zeng, Yingying Li, Zihua Wang, Ran Zhu, Tiancong Ma, and Mingyuan Gao. 2019. "Coordinatively Unsaturated Fe3+ Based Activatable Probes for Enhanced MRI and Therapy of Tumors." *Angewandte Chemie: International Edition* 58 (32): 11088–11096. doi:10.1002/anie.201904880.

Zhang, Xin, Lishan Chen, Chao Zhang, and Liqiong Liao. 2021. "Robust Near-Infrared-Responsive Composite Hydrogel Actuator Using Fe3+/Tannic Acid as the Photothermal Transducer." *ACS Applied Materials and Interfaces* 13 (15): 18175–18183. doi:10.1021/acsami.1c03999.

Zhang, Yaping, Lanbo Shen, Qi Zhi Zhong, and Jianhua Li. 2021. "Metal-Phenolic Network Coatings for Engineering Bioactive Interfaces." *Colloids and Surfaces. B, Biointerfaces* 205 (September). Colloids Surf B Biointerfaces. doi:10.1016/J.COLSURFB.2021.111851.

Zhang, Yulin, Kaiyan Xi, Xiao Fu, Haifeng Sun, Hong Wang, Dexin Yu, Zhiwei Li, et al. 2021. "Versatile Metal-Phenolic Network Nanoparticles for Multitargeted Combination Therapy and Magnetic Resonance Tracing in Glioblastoma." *Biomaterials* 278. Elsevier Ltd: 121163. doi:10.1016/j.biomaterials.2021.121163.

Zheng, Di Wei, Qi Lei, Jing Yi Zhu, Jin Xuan Fan, Chu Xin Li, Cao Li, Zushun Xu, Si Xue Cheng, and Xian Zheng Zhang. 2017. "Switching Apoptosis to Ferroptosis: Metal-Organic Network for High-Efficiency Anticancer Therapy." *Nano Letters* 17 (1): 284–291. doi:10.1021/acs.nanolett.6b04060.

Zheng, Huili, Baoxin Ma, Yesi Shi, Qixuan Dai, Dongsheng Li, En Ren, Jing Zhu, et al. 2021. "Tumor Microenvironment-Triggered MoS2@GA-Fe Nanoreactor: A Self-Rolling Enhanced Chemodynamic Therapy and Hydrogen Sulfide Treatment for Hepatocellular Carcinoma." *Chemical Engineering Journal* 406 (August 2020). Elsevier: 126888. doi:10.1016/j.cej.2020.126888.

Zheng, Yueyuan, Yuqing Liang, Depan Zhang, Xiaoyi Sun, Li Liang, Juan Li, and You Nian Liu. 2018. "Gelatin-Based Hydrogels Blended with Gellan as an Injectable Wound Dressing." *ACS Omega* 3 (5): 4766–4775. doi:10.1021/acsomega.8b00308.

Zhong, Qi Zhi, Shiyao Li, Jingqu Chen, Ke Xie, Shuaijun Pan, Joseph J. Richardson, and Frank Caruso. 2019. "Oxidation-Mediated Kinetic Strategies for Engineering Metal:

Phenolic Networks." *Angewandte Chemie: International Edition* 58 (36): 12563–12568. doi:10.1002/anie.201907666.

Zhou, Yaofeng, Siyu Fan, Lili Feng, Xiaolin Huang, and Xiaoyuan Chen. 2021. "Manipulating Intratumoral Fenton Chemistry for Enhanced Chemodynamic and Chemodynamic-Synergized Multimodal Therapy." *Advanced Materials* 33 (48): 1–28. doi:10.1002/adma.202104223.

# 5 Beneficial Effects of Essential Oils in the Management of Diabetes Mellitus and Obesity

*Debojyoti Mondal and Jeena Gupta*

## 5.1 INTRODUCTION

Diabetes mellitus, which is often referred to by its abbreviated form, DM, has emerged as one of the most common forms of chronic illness affecting at present people of all ages. Hyperglycaemia (an abnormally elevated blood sugar level) is the defining feature of diabetes mellitus, an endocrine illness that can be further subdivided into Type 1 and Type 2 forms (Ezhilarasu et al., 2020). Aging populations, dietary revolutions, and inactive lifestyles are all factors linked to a rise in DM (Ebrahimi et al., 2016; Harries et al., 2013). Prevalence estimates from the International Diabetes Federation (IDF) imply that there would be 537 million individuals with DM in the world in 2021, with that figure rising to 643 million by 2030 and 783 million by 2045. One out of every five people will lose their life to diabetes in 2025. The rise in worldwide health care costs attributable to diabetes has been significant, rising approximately USD 232 billion in 2007 to approximately USD 966 billion in 2021 for people aged 20–79 years. This is a growth of 316% over the course of the previous 15 years. According to projections made by the IDF, the overall cost of diabetes-related medical care will reach 1.03 trillion US dollars by the year 2030 and 1.05 trillion US dollars by the year 2045 (IDF, 2019). As a result, diabetes mellitus has arisen to be one of the most serious health concerns and a significant burden on society and the economy.

The accumulation of excessive quantities of body fat is often the key characteristic of obesity and it is prejudicated by a discrepancy between food consumption and energy expenditure. This discrepancy is exacerbated by social, psychological, and environmental variables (Romieu et al., 2017; Spinelli and Erminio, 2021). Obesity, as defined by the World Health Organization (WHO), is defined as a body mass index (BMI) score of 30 or higher (body mass index [BMI] is computed by dividing an individual's weight in kilogrammes by their height in square metres) (Rahman and Abbey, 2010). Because of persistent rise, especially in western countries, obesity has emerged as one of the most serious societal health concerns of today (Visscher et al., 2001). Diseases like Type 2 diabetes, coronary heart disease,

DOI: 10.1201/9781003389774-5

and lung diseases are only some of the many significant chronic diseases that obesity is linked to (Boutayeb et al., 2005; Apovian, 2016). According to the information that has been made available by WHO, the percentage of overweight people has risen dramatically (three times almost) since 1975 (Haththotuwa et al., 2020). There are more than twenty different types of persistent diseases and health problems, which include elevated blood pressure, DM type II, rheumatoid arthritis, dyslipidaemia, elevated blood cholesterol, strokes, obstructive sleep apnoea, and several malignancies, are linked to obesity (Rubenstein, 2005). A reduction in body weight has been shown to be effective in preventing or treating a number of these disorders (Reilly and Kelly, 2011). The rising rates of overweight and obesity, as well as health-related issues, have significant financial repercussions for the nation's medical care network (Christou et al., 2004).

An essential oil is a hydrophobic liquid that is extremely concentrated and comes from plants and contains volatile aromatic chemicals (Mulvaney, 2012). Essential oils have already been utilized as a treatment for everything from small scrapes to major mental health conditions including depression and anxiety for thousands of years (Ali et al., 2015; Eric Zielinski, 2018). They have witnessed a meteoric rise in popularity in the modern era as more and more individuals look for cheaper alternatives to costly prescription drugs. Extracting oils from plants results in the production of essential oils. This can be accomplished using a method called cold pressing or steam distillation (Eric Zielinski, 2018).

Essential oils have been utilized to improve health and well-being in a variety of cultures for centuries. These oils are well-known for their sedative properties, but they also have purported therapeutic uses (Ali et al., 2015). Essential oils, for instance, have been linked to a reduction in the symptoms of health problems like ulcers and loss of skin suppleness. In addition, they may aid among the fight against infections, which are more common in diabetics (Happy et al., 2021). Dill, cinnamon, coriander, and ylang ylang are just few of the essential oils that have been found to have a favourable impact on diabetic conditions. Although there is currently no known cure for diabetes, essential oils have been shown to alleviate some of its symptoms (Tisserand and Young, 2013).

## 5.2   ESSENTIAL OIL (EOS)

An essential oil is a supersaturated viscous liquid that comes from plants and contains chemical components that are volatile, implying they can rapidly evaporate at room temperature. Essential oils (EOs) are a complicated combination of different chemical compounds that are often the source of a plant's unique scent (Pavela and Benelli, 2016). These molecules are created during the secondary plant metabolism. Floral petal, pericarp, resins, tree bark, even herbaceous plant roots all contain essential oils (EOs). They get their common name, "essences," from the existence of volatile substances at ambient temperature that give them their distinctive aromas (Sharmeen and Mahomoodally, 2021). Therefore, it is not a coincidence that essential oils are referred to as "volatile oils," nor is it a coincidence that their constituents are classified as "aromatic," which is where the phrase "aromatic plants" comes from. The production and acquisition of such ingredients occurs within various secretion frameworks in the various plant families, such as the secretory chambers of the *Myrtaceae* and the *Rutaceae* families, the glandular trichomes of the *Lamiaceae*, the resin ducts of the *Asteraceae* and *Apiaceae*, and so on (Vigan, 2010).

Because of their antimicrobial, antifungal, and pesticidal action, essential oils play an important part in the safeguarding of plants. In addition, they can operate as an enticement toward pollen insects, which helps to encourage the dispersal of seeds as well as pollen. EOs typically have anywhere from 20 to 60 distinct compounds, but just two or three of those compounds account for 20–70% of the essence. The remaining compounds are only present in residues (Bakkali et al., 2008). Monoterpenes and sesquiterpenes make up the bulk of essential oils, although EOs also have trace amounts of aromatic molecules generated from phenylpropane. Because of their low molecular weight, all of the components can exist in liquid form even when the temperature is normal (Ni et al., 2021). Through the use of redox reactions, monoterpenes can be transformed into either linear or cyclic compounds. Additionally, monoterpenes have the ability to generate additional compounds that contain functional groups, the characteristics that are common to alcohols, alkynes, esters, ketones, and ether (Spalletta et al., 2018; Chung et al., 2018; Vieira et al., 2018; Kang et al., 2018).

The extraction of essential oil is generally carried out from various plant parts via the distillation (water or dry) or cold pressing methods (Baptista-Silva et al., 2020). By using a cold press on the exocarps of fruits like citrus, one can extract the essences that are contained within the fruit (Regnault-Roger et al., 2012). Hydrodistillation is a process that is quite similar to steam distillation. In hydrodistillation, plant matter is immersed in water and then the water is heated to a boil. The essential oil is carried by a stream into the compressor and finally into the fractional distillation system, where it is produced (Babu and Kaul, 2005; Schmidt, 2020).

Essential oils are now mostly employed in alternative medicine, cosmetics, and aromatherapy. Tea tree oil, rosemary oil, and lavender oil are examples of some of the essential oils that are utilized most frequently.

## 5.3 OBESITY

Obesity is a multifaceted illness caused by carrying around too much fat. It is important to remember that obesity is more of a medical than an aesthetic issue, because it raises the risk of serious diseases like coronary artery disease and hypertension, as well as several malignancies (Chooi et al., 2019). An abnormal or excessive buildup of fat is defined as a health risk by the World Health Organization (WHO), and both overweight and obesity fall under this definition (Chooi et al., 2019). One simple indicator of general body fatness is the body mass index (BMI). According to United States Centers for Disease Control and Prevention (CDC) and World Health Organization (WHO), adults with a body mass index (BMI) between 18.5 and 24.9 are considered to be within the healthy range, while those with a BMI of 25 kg/m$^2$ or above are classified as overweight, those with a BMI of 30 kg/m$^2$ or higher are classified as obese, and those with a BMI of 40 kg/m$^2$ or higher are classified as severely obese (Buttar et al., 2005).

Obesity is a multifactorial disease that occurs from persistent positive energy balance, which can be defined as daily nutrient consumption surpassing calorie expenditure. Despite the seeming simplicity of this definition, obesity is a medical condition that is caused by a combination of factors (Chooi et al., 2019). Weight gain and increased body fat occur when excess energy is transformed into triglyceride and then deposited in adipose tissue repositories. Although a decline in physical activity due to the advancement of lifestyles is also likely involved, the globalization of food systems that provide more packaged and affordable food and encourage silent excessive usage from energy-dense, nutritionally poor foods and beverages has already been identified as a significant driver of the obesity epidemic (Romieu et al., 2017; Colchero et al., 2019; Ladabaum et al., 2014).

### 5.3.1 Relevance of Essential Oils as an Obesity-Fighting Substance

Essential oils (EOs) have been proven to reduce fat mass and have anti-obesity benefits due to their ingredients, which have recently been the focus of scientific inquiry (Table 5.1 and Figure 5.1). Notably, EOs can have these effects whether they are ingested or inhaled (De Blasio et al., 2021). The volatile compounds that are present in EOs have the ability to interact with specific olfactory receptors, which in turn stimulates the central nervous system (CNS) to govern metabolic activity. This, in turn, regulates the stability between lipolysis and lipogenesis through the regulation of appetite. Hormones like leptin and insulin, together with the parasympathetic and sympathetic nervous systems' activation, are responsible for bringing about these results (Kelly et al., 2008).

### TABLE 5.1
### Essential Oils as Anti-Obesity Agents

| Oil Name | Mechanism/Importance | Model | References |
|---|---|---|---|
| Garlic essential oil | Effectiveness against nonalcoholic fatty liver disease by the downregulation of genes such as sterol regulatory element binding protein-1c, acetyl-CoA carboxylase, fatty acid synthase, etc. | Obese mice | Lai et al., 2014 |
| Mentha spicata essential oils | Effective as an obesity fighter and preventative. | NA | Ali-Shtayeh et al., 2019 |
| Patchouli essential oil (PEO) | PEO had an effect on specific indicators that are connected to metabolic disorders when it was inhaled. | NA | Hong et al., 2020 |
| Citronella oil | The rate of gain in weight slowed down and cholesterol levels in the blood were lowered. | Rat species: male Sprague-Dawley | Batubara et al., 2015 |

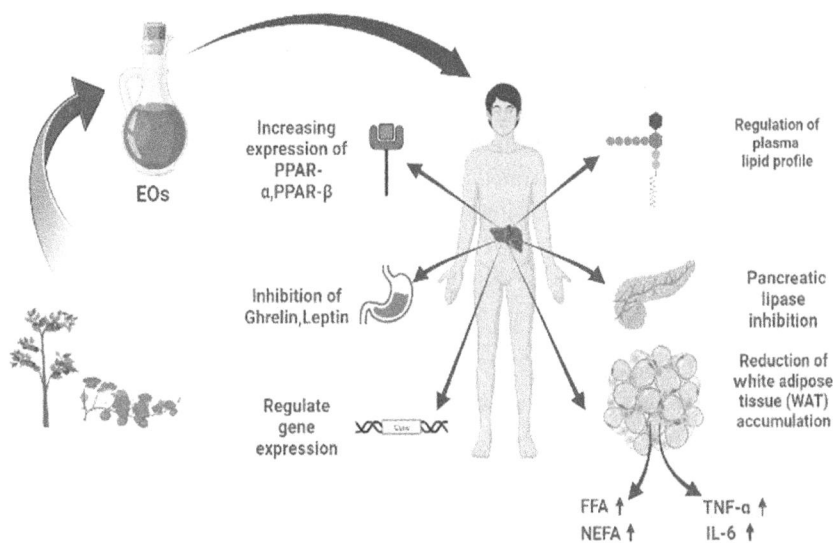

**FIGURE 5.1**    Target and mechanism of action of EOs against obesity.

Grapefruit (*Citrus paradisi*) essential oils (GEO) have been found in animal studies to stimulate the function of the sympathetic nervous system that primarily affect fat cells, the adrenal glands, and the kidneys when applied through the nasal route. This results in a reduction in hunger, an increase in thermogenesis and lipolysis, and a subsequent decrease in overall body weight. In addition to this, the GEO reduces the stimulation of the vagal nerves that control the stomach (Shen et al., 2005; Tanida et al., 2008; Nagai et al., 2014). According to the findings of Shen and colleagues (Provensi et al., 2014), GEO, and more specifically the limonene constituent, has this effect by triggering a histaminergic reaction. Histamines help control appetite by activating presynaptic H3 receptors, which reduces food intake (Musilli et al., 2014) and works together with thyroid hormones to reduce hyperlipidaemia and the risk of cardiovascular disease (Shen et al., 2007).

Yi-Syuan Lai and colleagues looked into the potential protective effects of garlic essential oil (GAEO) and its primary organosulfur component, diallyl disulfide (DADS), against the progression of nonalcoholic fatty liver disease (NAFLD). They did this for a period of 12 weeks, during which time they fed either a regular diet or a high-fat diet (HFD), with or without DADS. The findings demonstrated that GAEO and DADS showed anti-obesity as well as antihyperlipidemic activities in a dose-dependent manner by attenuating the increases in body weight, adipose tissue weight, and total cholesterol caused by the HFD. Furthermore, the outcomes demonstrated that GAEO and DADS protected obese mice with long-term HFD-induced NAFLD against lipogenesis, inflammatory processes, and oxidative metabolism by reducing lipid metabolic abnormalities and oxidative stress (Lai et al., 2014).

Using adult male Sprague Dawley rats as a model, Batubara et al. found that inhaling citronella EOs derived from *Cymbopogon nardus* stimulated the sympathetic nervous system, resulting in a reduction in body weight. Specifically, β-citronellol was the agent that was responsible for mediating the effect (Batubara et al., 2015). Patchouli essential oils (PEO) have been shown to have a similar impact when inhaled, with studies showing that doing so reduces food intake, helps to lose weight, and lowers serum leptin levels. PEO's primary ingredient is citronellol, a pungent molecule that has been demonstrated to cut down on food consumption, and thus, the probability of becoming obese (Hong et al., 2020).

Complexity abounds in attempting to understand essential oils' potential to combat weight gain. In a study, the mice group treated with citrus essential oil lost much more weight and ate significantly less than control group during the course of the study's 45-day duration. In mouse models of drug-induced obesity, citrus essential oil had been discovered to be beneficial in reducing body weight and preventing further weight gain (Asnaashari et al., 2010). Other plant seed oils, such as pomegranate seed oil, rapeseed oil, and calendula seed oil, have also been shown to decrease body fat mass when studied in animal models (Carvalho et al., 2014; Rashed et al., 2017).

The essential oils that are derived from sweet oranges (SO) (*Citrus sinensis*) possess anti-obesity abilities, which have been demonstrated with experimental models both *in vivo* and *in vitro*. In particular, it has been observed that microencapsulated SO induces weight loss in obese SD rats, which is accompanied by a decrease in the expression of the peroxisome proliferators activated receptor (PPAR) and ACC, which promotes lipogenesis of the subcutaneous adipose tissue, and an increase in the expression of UCP2, HSL, and carnitine palmitoyl transferase I, which promotes the entry of fatty acids (Jing et al., 2013). The anti-obesity efficacy of stachys EOs was evaluated. The essential oil has shown remarkable promise as an anti-obesity therapeutic, an effect attributed to the existence of chemical compositions (such as germacrene D, α-pinene, germacrene D, β-pinene, valeranone, and hexahydrofarnesyl acetone) that vary among species (Bahadori et al., 2020).

Oregano essential oils (OEO) have found widespread applications. In reality, the high levels of mono- and sesquiterpenes found in OEO are responsible for its impressive biological activity. Carvacrol, thymol, terpinen-4-ol, and linalool seem to be of specific importance among the primary components of OEO. The amounts of these constituents vary, depending on the variety of oregano that was used to make the essential oil. Specifically, oregano species rich in carvacrol have been the focus of numerous investigations due to their ability to combat obesity (Diniz et al., 2020; Levya-Lopez et al., 2017; Zou et al., 2016). Carvacrol has been shown to inhibit the accumulation of lipids in many cell lines undergoing adipogenic development. Modulation of genes involved in adipogenesis, like the transcription factor ChREBP, appears to be responsible for the observed effects. Carvacrol has been reported to decrease inflammation and hypercholesterolaemia in obese people (Cho et al., 2012; Spalletta et al., 2018).

The essential oil of *Lippia alba* has shown potential as a possible obesity-fighting therapeutic. In normal rats, consumption of EO results in a regulation of body weight gain as well as a reduction in both glucose and cholesterol levels (Acevedo-Estupinan et al., 2019).

## 5.4   DIABETES MELLITUS

Diabetes mellitus (DM), more commonly referred to by its medical term diabetes, is sickness that affects a large percentage of the population worldwide. DM develops when the body either develops insulin-resistance or insulin-insufficiency (American Diabetes Association, 2009). The genesis of this phenomenon is mostly attributable to a conjunction of two primary factors. The failure of the pancreas's beta cells to properly produce insulin is the primary cause. A secondary reason is when cells that are normally responsive to insulin are unable to react to insulin (Galicia-Garcia et al., 2020). Diabetes is among the diseases that are rising at the quickest rate all over the world. According to projections made by the International Diabetes Federation (IDF), there will be 537 million people in the world aged 20 to 79 who have diabetes mellitus (DM) in the year 2021. This number is projected to reach 643 million by the year 2030, and 783 million by the year 2045, according to current projections and forecasts (International Diabetes Federation, 2019). The rise in worldwide health care expenses owing to diabetes has been enormous, increasing from roughly USD 232 billion in 2007 to nearly USD 966 billion in 2021 for those aged 20–79 years old. This increase is due to diabetes. Over the course of the past 15 years, this represents an increase of 316% ("IDF diabetes atlas," 2019). To date, there is no cure for diabetes; however, the disease can be managed with treatment. Keeping blood sugar levels as close to normal as feasible and delaying or preventing the onset of diabetes-related medical issues may necessitate the use of pharmaceutical drugs and/or insulin (Artasensi et al., 2020).

### 5.4.1   Relevance of Essential Oils as Anti-Diabetic Agents

Hyperglycaemia, which is a defining characteristic of diabetes, is the end result of insulin sensitivity, inappropriate secretion of insulin, or improper glucagon production (Zimmet et al., 2014; Olokoba et al., 2012). Studies on the possible anti-diabetic activities of phytochemicals including polyphenols and EOs have been expanded (Table 5.2 and Figure 5.2). The hypoglycaemic effect of polyphenol has been the

**TABLE 5.2**
**Essential Oils for Anti-Diabetic Agents**

| Oil name | Mechanism/Importance | Model | References |
|---|---|---|---|
| *Pelargonium graveolens* L'Hér | reducing the risk of oxidative stress | Alloxan induced diabetic rats | Boukhris et al., 2012 |
| *Nigella sativa* | lowering free radicals and increasing antioxidant capability | Sprague Dawley rats streptozotocin (STZ) induced | Sultan et al., 2014 |
| *Melissa officinalis* | upregulating glucose metabolism-related genes, e.g., hepatic glucokinase and GLUT4, as well as adipocyte GLUT4, PPAR-γ, PPAR-α, and SREBP-1c expression | Mice | Chung et al., 2010; Hasanein and Riahi, 2015 |

*(Continued)*

**TABLE 5.2 (*Continued*)**

**Essential Oils for Anti-Diabetic Agents**

| Oil name | Mechanism/Importance | Model | References |
|---|---|---|---|
| *Foeniculum vulgare* Mill | antioxidative action and ability to restore redox equilibrium | α | Abou El-Soud et al., 2011 |
| fenugreek, cinnamon, cumin, oregano essential oil combination | eliminating or reducing blood sugar | Zucker fatty rats, hypertensive rats | Talpur et al., 2005 |
| rosemary (*Rosmarinus officinalis* L.) | in alloxan-induced hyperglycaemia, essential oils show preventive benefits | rats | Selmi et al., 2017 |
| *Citrus sinensis* (L.) | decrease in blood sugar levels elevated GLUT4 and insulin receptor signalling molecule expression in adipose tissue | albino rats streptozotocin-induced insulin-resistant diabetic rats | Muhammad et al., 2013; Sathiyabama et al., 2018 |
| black pepper (*Piper guineense*) seeds | in a concentration-dependent fashion, essential oil reduced the activity of the α-amylase, α-glucosidase, and ACE enzymes | in vitro | Oboh et al., 2013 |

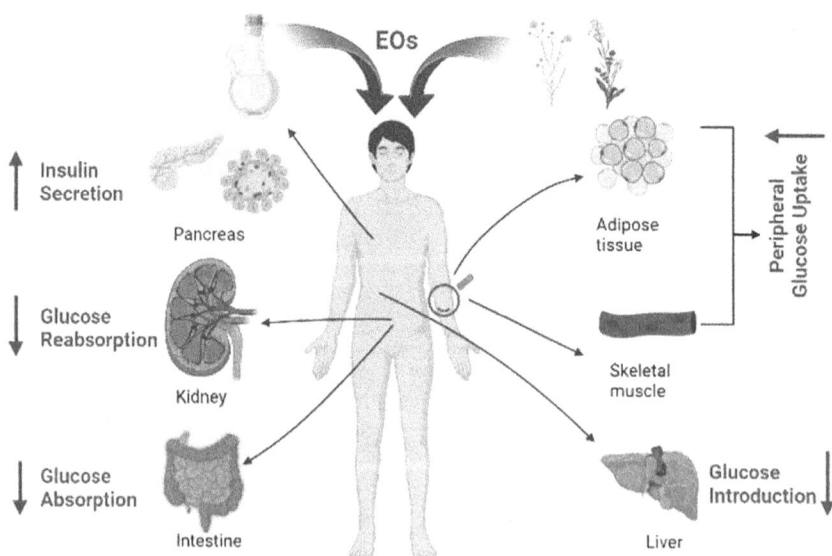

**FIGURE 5.2**   Targeting tissue and mechanism of action of EOs against diabetes.

primary focus of this research, but the possible inhibitory effect of substances like EOs has been largely overlooked (Kulisic et al., 2004). Furthermore, there is evidence from a few studies that EOs from a wide variety of plants may have an important role in helping to alleviate a few components of the metabolic syndrome that are linked to diabetes (Vujosevic et al., 2014).

The effects of lemon balm (*Melissa officinalis*) essential oil (LO) on mice's blood sugar levels were studied. LO therapy studies of genes involved in glucose metabolism. The expression of hepatic glucokinase, GLUT4, PPAR-, PPAR-, and SREBP-1c were all significantly increased. Expression of glucose-6-phosphatase and phosphoenolpyruvate carboxykinase, on the other hand, was suppressed. Improved glucose absorption and consumption in the liver and adipose tissue, and suppression of gluconeogenesis in the liver, are thought to be the primary mechanisms responsible for the hypoglycaemic effect (Chung et al., 2010).

*Foeniculum vulgare* essential oil (FVEO) was tested for its ability to lower blood sugar levels and shown to have anti-diabetic properties. This antioxidative impact and restoration of redox equilibrium may explain why FVEO improved hyperglycaemia and histological impairments in hyperglycaemia-induced rats (Abou El-Soud et al., 2011).

Diabetic rats were given a formulation of omega-3 fatty acids with fenugreek terpenes (fenugreek essential oil). Inhibitory effects of this oil were tested by measuring its ability to reduce levels of α-amylase, maltase, and plasma angiotensin-converting enzyme (ACE) in animals. Results showed that key enzymes related to diabetes, including α-amylase activity (inhibited by 46% and 52% in the pancreas and plasma, respectively) and maltase activity (inhibited by 37% and 35%), were significantly suppressed following administration of the formulation of omega-3 with fenugreek terpenes (essential oil). The results also showed that this supplement reduced death and damage to the rats' β-cells (Kawamoto et al., 2010). Similarly, the phytoconstituents and anti-diabetic prospects of *Salvia sclarea* L. essential oils (SCEO) were analyzed by Raafat et al. (2018), and probable anti-diabetic benefits of SCEOs were observed (Raafat and Habib, 2018).

In relation to the foregoing, Yen et al., (2015) used 3T3-L1 adipocytes to examine the glucose-consuming and lipid-drop-accumulating activities of EOs purchased on the Taiwanese market. Remarkably, they discovered that treating 3T3-L1 adipocytes with EOs from *Melissa officinalis* significantly enhanced glucose consumption and inhibited fat build-up. The acetyl-CoA carboxylase and AMP-activated protein kinase (AMPK) pathway has been linked to ATP replenishment and regulation of glucose metabolism by *M. officinalis* EOs. The anti-diabetic efficacy of *Nigella sativa* fixed oil (NFO) and essential oil (NEO) was investigated in three groups of experimental rats by Muhammad Tauseef Sultan et al. The formulations were able to alter the lipid profile while simultaneously reducing the harm caused by the antioxidants. The use of oils extracted from *N. sativa* was found to be beneficial to health and exhibited some encouraging anti-diabetic benefits (Sultan et al., 2014).

With reference to the traditional methods of medicine used in Turkey, *Myrtus communis* essential oil (MCO) was utilized by Aylin Sepici and colleagues to reduce the amount of glucose in the blood of Type 2 diabetic samples. They intended to examine the oral hypoglycaemic activity of a single dosage and several doses of MCO in both standard and alloxan-treated diabetic rabbits as part of their study. After administering MCO to diabetic animals at a dose of 50 mg/kg for four hours, a good hypoglycaemic activity was found in the animals. The reduction in blood glucose level may be attributable to the reversible inhibition of α-glucosidases that are present in the small intestinal mucosa, a higher rate of glycolysis as envisioned by the increased activity of glucokinase, as one of the specific enzymes of glycolysis, and an improved level of glycogenesis as demonstrated by greater quantity of glycogen in the liver present after MCO administration (Sepici et al., 2004). Several essential oils from different sources like *Citrus sinensis*, *Citrus limon* (Oboh et al., 2013), *Laurus nobilis* (Basak et al., 2013), and *Tanacetum praeteritum* (Özek, 2018) were tested in a number of studies aimed at determining their effects on the Type 2 diabetes-related enzymes α-amylase and α-glucosidase.

Therapeutically useful components including strong antioxidant properties have been identified in the essential oil of *Rhaponticum acaule* (REO), as noted by Mosbah et al. In this instance, REO has been demonstrated to inhibit alpha glucosidase, xanthine oxidase, and pancreatic lipase in enzymatic kinetic experiments. One approach in diabetic patients is the suppression of alpha glucosidase (Belhadj et al., 2018). *Salvia officinalis* L. essential oils (SOEO) have been found to reduce blood sugar and fight obesity. Indeed, it has been established that oral treatment of SOEO in alloxan-induced diabetes in male Wistar mice reduces glycemia and the amount of glycogen deposited in the liver through inhibiting α-amylase and lipase. It has also been demonstrated that taking SOEO as a dietary supplement can be advantageous in the treatment of diabetes mellitus by reducing the glucose concentration (Behradmanesh et al., 2013; Lima et al., 2006).

## 5.5  FUTURE PERSPECTIVES

The effectiveness of essential oil for a variety of therapeutic activities, such as treating diabetes and obesity, is appealing. Essential oil has been shown to be effective in treating diabetes and preventing obesity in a variety of trials, both in *in vitro* and *in vivo* studies. Several of the studies that were described additionally mentioned a variety of target techniques. The positive effects of essential oil consumption, whether through inhalation or ingestion, can be amplified in an individual who maintains a healthy lifestyle by adhering to a proper diet, engaging in consistent physical exercise, and avoiding a sedentary lifestyle. Yet, there have been reports that essential oils derived from oregano and other sources can have negative consequences, despite the fact that these oils have a wide range of positive applications. As a direct result of this, pre-clinical studies are required in order to assure that the utilization of these chemicals in people is risk-free. In a similar vein, administration strategies ought to be investigated in order to maximize the efficacy of such substances.

## 5.6  CONCLUSION

In an effort to enlighten on essential oils' and associated compounds' potential in prevention and treatment of diabetes and obesity, this review compiles relevant research. This article's results are meant to pique the interest of scientists on the lookout for new medications derived from natural sources and of those exploring the pharmacological versatility of essential oils in the treatment of diabetes and obesity. So, essential oils and their components can be taken into consideration in the future for more clinical assessments and potential uses, as well as for use as adjuvants to existing treatments.

## REFERENCES

Abou El-Soud, Neveen, Nabila El-Laithy, Gamila El-Saeed, Mohamed Salah Wahby, Mona Khalil, Fatma Morsy, and Nermeen Shaffie. "Antidiabetic activities of Foeniculum vulgare Mill. essential oil in streptozotocin-induced diabetic rats." *Macedonian Journal of Medical Sciences (Archived)* 4, no. 2 (2011): 139–146.

Acevedo-Estupinan, Maria Victoria, Elena Stashenko, and Fernando Rodríguez-Sanabria. "Effect of Lippia alba essential oil administration on obesity and T2DM markers in Wistar rats." *Revista Colombiana de Ciencias Químico-Farmacéuticas* 48, no. 2 (2019): 411–424.

Ali, Babar, Naser Ali Al-Wabel, Saiba Shams, Aftab Ahamad, Shah Alam Khan, and Firoz Anwar. "Essential oils used in aromatherapy: A systemic review." *Asian Pacific Journal of Tropical Biomedicine* 5, no. 8 (2015): 601–611.

Ali-Shtayeh, Mohammed S., Rana M. Jamous, Salam Y. Abu-Zaitoun, Ahmad I. Khasati, and Samer R. Kalbouneh. "Biological properties and bioactive components of Mentha spicata L. essential oil: Focus on potential benefits in the treatment of obesity, Alzheimer's disease, dermatophytosis, and drug-resistant infections." *Evidence-Based Complementary and Alternative Medicine* 2019 (2019).

American Diabetes Association. "Diagnosis and classification of diabetes mellitus." *Diabetes Care* 32, no. Suppl 1 (2009): S62.

Apovian, Caroline M. "Obesity: Definition, comorbidities, causes, and burden." (2016).

Artasensi, Angelica, Alessandro Pedretti, Giulio Vistoli, and Laura Fumagalli. "Type 2 diabetes mellitus: A review of multi-target drugs." *Molecules* 25, no. 8 (2020): 1987.

Asnaashari, Solmaz, Abbas Delazar, Bohlol Habibi, Roghayeh Vasfi, Lutfun Nahar, Sanaz Hamedeyazdan, and Satyajit D. Sarker. "Essential oil from Citrus aurantifolia prevents ketotifen-induced weight-gain in mice." *Phytotherapy Research* 24, no. 12 (2010): 1893–1897.

Atlas Diabetes. "IDF diabetes atlas." *International Diabetes Federation* (9th edition). Available online: www.idf.org/about-diabetes/facts-figures (2019).

Babu, Kiran G. D, and V. K. Kaul. "Variation in essential oil composition of rose-scented geranium (Pelargonium sp.) distilled by different distillation techniques." *Flavour and Fragrance Journal* 20, no. 2 (2005): 222–231.

Bahadori, Mir Babak, Filippo Maggi, Gokhan Zengin, Behvar Asghari, and Morteza Eskandani. "Essential oils of hedgenettles (Stachys inflata, S. lavandulifolia, and S. byzantina) have antioxidant, anti-Alzheimer, antidiabetic, and anti-obesity potential: A comparative study." *Industrial Crops and Products* 145 (2020): 112089.

Bakkali, Fadil, Simone Averbeck, Dietrich Averbeck, and Mouhamed Idaomar. "Biological effects of essential oils: A review." *Food and Chemical Toxicology* 46, no. 2 (2008): 446–475.

Baptista-Silva, Sara, Sandra Borges, Oscar L. Ramos, Manuela Pintado, and Bruno Sarmento. "The progress of essential oils as potential therapeutic agents: A review." *Journal of Essential Oil Research* 32, no. 4 (2020): 279–295.

Basak, Serap Sahin, and Ferda Candan. "Effect of laurus nobilis L. essential oil and its main components on α-glucosidase and reactive oxygen species scavenging activity." *Iranian Journal of Pharmaceutical Research: IJPR* 12, no. 2 (2013): 367.

Batubara, Irmanida, Irma H. Suparto, Siti Sa'diah, Ryunosuke Matsuoka, and Tohru Mitsunaga. "Effects of inhaled citronella oil and related compounds on rat body weight and brown adipose tissue sympathetic nerve." *Nutrients* 7, no. 3 (2015): 1859–1870.

Behradmanesh, Saeed, Fatemeh Derees, and Mahmoud Rafieian-Kopaei. "Effect of Salvia officinalis on diabetic patients." *Journal of Renal Injury Prevention* 2, no. 2 (2013): 51.

Belhadj, Sahla, Olfa Hentati, Majdi Hammami, Aida Ben Hadj, Tahia Boudawara, Mohamed Dammak, Sami Zouari, and AbdelFattah El Feki. "Metabolic impairments and tissue disorders in alloxan-induced diabetic rats are alleviated by Salvia officinalis L. essential oil." *Biomedicine & Pharmacotherapy* 108 (2018): 985–995.

Boukhris, Maher, Mohamed Bouaziz, Ines Feki, Hedya Jemai, Abdelfattah El Feki, and Sami Sayadi. "Hypoglycemic and antioxidant effects of leaf essential oil of Pelargonium graveolens L'Hér. in alloxan induced diabetic rats." *Lipids in Health and Disease* 11 (2012): 1–10.

Boutayeb, Abdesslam, and Saber Boutayeb. "The burden of non communicable diseases in developing countries." *International Journal for Equity in Health* 4 (2005): 1–8.

Buttar, Harpal S., Timao Li, and Nivedita Ravi. "Prevention of cardiovascular diseases: Role of exercise, dietary interventions, obesity and smoking cessation." *Experimental & Clinical Cardiology* 10, no. 4 (2005): 229.

Carvalho Filho, Jorge Mancini. "Pomegranate seed oil (Punica granatum L.): A source of punicic acid (conjugated α-linolenic acid)." *J Human Nutri Food Sci* 2, no. 1 (2014): 1–11.

Cho, Soomin, Youngshim Choi, Soyoung Park, and Taesun Park. "Carvacrol prevents diet-induced obesity by modulating gene expressions involved in adipogenesis and inflammation in mice fed with high-fat diet." *The Journal of Nutritional Biochemistry* 23, no. 2 (2012): 192–201.

Chooi, Yu Chung, Cherlyn Ding, and Faidon Magkos. "The epidemiology of obesity." *Metabolism* 92 (2019): 6–10.

Christou, Nicolas V., John S. Sampalis, Moishe Liberman, Didier Look, Stephane Auger, Alexander PH McLean, and Lloyd D. MacLean. "Surgery decreases long-term mortality, morbidity, and health care use in morbidly obese patients." *Annals of Surgery* 240, no. 3 (2004): 416.

Chung, Jin, Sumi Kim, Hyun Ah Lee, Mi Hee Park, Seyeon Kim, Yu Ri Song, and Hee Sam Na. "Trans-cinnamic aldehyde inhibits Aggregatibacter actinomycetemcomitans-induced inflammation in THP-1-derived macrophages via autophagy activation." *Journal of Periodontology* 89, no. 10 (2018): 1262–1271.

Chung, Mi Ja, Sung-Yun Cho, Muhammad Javidul Haque Bhuiyan, Kyoung Heon Kim, and Sung-Joon Lee. "Anti-diabetic effects of lemon balm (Melissa officinalis) essential oil on glucose-and lipid-regulating enzymes in type 2 diabetic mice." *British Journal of Nutrition* 104, no. 2 (2010): 180–188.

Colchero, M. Arantxa, Carlos M. Guerrero-López, Mariana Molina, and Mishel Unar-Munguía. "Affordability of food and beverages in Mexico between 1994 and 2016." *Nutrients* 11, no. 1 (2019): 78.

De Blasio, Anna, Antonella D'Anneo, Marianna Lauricella, Sonia Emanuele, Michela Giuliano, Giovanni Pratelli, Giuseppe Calvaruso, and Daniela Carlisi. "The beneficial effects of essential oils in anti-obesity treatment." *International Journal of Molecular Sciences* 22, no. 21 (2021): 11832.

Diniz do Nascimento, Lidiane, Angelo Antônio Barbosa de Moraes, Kauê Santana da Costa, João Marcos Pereira Galúcio, Paulo Sérgio Taube, Cristiane Maria Leal Costa, Jorddy Neves Cruz, Eloisa Helena de Aguiar Andrade, and Lênio José Guerreiro de Faria. "Bioactive natural compounds and antioxidant activity of essential oils from spice plants: New findings and potential applications." *Biomolecules* 10, no. 7 (2020): 988.

Ebrahimi, Hossein, Mohammad Hassan Emamian, Mohammad Shariati, Hassan Hashemi, and Akbar Fotouhi. "Diabetes mellitus and its risk factors among a middle-aged population of Iran, a population-based study." *International Journal of Diabetes in Developing Countries* 36 (2016): 189–196.

Eric Zielinski, D. C. *The Healing Power of Essential Oils: Soothe Inflammation, Boost Mood, Prevent Autoimmunity, and Feel Great in Every Way.* Harmony, 2018.

Ezhilarasu, Hariharan, Dinesh Vishalli, S. Thameem Dheen, Boon-Huat Bay, and Dinesh Kumar Srinivasan. "Nanoparticle-based therapeutic approach for diabetic wound healing." *Nanomaterials* 10, no. 6 (2020): 1234.

Galicia-Garcia, Unai, Asier Benito-Vicente, Shifa Jebari, Asier Larrea-Sebal, Haziq Siddiqi, Kepa B. Uribe, Helena Ostolaza, and César Martín. "Pathophysiology of type 2 diabetes mellitus." *International Journal of Molecular Sciences* 21, no. 17 (2020): 6275.

Happy, Afroza Akter, Ferdoushi Jahan, and Md Abdul Momen. "Essential oils: Magical ingredients for skin care." *Journal of Plant Sciences* 9, no. 2 (2021): 54.

Harries, A. D., S. Satyanarayana, A. M. V. Kumar, S. B. Nagaraja, P. Isaakidis, S. Malhotra, S. Achanta et al. "Epidemiology and interaction of diabetes mellitus and tuberculosis and challenges for care: A review." *Public Health Action* 3, no. 1 (2013): 3–9.

Hasanein, P., and Riahi, H. "Antinociceptive and antihyperglycemic effects of Melissa officinalis essential oil in an experimental model of diabetes." *Medical Principles and Practice* 24, no. 1 (2015): 47–52.

Haththotuwa, Rohana N., Chandrika N. Wijeyaratne, and Upul Senarath. "Worldwide epidemic of obesity." In *Obesity and Obstetrics*, pp. 3–8. Elsevier, 2020.

Hong, Seong Jun, Jinju Cho, Chang Guk Boo, Moon Yeon Youn, Jeong Hoon Pan, Jae Kyeom Kim, and Eui-Cheol Shin. "Inhalation of Patchouli (Pogostemon Cablin Benth.) essential oil improved metabolic parameters in obesity-induced Sprague Dawley rats." *Nutrients* 12, no. 7 (2020): 2077.

International Diabetes Federation. IDF Diabetes Atlas 10th Edition 2019, Global Estimates for the Prevalence of Diabetes for 2019, 2030 and 2045. Available online: www.diabetesatlas.org/ (accessed on 30 January 2023).

Jing, Li, Yu Zhang, Shengjie Fan, Ming Gu, Yu Guan, Xiong Lu, Cheng Huang, and Zhiqin Zhou. "Preventive and ameliorating effects of Citrus D-limonene on dyslipidemia and hyperglycemia in mice with high-fat diet-induced obesity." *European Journal of Pharmacology* 715, no. 1–3 (2013): 46–55.

Kang, Nam Hyeon, Sulagna Mukherjee, Taesun Min, Sun Chul Kang, and Jong Won Yun. "Trans-anethole ameliorates obesity via induction of browning in white adipocytes and activation of brown adipocytes." *Biochimie* 151 (2018): 1–13.

Kawamoto, Ryuichi, Yasuharu Tabara, Katsuhiko Kohara, Tetsuro Miki, Tomo Kusunoki, Shuzo Takayama, Masanori Abe, Tateaki Katoh, and Nobuyuki Ohtsuka. "Low-density lipoprotein cholesterol to high-density lipoprotein cholesterol ratio is the best surrogate marker for insulin resistance in non-obese Japanese adults." *Lipids in Health and Disease* 9, no. 1 (2010): 1–6.

Kelly, AM Clare, Lucina Q. Uddin, Bharat B. Biswal, F. Xavier Castellanos, and Michael P. Milham. "Competition between functional brain networks mediates behavioral variability." *Neuroimage* 39, no. 1 (2008): 527–537.

Kulisic, T., A. Radonic, V. Katalinic, and M. Milos. "Use of different methods for testing antioxidative activity of oregano essential oil." *Food Chemistry* 85, no. 4 (2004): 633–640.

Ladabaum, Uri, Ajitha Mannalithara, Parvathi A. Myer, and Gurkirpal Singh. "Obesity, abdominal obesity, physical activity, and caloric intake in US adults: 1988 to 2010." *The American Journal of Medicine* 127, no. 8 (2014): 717–727.

Lai, Yi-Syuan, Wei-Cheng Chen, Chi-Tang Ho, Kuan-Hung Lu, Shih-Hang Lin, Hui-Chun Tseng, Shuw-Yuan Lin, and Lee-Yan Sheen. "Garlic essential oil protects against obesity-triggered nonalcoholic fatty liver disease through modulation of lipid metabolism and oxidative stress." *Journal of Agricultural and Food Chemistry* 62, no. 25 (2014): 5897–5906.

Leyva-López, Nayely, Erick P. Gutiérrez-Grijalva, Gabriela Vazquez-Olivo, and J. Basilio Heredia. "Essential oils of oregano: Biological activity beyond their antimicrobial properties." *Molecules* 22, no. 6 (2017): 989.

Lima, Cristovao F., Marisa F. Azevedo, Rita Araujo, Manuel Fernandes-Ferreira, and Cristina Pereira-Wilson. "Metformin-like effect of Salvia officinalis (common sage): Is it useful in diabetes prevention?" *British Journal of Nutrition* 96, no. 2 (2006): 326–333.

Muhammad, N. O., O. Soji-Omoniwa, L. A. Usman, and B. P. Omoniwa. "Antihyperglycemic activity of leaf essential oil of Citrus sinensis (L.) Osbeck on alloxan-induced diabetic rats." *Annual Research & Review in Biology* (2013): 825–834.

Mulvaney, Jill. "Essential oils and steam distillation." *Australian Journal of Herbal Medicine* 24, no. 4 (2012): 140–142.

Musilli, Claudia, Gaetano De Siena, Maria Elena Manni, Andrea Logli, Elisa Landucci, Riccardo Zucchi, Alessandro Saba et al. "Histamine mediates behavioural and metabolic effects of 3-iodothyroacetic acid, an endogenous end product of thyroid hormone metabolism." *British Journal of Pharmacology* 171, no. 14 (2014): 3476–3484.

Nagai, Katsuya, Akira Niijima, Yuko Horii, Jiao Shen, and Mamoru Tanida. "Olfactory stimulatory with grapefruit and lavender oils change autonomic nerve activity and physiological function." *Autonomic Neuroscience* 185 (2014): 29–35.

Ni, Zhi-Jing, Xin Wang, Yi Shen, Kiran Thakur, Jinzhi Han, Jian-Guo Zhang, Fei Hu, and Zhao-Jun Wei. "Recent updates on the chemistry, bioactivities, mode of action, and industrial applications of plant essential oils." *Trends in Food Science & Technology* 110 (2021): 78–89.

Obesity, W. H. O. "Overweight Fact Sheet N 311. January 2015." Retrieved 2nd February (2016).

Oboh, Ganiyu, Ayokunle O. Ademosun, Oluwatoyin V. Odubanjo, and Ifeoluwa A. Akinbola. "Antioxidative properties and inhibition of key enzymes relevant to type-2 diabetes and hypertension by essential oils from black pepper." *Advances in Pharmacological Sciences* 2013 (2013).

Olokoba, A. B., O. A. Obateru, and L. B. Olokoba. "Type 2 diabetes mellitus: A review of current trends." *Oman Medical Journal* 27 (2012): 269–273.

Özek, Gülmira. "Chemical diversity and biological potential of Tanacetum praeteritum subsp. praeteritum essential oils." *Journal of the Turkish Chemical Society Section A: Chemistry* 5, no. 2 (2018): 493–510.

Pavela, Roman, and Giovanni Benelli. "Essential oils as ecofriendly biopesticides? Challenges and constraints." *Trends in Plant Science* 21, no. 12 (2016): 1000–1007.

Provensi, Gustavo, Roberto Coccurello, Hayato Umehara, Leonardo Munari, Giacomo Giacovazzo, Nicoletta Galeotti, Daniele Nosi et al. "Satiety factor oleoylethanolamide recruits the brain histaminergic system to inhibit food intake." *Proceedings of the National Academy of Sciences* 111, no. 31 (2014): 11527–11532.

Raafat, Karim, and Jean Habib. "Phytochemical compositions and antidiabetic potentials of Salvia sclarea L. essential oils." *Journal of Oleo Science* 67, no. 8 (2018): 1015–1025.

Rahman, Mahbubur, and Abbey B. Berenson. "Accuracy of current body mass index obesity classification for white, black and Hispanic reproductive-age women." *Obstetrics and Gynecology* 115, no. 5 (2010): 982.

Rashed, Aswir Abd, Mohd Naeem Mohd Nawi, and Kasmawati Sulaiman. "Assessment of essential oil as a potential anti-obesity agent: A narrative review." *Journal of Essential Oil Research* 29, no. 1 (2017): 1–10.

Regnault-Roger, Catherine, Charles Vincent, and John Thor Arnason. "Essential oils in insect control: Low-risk products in a high-stakes world." *Annual Review of Entomology* 57 (2012): 405–424.

Reilly, John J., and Joanna Kelly. "Long-term impact of overweight and obesity in childhood and adolescence on morbidity and premature mortality in adulthood: Systematic review." *International Journal of Obesity* 35, no. 7 (2011): 891–898.

Romieu, Isabelle, Laure Dossus, Simón Barquera, Hervé M. Blottière, Paul W. Franks, Marc Gunter, Nahla Hwalla et al. "Energy balance and obesity: What are the main drivers?" *Cancer Causes & Control* 28 (2017): 247–258.

Rubenstein, Arthur H. "Obesity: A modern epidemic." *Transactions of the American Clinical and Climatological Association* 116 (2005): 103.

Sathiyabama, Rajiv Gandhi, Gopalsamy Rajiv Gandhi, Marina Denadai, Gurunagarajan Sridharan, Gnanasekaran Jothi, Ponnusamy Sasikumar, Jullyana de Souza Siqueira Quintans et al. "Evidence of insulin-dependent signalling mechanisms produced by Citrus sinensis (L.) osbeck fruit peel in an insulin resistant diabetic animal model." *Food and Chemical Toxicology* 116 (2018): 86–99.

Schmidt, Erich. "Production of essential oils." In *Handbook of Essential Oils*, pp. 125–160. CRC Press, 2020.

Selmi, Slimen, Kais Rtibi, Dhekra Grami, Hichem Sebai, and Lamjed Marzouki. "Rosemary (Rosmarinus officinalis) essential oil components exhibit anti-hyperglycemic, anti-hyperlipidemic and antioxidant effects in experimental diabetes." *Pathophysiology* 24, no. 4 (2017): 297–303.

Sepici, Aylin, Ilhan Gürbüz, Cemal Çevik, and Erdem Yesilada. "Hypoglycaemic effects of myrtle oil in normal and alloxan-diabetic rabbits." *Journal of Ethnopharmacology* 93, no. 2–3 (2004): 311–318.

Sharmeen, Jugreet B., Fawzi M. Mahomoodally, Gokhan Zengin, and Filippo Maggi. "Essential oils as natural sources of fragrance compounds for cosmetics and cosmeceuticals." *Molecules* 26, no. 3 (2021): 666.

Shen, J., Akira Niijima, Mamoru Tanida, Y. Horii., K. Maeda, and Katsuya Nagai. (2005). Olfactory stimulation with scent of grapefruit oil affects autonomic nerves, lipolysis and appetite in rats. *Neuroscience Letters*, 380(3), 289–294.

Shen, Jiao, Mamoru Tanida, Akira Niijima, and Katsuya Nagai. "In vivo effects of leptin on autonomic nerve activity and lipolysis in rats." *Neuroscience Letters* 416, no. 2 (2007): 193–197.

Spalletta, Sonia, Vincenzo Flati, Elena Toniato, Jacopo Di Gregorio, Antonio Marino, Laura Pierdomenico, Marco Marchisio, Gabriella D'Orazi, Ivana Cacciatore, and Iole Robuffo. "Carvacrol reduces adipogenic differentiation by modulating autophagy and ChREBP expression." *PLoS One* 13, no. 11 (2018): e0206894.

Spinelli, Sara, and Erminio Monteleone. "Food preferences and obesity." *Endocrinology and Metabolism* 36, no. 2 (2021): 209–219.

Sultan, Muhammad Tauseef, Masood Sadiq Butt, Roselina Karim, M. Zia-Ul-Haq, Rizwana Batool, Shakeel Ahmad, Luigi Aliberti, and Vincenzo De Feo. "Nigella sativa fixed and essential oil supplementation modulates hyperglycemia and allied complications in streptozotocin-induced diabetes mellitus." *Evidence-Based Complementary and Alternative Medicine* 2014 (2014).

Talpur, N., B. Echard, C. Ingram, D. Bagchi, and H. Preuss. "Effects of a novel formulation of essential oils on glucose-insulin metabolism in diabetic and hypertensive rats: A pilot study." *Diabetes, Obesity and Metabolism* 7, no. 2 (2005): 193–199.

Tanida, Mamoru, Jiao Shen, Takuo Nakamura, Akira Niijima, and Katsuya Nagai. "Day-night difference in thermoregulatory responses to olfactory stimulation." *Neuroscience Letters* 439, no. 2 (2008): 192–197.

Tisserand, Robert, and Rodney Young. *Essential Oil Safety: A Guide for Health Care Professionals.* Elsevier Health Sciences, 2013.

Vieira, Ana Julia, Fernando Pereira Beserra, M. C. Souza, B. M. Totti, and A. L. Rozza. "Limonene: Aroma of innovation in health and disease." *Chemico-Biological Interactions* 283 (2018): 97–106.

Vigan, Martine. "Essential oils: Renewal of interest and toxicity." *European Journal of Dermatology* 20, no. 6 (2010): 685–692.

Visscher, Tommy L. S, and Seidell, Jacob C. "The public health impact of obesity." *Annual Review of Public Health* 22, no. 1 (2001): 355–375.

Vujosevic, S., Borozan, S., Radojevic, N., Aligrudic, S., and Bozovic, D. (2014). "Relationship between 25-hydroxyvitamin D and newly diagnosed type 2 diabetes mellitus in post-menopausal women with osteoporosis." *Medical Principles and Practice* 23, no. 3 (2014): 229–233.

Yen, Hsiu-Fang, Chi-Ting Hsieh, Tusty-Jiuan Hsieh, Fang-Rong Chang, and Chin-Kun Wang. "In vitro anti-diabetic effect and chemical component analysis of 29 essential oils products." *Journal of Food and Drug Analysis* 23, no. 1 (2015): 124–129.

Zimmet, Paul Z., Dianna J. Magliano, William H. Herman, and Jonathan E. Shaw. "Diabetes: A 21st century challenge." *The Lancet Diabetes & Endocrinology* 2, no. 1 (2014): 56–64.

Zou, Yi, Quanhang Xiang, Jun Wang, Hongkui Wei, and Jian Peng. "Effects of oregano essential oil or quercetin supplementation on body weight loss, carcass characteristics, meat quality and antioxidant status in finishing pigs under transport stress." *Livestock Science* 192 (2016): 33–38.

# 6 Essential Oils for Insomnia

## *Power in Health Promoting and Quality of Life*

*Alev Önder and Antoaneta Trendafilova*

## 6.1 INTRODUCTION

Sleep is a complicated biological process that can be defined by behavioral, physiological, and electrophysiological parameters (Eban-Rothschild et al., 2018). Sleep represents a period that affects many physiological systems, especially under neurobiological regulation, is essential in people's daily lives and takes about 30% of the day (Grandner, 2017). However, stress and pressures make sleep disorder problems increasingly common (Bhaskar et al., 2016).

A common sleep disorder, insomnia (Dool-Ri et al., 2019), is described as difficulty perceiving things objectively related to the initiation, length, reinforcement, or quality of sleep that happens despite sufficient sleep opportunities. In this case, the patient is dissatisfied with the duration and/or quality of sleep, which affects the individual's ability to function in society throughout the day (Buysse, 2013; Fernandez-Mendoza, 2017), due to different degrees of depression and anxiety accompanying patients simultaneously who have insomnia (Everitt et al., 2018). While insomnia may seem medically the most common public health issue, it was initially thought of as a symptom but is now defined as an ailment (Bollu and Kaur, 2019). It is a known fact that insomnia increases with age, but sleep dissatisfaction and diagnosis rates vary little with age. Lots of factors can initiate, continue, or increase the risk of insomnia, most frequently as mental disorders, acute stress, environmental changes, and deterioration of immune function (Ohayon, 2002; Varkevisser et al., 2007; Han et al., 2012; Morin and Jarrin, 2022). Moreover, genetic factors and genes associated with insomnia have also been identified (Bollu and Kaur, 2019). Insomnia remarked with clinical signs as dysfunctions in the sleep process, daytime cognition, limbic system, and peripheral nerve system, all of which not only cause anxiety, depression, or fear but also reduce mental training and productivity, as well as cardiovascular and mental diseases also increases with its incidences (Taylor et al., 2003; Doghramji, 2010; Sarris and Byrne, 2011).

Currently, two main methods are mentioned to help patients improve their symptoms of insomnia treatment, such as difficulty falling and keeping asleep. The first one is the treatment of health education, light therapy, psychological, cognitive, and behavioral therapy, which are called non-drug treatments (Riemann et al., 2015);

the second one is the treatment of drug therapy, including benzodiazepine receptor agonists, non-benzodiazepine receptor agonists, selective melatonin receptor agonists, sedatives, anti-anxiety, and antidepressant drugs (Winkler et al., 2014), mainly with the target of serotonin (5-HT) receptors (Monti, 2011) and γ-aminobutyric acid (GABA) receptors (Shi et al., 2014).

General approaches to treating insomnia include pharmacological therapy and pharmaceutical hypnotics (Lie et al., 2015). However, these drugs, prescribed for insomnia, may also have various inconveniences and toxic effects. For all these reasons, people tend to find natural solutions to improve or alleviate insomnia symptoms (Tariq and Pulisetty, 2008; Abad and Guilleminault, 2018).

The essential oils and their components have antimicrobial, antiviral, antibiotic, anti-inflammatory, anticancer, and antioxidant properties, besides psychogenic effects such as reducing stress, treating depression, and helping insomnia, but require careful use (Ramsey et al., 2020). Essential oils can often be used in complementary therapies to prevent and alleviate symptoms related to CNS (central nervous system)-based disorders, including insomnia (Soares et al., 2021). There are some popular essential oils on this topic, and those used for insomnia have been discussed frequently and extensively in some publications (Borrás et al., 2021). The scope and purpose of this chapter are to highlight the mechanisms of the sleep process and essential oils in preventing insomnia, the importance of aromatherapy, and some prominent essential oils used in insomnia with *in vivo* and *in vitro* examples.

## 6.2 ACTIVITY MECHANISMS OF ESSENTIAL OILS IN INSOMNIA

The sedative agents exhibited sedation, hypnosis, anti-anxiety, and antidepressant effects as the main pharmacological effects. The mechanisms of action stand out as promoting central neurotransmitters, affecting sleep-related cytokines, and restoring the structure of the CNS (Shi et al., 2016). Especially in mammals, the hypothalamic-pituitary-adrenal axis, sympathetic nervous system, and efferent vagus nerve are responsible for the CNS response to stress (Chung et al., 2017). Activation of the GABA receptor system and blockade of neuronal voltage-gated sodium channels ($Na^+$ channels) are required to balance neuronal excitation and inhibition, which are vital for normal brain function and critical for CNS disorders (Semyanov et al., 2004). The medicines used to treat insomnia have undesirable side effects (Suzana et al., 2010; Winkler et al., 2014). However, the most recent intention to create drugs for treating insomnia is serotonin (5-HT) (Monti, 2011) and GABA receptors (Shi et al., 2014; Zhong et al., 2019) which have more or fewer side effects. Psychological stress, chronic pain, and medications with varying degrees of depression and anxiety cause insomnia, sometimes accompanied by mental activity problems (Jolanta, 2010; Everitt et al., 2018). In sleep physiology, noradrenalin, histamine, dopamine, glutamate, and GABA play an important role in the process, besides other neurotransmitters such as orexins A and B, adenosine, glycine, ACh (acetylcholine), serotonin (5-HT), and melatonin (Borrás et al., 2021). It should be known that the molecular factors responsible for the regulation of sleep–wake-up (Figure 6.1) contain chemicals that promote wakefulness, such as orexin, norepinephrine, and histamine, and sleep-promoting chemicals, such as GABA (γ-aminobutyric acid), adenosine, melatonin, and prostaglandin D2, etc. (Bollu and Kaur, 2019). In this context, benzodiazepines and benzodiazepine receptor agonists or non-benzodiazepine receptor

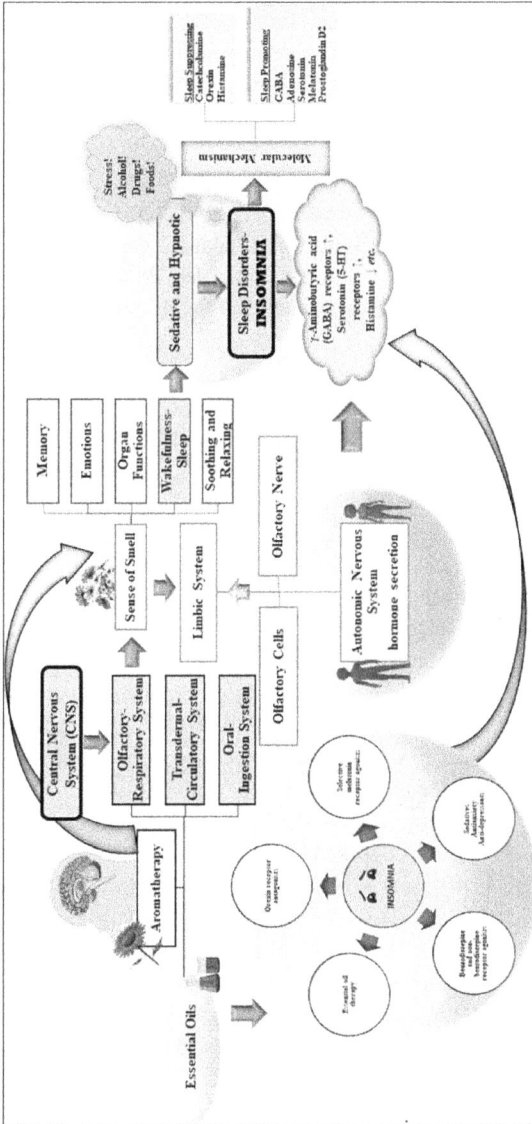

**FIGURE 6.1** Schematic representation of insomnia and its mechanisms with essential oils.

agonists act on GABA receptor sites, acting as a sedative, anxiolytic, muscle relaxant, and hypnotic (Nutt and Stahl, 2010). The natural hormone melatonin, produced by the pineal gland, is available over the counter and is FDA-approved for treating insomnia, specifically in older adults (Kato et al., 2005). Melatonin reaches its highest level at night to balance the body's natural circadian rhythm (Siegel, 2004; Lie et al., 2015). Orexin receptor antagonists also act as dual orexin receptor antagonists (OX1 and OX2 receptor), which inactivates the orexin/hypocretin system, which plays a critical role in wakefulness (Citrome, 2014) and also the histamine-1 receptor antagonist (Yeung et al., 2015). The neurons in the forebrain and hypothalamus release GABA and histamine. These neurotransmitters have opposite effects, such as increasing GABA and decreasing histamine to induce sleep. The other neurotransmitters released by reticular activating system neurons, such as norepinephrine, acetylcholine, and serotonin, contribute to maintaining wakefulness. Orexin from the hypothalamus is a neuropeptide that plays a significant role in maintaining wakefulness. The effect of orexin is hypothesized to alter the activity of neurotransmitters involved in regulating sleep/wake states (Siegel, 2004; Lie et al., 2015).

The secondary metabolites are the majority of bioactive phytochemicals with various pharmacological effects (Twaij and Hasan, 2022). Essential oils, a group of secondary metabolites, are defined by the European Pharmacopeia seventh edition as "Odorant products, which have a complex composition, and obtained from plant raw extract, either extracted by the steam of water, dry distillation or a suitable mechanical method without heating. Generally, a physical method separates the essential oil from the aqueous phase, which has no significant change in its chemical composition" (El Asbahani et al., 2009). Essential oils have been used to treat many diseases since ancient times due to their diverse biological activities (Perricone et al., 2015; Elshafie and Camele, 2017). There is some evidence about the pharmacological properties of essential oils/components and the mechanisms underlying their effects (Bakkali et al., 2008; Koyama and Heinbockel, 2020; Ramsey et al., 2020). The neuropharmacological activity mechanism of essential oils *in vitro* and *in vivo* models has also been investigated on psychiatric disorders, including evidence from a limited number of published clinical studies (Perry and Perry, 2006). The pharmacological and/or psychological effects of essential oils are now recognized, and their use is widely extended. There are many studies on the effects of essential oils on the CNS. Preclinical and clinical studies have recently focused on the emergence of essential oils as a promising source for the modulation of the GABAergic system and $Na^+$ ion channels, for their antinociceptive, anxiolytic, and anticonvulsant properties. Some studies mention that the essential oil and its components may interact with therapeutic target proteins, for example inhibiting the function of $Na^+$ channels and also activating $GABA_A$ receptors ($GABA_AR$) so that the effect can occur (Wang and Heinbockel, 2018; Lizarraga-Valderrama, 2021).

Lizarraga-Valderrama explained that essential oils have an interrelation with anti-inflammatory and pro-inflammatory responses in the CNS against stress. For example, frankincense, ylang-ylang, neroli and bergamot, sweet orange, geranium, and rose oils can affect the hypothalamic-pituitary-adrenal axis by lowering glucocorticoid levels, creating a calming effect. On the other hand, the pro-inflammatory response can be suppressed by downregulating NF-κB, as in cinnamon essential oil, resulting in an anxiolytic effect. It also produces calming effects by increasing serotonin levels while reducing glucocorticoids, as in the case of ylang-ylang oil. In addition, the essential oils of bergamot, lemongrass, and lavender may exert their anxiolytic effects by activating the GABAergic system (Lizarraga-Valderrama, 2021). All these mechanisms, directly or indirectly, positively affect insomnia.

In a previous study, inhalation of *Perilla frutescens* essential oil [perillaldehyde (54.37%), 1,4-cineole (7.42%), acetaldehyde diethyl acetal (6.61%), D-limonene (5.09%), eucalyptol (4.94%)] significantly reduces the autonomic activity in para-chlorophenylalanine insomnia mice. The oil also demonstrated sedative and hypnotic effects in rats, increasing the rate of falling asleep, shortening sleep delay, and prolonging sleep time. The enzyme-linked immunosorbent assay showed that *P. frutescens* oil increases the content of 5-HT and GABA in the hypothalamus and cerebral cortex; this may be sedative and hypnotic effects via the GABAergic pathway, via inhalation increasing the expression of $GABA_A\alpha1$ and $GABA_A\alpha2$ positive cells, the level of $GABA_A\alpha1$ and $GABA_A\alpha2$ proteins, and also the level of $GABA_A\alpha1$ mRNA and $GABA_A\alpha2$ mRNA in the hypothalamus and cerebral cortex (Zhong et al., 2021).

Experimental studies in animal models have proven that multiple neurotransmitter systems are involved in the mode of action of essential oils, resulting in measurable physiological effects in the brain. It is important to treat depression, anxiety, and dementia as some mental illnesses, mainly with anxiolytic, antidepressant, and sedative effects (Lizarraga-Valderrama, 2021).

## 6.3 IMPORTANCE OF AROMATHERAPY IN INSOMNIA

Aromatherapy aims at the controlled use of herbal essential oils for healing purposes (Cooke and Ernst, 2000). Aromatherapy or "essential oil therapy" has been defined as the art and science of using aromatic essential oils naturally extracted from plants to balance, harmonize, and enhance body, mind, and spirit health (National Association for Holistic Aromatherapy, 2016). The essential oils mainly contain terpenes, aldehydes, esters, alcohols, and other chemical components. The oils can be inhaled directly, bathed, or used in massages, and have been used to reduce insomnia, anxiety, pain, fatigue, and other symptoms (Ren et al., 2019). Nevertheless, the therapeutic usage of essential oils must be done with clinical safety standards (Stea et al., 2014). Essential oils can be absorbed into the body through the olfactory and respiratory systems (by steam breathing); transdermal (lotions or compresses during massage and bathing); or orally (ingesting essential oils in capsules or as an additive to food or medicinal preparations; however, this last option may be considered herbal medicine rather than aromatherapy) (Gnatta et al., 2016; Acimovic, 2021; Cui et al., 2022). The olfactory pathway not only transmits the sense of smell but also serves to regulate memory, emotions, internal organs, and advanced functions of the brain, such as wakefulness and sleep through olfactory regulation (Masuo et al., 2021; Fung et al., 2021).

The primary mechanism of aromatherapy is related to the limbic system of the brain. Fragrance components stimulate olfactory cells, which deliver signals to the brain and affect the autonomic nervous system and hormone secretion (Kagawa et al., 2003). After reaching the limbic system via the olfactory nerve, the odor molecules produce calming and relaxing effects, affecting blood pressure, heart rate, memory, and stress response (Buckle, 2007). The essential oils transmit directly to the respiratory, circulatory, and CNS through the skin and respiratory tracts (Fung et al., 2021). Essential oils have sedative and hypnotic effects, but investigations on these effects of essential oils and their components are pretty limited (Lillehei and Halcon, 2014). While using essential oils reduces excessive drug use, it can also cure sleep disorders that can cause various health problems in the long term. Inhalation is a fast and effective form of aromatherapy that induces CNS response in a few seconds. Volatile molecules enter the circulatory system after gas exchange to the lungs (Cui et al., 2022). Neurotransmitters that transfer the odor transmission information and the orexin (hypocretin) neuronal system stimulate neurons in the brain stem, basal forebrain, and hypothalamus in the lateral region of the hypothalamus, producing GABA, serotonin (5-HT), etc. (Figure 6.1). These transmitters are closely related to the pathogenesis of insomnia and other diseases (Christen-Zaech et al., 2003).

Essential oils are presumed to improve sleep quality. In addition, a recent study emphasized that the fragrance of essential oils can be used to improve subjective and objective sleep quality in healthy people, and it can be a potential solution to poor sleep quality and insomnia (Ko et al., 2021). Essential oils were tested daily for air diffusion to detect the therapeutic effect of central fatigue. It was determined that there was a significant decrease in sleep deprivation after 21 days of administration in rats separated into a control group, a chronic sleep deprivation group, and an essential oil inhalation group. Thus, it has been noted that there is a positive result that essential oil formulations can reduce central fatigue in rats and can be used in conditions such as insomnia and depression (Han et al., 2018). For example, sleeping people exposed to the aroma of lavender have better sleep quality and energy during the daytime (Ko et al., 2021). Linalool and linalyl acetate are the major components of lavender essential oil in coriander essential oils. Low-dose linalool has been reported to have a sedative effect on the human body by inhalation (Hosseini et al., 2021; Xu et al., 2021, 2023). It has even been reported that essential oils can help in the care of cancer patients by helping manage side effects such as insomnia and nausea. Lavender, peppermint, and orange are well-known essential oils used to support cancer patients experiencing insomnia, nausea, and anxiety (Reis and Jones, 2017). Previous studies have indicated that some essential oils, including bergamot, sweet orange, valerian, lemon, rose, cedar, etc., have sedative and hypnotic effects (Lillehei and Halcon, 2014). Anshen essential oil, compatible with lavender, sweet orange, and sandalwood essential oil, has been investigated for people living with insomnia, often accompanied by varying degrees of depression and anxiety symptoms based on the aromatherapy theory of traditional Chinese medicine. The inhalation of Anshen essential oil [D-limonene (24.07%), linalool (21.98%), linalyl acetate (15.37%), α-pinene (5.39%), and α-santalol (4.8%)] was contributed to reduce the latency and prolong sleep time in mice. The results of the enzyme-linked immunosorbent test indicated that the Anshen essential oil could increase the content of 5-HT and GABA in the mouse brain (Zhong et al., 2019).

In this context, aromatherapy is mainly used in the treatment of disorders related to chronic pain, healing wounds, depression, anxiety, increasing cognitive efficiency, reducing stress, and other psychological and physiological conditions, including insomnia (Perry and Perry, 2006; Cho et al., 2013; Reis and Jones, 2017). Aromatherapy is beneficial for improving sleep (Hwang and Shin, 2015). Especially *Lavandula officinalis*, *Citrus sinensis*, *Rosa damascena*, Neroli (*Citrus aurantium*), and *Anthemis nobilis* reduce anxiety in surgical patients (Stea et al., 2014).

As a result, aromatherapy seems to be a remarkable field for treating insomnia, or at least difficulty falling asleep, because it reports the beneficial effects of essential oils in terms of relaxing, calming, or sleep-inducing activities.

## 6.4　ESSENTIAL OILS USED IN INSOMNIA

Relaxation is described as an emotional state without anger, anxiety, fear, or similar arousal. The sedative effect is to calm the functions of the central nervous system. However, sleep is an unconscious, natural, repetitive state in which sensory and motor activities are temporarily inactive. Therefore, the agents used to achieve these effects are known as sedative or hypnotic, and these effects overlap (Dobetsberger and Buchbauer, 2011). In this section, the essential oils, which are thought to be directly effective in insomnia, will be emphasized.

Essential oils effectively relieve symptoms of depression, anxiety, and stress in adults. It has been suggested that anxiolytic and antidepressant effects may be related to suppressing sympathetic nervous system activity (Fung et al., 2021). Some essential oils that are already quite popular as anxiolytic, sedative, and relaxing oils obtained from lavender (*Lavandula angustifolia* Mill., Lamiaceae), rose (*Rosa damascena* Mill., Rosaceae), orange (*Citrus sinensis* L., Rutaceae), bergamot (*Citrus bergamia* Risso., Rutaceae), lemon (*Citrus limon* L., Rutaceae), sandalwood (*Santalum album* RBr., Santalaceae), sage (*Salvia sclarea* L., Lamiaceae), roman chamomile (*Anthemis nobilis* L., Asteraceae), and geranium (*Pelargonium* spp., Geraniaceae) (Setzer, 2009; Dobetsberger and Buchbauer, 2011), were mentioned in some articles.

Animal studies (Belovicova et al., 2017; Slattery and Cryan, 2012) have also assisted in investigating the underlying mechanisms of essential oils. It has been found that the anxiolytic effects of essential oils are associated with increased serotonin (5-HT) levels or dopamine (DA) levels. In contrast, their antidepressant effect is related to increased brain-derived neurotrophic factor (Fung et al., 2021). Although most essential oils can interact with several neurotransmitter pathways, such as the noradrenergic, 5-HTergic, GABAergic, and DAergic systems, the action of essential oils mainly depends on the efficacy of their active components. Some major oil compounds, such as linalool, limonene, benzyl benzoate, and benzyl alcohol, have been reported to exert anxiolytic and antidepressant effects. For example, the benzyl benzoate in ylang-ylang activates the 5-HTergic and DAergic pathways that are effective on anxiety (Zhang et al., 2016). Other study results showed that linalool and β-pinene produced an effect through interaction with the GABAergic pathway. Because lavender and bergamot oils contain linalool, they can act on GABA receptors to claim an anxiolytic and antidepressant effect (Wang and Heinbockel, 2018). In addition, cinnamon oil also has an anxiolytic effect by inhibiting the release of pro-inflammatory cytokines (Lizarraga-Valderrama, 2021). Sweet orange, rose, and lavender essential oils produce a calming effect by interacting with the hypothalamic-pituitary-adrenal (HPA) axis to reduce cortisol concentration in serum (Lizarraga-Valderrama, 2021).

As the first example, the essential oil of *Acorus tatarinowii* Schott/Shi Chang Pu/ rhizomes from the Acoraceae family reduced locomotor activity times. When administered intraperitoneally, it increased subthreshold barbiturate-induced sedative and hypnotic effects on male and female Kunming mice. This result is thought to be based on the mechanism of protecting neurons and increasing the permeability of the blood-brain barrier (Kim et al., 2022). *Aloysia citriodora* Paláu (*Lippia citriodora* Kunth) from Verbenaceae, "Lemon Verbena", has long been used in traditional medicine with different populations for the treatment of sedation and insomnia in the history (Bahramsoltani et al., 2018). *A. citriodora* (total essential oil 1.66 mg/10 mL and total flavonoid amount as quercetin 3.22 mg/10 ml syrup) was given to 100 randomly selected patients with insomnia, and placebo was administered to the other group to evaluate the efficacy of this plant. This study was evaluated using the Pittsburgh Sleep Quality Index (PSQI) and Insomnia Severity Index (ISI) questionnaires. In the *A. citriodora* group, significant improvement was observed after 4 weeks of treatment (p < 0.001 for all), and it concluded that oral intake could be recommended as a complementary therapy in patients suffering from insomnia (Afrasiabian et al., 2019). A significant species in the history of medicine, *Artemisia absinthium*/wormwood from Asteraceae is formerly known as a medicinal herb in medieval Europe famous for its use against fatigue, but now it is known as an effective agent in the treatment of insomnia in traditional Asian and European medicine (Ahamad et al., 2019; Szopa et al., 2020). Moreover, in homeopathy, this plant is recommended for hallucinations, nightmares, irritability, insomnia, dizziness, and epileptic seizures (Lockie, 2006).

*Citrus aurantium* L. (Rutaceae) is widely used to treat insomnia, anxiety, and epilepsy. The pericarpium essential oil and the ethanol (70% w/v) extract from the leaves were used in the experiments on Swiss male mice to evaluate sedative/hypnotic, anxiolytic, and anticonvulsant effects. The results revealed that the essential oil from the pericarp increased the latency of prolonging the sleep time induced by barbiturates in a non-dose-dependent manner. The anxiety and sedation model was suitable for the ethnopharmacological use of *C. aurantium*, which may be helpful in primary care after the toxicological examination (Carvalho-Freitas and Costa, 2002). According to ethnopharmacological information, *Citrus* species have beneficial effects in reducing anxiety or insomnia symptoms. Based on these outcomes, *C. aurantium* has been suggested as an adjuvant to antidepressants. The obtained data showed that the anxiolytic-like activity observed in the light/dark box procedure after acute (5 mg/kg) or 14 days of repeated (1 mg/kg/day) dosing was mediated by the serotonergic system (5-HT1A receptors). Also, after oil application, toxicity was not observed (Costa et al., 2013). *Coriandrum sativum* L. or coriander (Apiaceae) is an herb cultivated worldwide as a culinary, medicinal, or fundamental crop (Önder, 2018). It is used in traditional medicine to relieve anxiety and insomnia. Hydroalcoholic and aqueous extracts from the aerial parts and fruits are known to have anxiolytic and sedative effects in rodents. The effects of intracerebroventricular (i.c.v.) administration of coriander fruits oil and its main component, linalool, were also investigated on locomotor activity and emotionality of newly hatched chicks. The essential oil obtained from *C. sativum* fruits produces a sedative effect at 8.6 and 86 mg/chick doses by i.c.v. The injection may be due to the monoterpene linalool, which also induces a calming effect and can be considered a potential therapeutic agent identical to diazepam (Gastón et al., 2016). The leaves and stem bark of *Croton conduplicatus* Kunth (Euphorbiaceae), a Brazilian aromatic medicinal plant commonly known as "quebra-faca", are used as a natural analgesic in treating headaches in folk medicine. Different experimental models were used to evaluate several activities, including the anxiolytic (elevated plus maze and hole board tests) and sedative (thiopental-induced sleep time) effects of the essential oil. Studies have supported that essential oil has proven to be a multi-targeted agent, showing not only anxiolytic and sedative effects depending on the dose (Oliveira Júnior et al., 2018).

The leaves, fruits, and seeds essential oil of *Dennettia tripetala* G. Baker's (Annonaceae) have a component named 1-nitro-2-phenylethane responsible for its effect. The hypnotic, anticonvulsant, and anxiolytic effects of this compound were dose-related (the acute toxicity, $LD_{50}$=490 mg/kg intraperitoneally) as observed in mice (Oyemitan et al., 2013).

*Lantana camara* L. (Verbenaceae) oil from West Africa was evaluated for sedative activity in rats by inhalation administration. Inhaled oil, including sabinene (38.81%) and 1,8-cineole (28.90%) as major components, significantly reduced the locomotor course in a dose-dependent manner in rats, specifically at doses of 0.0004 and 0.04 mg per 400 µL triethyl citrate (TEC) (Dougnon and Ito, 2020). The efficacy of Silexan (standardized lavender essential oil for oral use) was compared with lavender essential oil by breathing for sleep delay, duration, quality, disturbed sleep, and anxiety in adult patients, and no evidence was found in the literature according to this point (Greenberg and Slyer, 2018). Although the available evidence shows promising results, lavender treats behavioral problems in older adults, especially sleep disorders. It is also stated that no side effects were observed in patients during application sessions (Velasco-Rodríguez et al., 2019). *Lavandula angustifolia* Mill. (lavender) from Lamiaceae has traditionally been used for sleep improvement. The efficacy of inhaled *L. angustifolia* in diabetic patients treated with inhaled lavender or placebo for two days as a complementary therapy was demonstrated that inhaled lavender could improve sleep quality and quantity, quality of life, and mood without significant effect on metabolic status in diabetic patients suffering from insomnia (Nasiri et al., 2020). The result of inhalation of *L. angustifolia* essential oil on sleep and menopausal symptoms in postmenopausal women who have insomnia was also evaluated and measured by the Pittsburgh Sleep Quality Index. The essential oil inhalation improved the overall sleep patterns, quality, and sleep efficiency of the participants in the group (Dos Reis Lucena et al., 2021). There are claims that *L. angustifolia* essential oil has particularly anxiolytic and sedative properties, with a long history of medicinal use. Lavender oil has been used to reduce nuisance and as a natural cure for insomnia. Increasing evidence has found similarities between the effects of lavender oil and anxiolytic drugs such as benzodiazepines. Lavender oil inhalation reduced the number of waking episodes but maintained the normal time spent in wakefulness, non-rapid eye movement, and rapid eye movement sleep may suggest beneficial anxiolytic-like effects of lavender oil for sleep improvement purposes, which is marked anxiolytic-like effect on sleep (Manor et al., 2021).

*Nelumbo nucifera* from Nelumbonaceae, or sacred lotus, has been a valuable vegetable as a functional food and herbal medicine for over 2000 years. It was declared that this herb had been used in traditional medicine to treat chronic dyspepsia, hematuria, nervous disorders, cardiovascular diseases, hyperlipidemia, and insomnia (Chen et al., 2019).

*Origanum* species (Lamiaceae), distributed in the Mediterranean, Euro-Siberian, and Iran-Siberian regions, is a spice known as "thyme" or "pizza-spice" in southern Europe and the Americas with important biological activities including insomnia

(Sharifi-Rad et al., 2021). Especially in Cuba, there are records of using *O. majorana* in insomnia (Cano and Volpato, 2004). Rosemary (*Rosmarinus officinalis* L.) from Lamiaceae is a bushy evergreen shrub that grows in regions from the Mediterranean to the Himalayas. In traditional medicine, the plant has improved intercostal neuralgia, headache, migraine, insomnia, emotional disturbance, and depression. Different studies highlighted the neuropharmacological effects of rosemary and some clinical effects supported in animal studies (Ghasemzadeh Rahbardar and Hosseinzadeh, 2020).

An oil blend called Anshen essential oil is used to treat insomnia and consists of several essential oils, including sandalwood, aloe, rose, and lavender, with a soothing-calming effect. However, it was indicated that further research on the mechanism of this oil requires new therapeutic ideas and methods (Ren et al., 2019). It has also been shown that a 6:2:0.5 mixture of essential oils lavender (*Lavandula officinalis*), chamomile (*Anthemis nobilis*), and neroli (*Citrus aurantium*) can reduce anxiety, enhance sleep, and balance blood pressure in patients with stented hearts (Cho et al., 2013).

## 6.5   CONCLUSION

Recently, the discovery of new, primary, and reliable alternative or complementary solutions in treating insomnia has been considered with a stimulated momentum. It is possible to increase examples on this subject. Thus, only some more recent examples are covered here. Many essential oils show sedative, hypnotic, and anxiolytic effects. Especially some main chemical components in the composition of essential oils are also important in the emergence of these effects. However, scientific studies of essential oils on the sedative, hypnotic, and anxiolytic effects are relatively limited. Clinical applications of essential oils used in aromatherapy still attract much more attention, and detailed studies on the pharmacological activities of inhaled essential oils are ongoing. There are many preparations and formulations whose effects have been proven and turned into products in this regard.

For this reason, the number and reliability of essential oils used in some sleep disorders like insomnia are increasing. However, essential oils, which have a complex structure, still need to be used carefully and in a controlled manner. For all that, there is an undeniable truth with scientific evidence that essential oils are used against insomnia.

## REFERENCES

Abad, V.C., and Guilleminault, C. 2018. Insomnia in elderly patients: Recommendations for pharmacological management. *Drugs Aging.* 35:791–817.

Acimovic, M. 2021. Essential oils: Inhalation aromatherapy: A comprehensive review. *J. Agron. Technol. Eng. Manag.* 4:547–557.

Afrasiabian, F., Mirabzadeh Ardakani, M., Rahmani, K. et al. 2019. *Aloysia citriodora* Palau (*Lemon verbena*) for insomnia patients: A randomized, double-blind, placebo-controlled clinical trial of efficacy and safety. *Phytother Res.* 33:350–359.

Ahamad, J., Mir, S.R., Amin, S.A. 2019. Pharmacognostic review on *Artemisia absinthium*. *Int. Res. J. Pharm.* 10:25–31.

Bahramsoltani, R., Rostamiasrabadi, P., Shahpiri, Z. et al. 2018. *Aloysia citrodora* Paláu (*Lemon verbena*): A review of phytochemistry and pharmacology. *J Ethnopharmacol.* 222:34–51.

Bakkali, F., Averbeck, S., Averbeck, D., Idaomar, M. 2008. Biological effects of essential oils: A review. *Food Chem Toxicol.* 46:446–475.

Belovicova, K., Bogi, E., Csatlosova, K., Dubovicky, M. 2017. Animal tests for anxiety-like and depression-like behavior in rats. *Interdiscip. Toxicol.* 10:40–43.

Bhaskar, S., Hemavathy, D., Prasad, S. 2016. Prevalence of chronic insomnia in adult patients and its correlation with medical comorbidities. *J Family Med Prim Care.* 5:780–784.

Bollu, P.C., and Kaur, H. 2019. Sleep medicine: Insomnia and sleep. *Mo Med.* 116:68–75.

Borrás, S., Martínez-Solís, I., Ríos, J.L. 2021. Medicinal plants for insomnia related to anxiety: An updated review. *Planta Med.* 87:738–753.

Buckle, J. 2007. Literature review: Should nursing take aromatherapy more seriously. *Br J Nurs.* 16:116–20.

Buysse, D.J. 2013. Insomnia. *JAMA.* 309:706–16.

Cano, J.H., and Volpato, G. 2004. Herbal mixtures in the traditional medicine of eastern Cuba. *J. Ethnopharmacol.* 90:293–316.

Carvalho-Freitas, M.I., and Costa, M. 2002. Anxiolytic and sedative effects of extracts and essential oil from *Citrus aurantium* L. *Biol Pharm Bull.* 25:1629–1633.

Chen, G., Zhu, M., Guo, M. 2019. Research advances in traditional and modern use of *Nelumbo nucifera*: Phytochemicals, health promoting activities and beyond. *Crit Rev Food Sci Nutr.* 59(supl):S189-S209.

Cho, M.Y., Min, E.S., Hur, M.H., Lee, M.S. 2013. Effects of aromatherapy on the anxiety, vital signs, and sleep quality of percutaneous coronary intervention patients in intensive care units. *Evid Based Complement Alternat Med.* 2013:381381.

Christen-Zaech, S., Kraftsik, R., Pillevuit, O. et al. 2003. Early olfactory involvement in Alzheimer's disease. *Can J Neurol Sci.* 30:20–5.

Chung, S., Son, G.H., Kim, K. 2017. Circadian rhythm of adrenal glucocorticoid: Its regulation and clinical implications. *Biochimica et Biophysica Acta.* 1812:581–591.

Citrome, L. 2014. Suvorexant for insomnia: A systematic review of the efficacy and safety profile for this newly approved hypnotic-what is the number needed to treat, number needed to harm and likelihood to be helped or harmed? *Int J Clin Pract.* 68:1429–1441.

Cooke, B., and Ernst, E. 2000. Aromatherapy: A systematic review. *Br J Gen Pract.* 50:493–496.

Costa, C.A., Cury, T.C., Cassettari, B.O., Takahira, R.K., Flório, J.C., Costa, M. 2013. *Citrus aurantium* L. essential oil exhibits anxiolytic-like activity mediated by 5-HT(1A)-receptors and reduces cholesterol after repeated oral treatment. *BMC Complement Altern Med.* 13:42.

Cui, J., Li, M., Wei, Y. et al. 2022. Inhalation aromatherapy *via* brain-targeted nasal delivery: Natural volatiles or essential oils on mood disorders. *Front Pharmacol.* 13:860043.

Dobetsberger, C., and Buchbauer, G. 2011. Actions of essential oils on the central nervous system: An updated review. *Flavour Fragr. J.* 26:300–316.

Doghramji, K. 2010. The evaluation and management of insomnia. *Clin Chest Med.* 31:327e39.

Dool-Ri, O., Yujin, K., Ara, J., et al. 2019. Sedative and hypnotic effects of *Vaccinium bracteatum* thunb: Through the regulation of serotonergic and GABA-ergic systems: Involvement of 5-HT receptor agonistic activity. *Biomed. Pharmacother.* 109:2218–2227.

Dos Reis Lucena, L., Dos Santos-Junior, J.G., Tufik, S., Hachul, H. 2021. Lavender essential oil on postmenopausal women with insomnia: Double-blind randomized trial. *Complement Ther Med.* 59:102726.

Dougnon, G., and Ito, M. 2020. Sedative effects of the essential oil from the leaves of *Lantana camara* occurring in the Republic of Benin via inhalation in mice. *J Nat Med.* 74:159–169.

Eban-Rothschild, A., Appelbaum, L., de Lecea, L. 2018. Neuronal mechanisms for sleep/wake regulation and modulatory drive. *Neuropsychopharmacology.* 43:937–952.

El Asbahani, A., Miladi, K., Badri, W. et al. 2009. Essential oils: From extraction to encapsulation. *Int. J. Pharm.* 483:220–243.

Elshafie, H.S., and Camele, I. 2017. An overview of the biological effects of some Mediterranean essential oils on human health. *Biomed Res Int.* 2017:9268468.

Everitt, H., Baldwin, D.S., Stuart, B. et al. 2018. Antidepressants for insomnia in adults. *Cochrane Database Syst Rev.* 5:CD010753.

Fernandez-Mendoza, J. 2017. The insomnia with short sleep duration phenotype: An update on it's importance for health and prevention. *Current Opinion in Psychiatry.* 30:56–63.

Fung, T.K.H., Lau, B.W.M., Ngai, S.P.C., Tsang, H.W.H. 2021. Therapeutic effect and mechanisms of essential oils in mood disorders: Interaction between the nervous and respiratory systems. *Int J Mol Sci.* 22:4844.

Gastón, M.S., Cid, M.P., Vázquez, A.M. et al. 2016. Sedative effect of central administration of *Coriandrum sativum* essential oil and its major component linalool in neonatal chicks. *Pharm Biol.* 54:1954–1961.

Ghasemzadeh Rahbardar, M., and Hosseinzadeh, H. 2020. Therapeutic effects of rosemary (*Rosmarinus officinalis* L.) and its active constituents on nervous system disorders. Iran *J Basic Med Sci.* 23:1100–1112.

Gnatta, J.R., Kurebayashi, L.F., Turrini, R.N., and Silva, M.J. 2016. Aromatherapy and nursing: Historical and theoretical conception. *Rev. Esc. Enferm. USP.* 50:130–136.

Grandner, M.A. 2017. Sleep, health, and society. *Sleep Med Clin.* 12:1–22.

Greenberg, M.J., and Slyer, J.T. 2018. Effectiveness of Silexan oral lavender essential oil compared to inhaled lavender essential oil aromatherapy for sleep in adults: A systematic review. *JBI Database System Rev Implement Rep.* 16: 2109–2117.

Han, C., Li, F., Tian, S. et al. 2018. Beneficial effect of compound essential oil inhalation on central fatigue. *BMC Complement Altern Med.* 18:309.

Han, K.S., Kim, L., Shim, I. 2012. Stress and sleep disorder. *Exp Neurobiol.* 21:141–50.

Hosseini, M., Boskabady, M.H., Khazdair, M.R. 2021. Neuroprotective effects of *Coriandrum sativum* and its constituent, linalool: A review. *Avicenna J Phytomed* 11:436–450.

Hwang, E., and Shin, S. 2015. The effects of aromatherapy on sleep improvement: A systematic literature review and meta-analysis. *J Altern Complement Med.* 21:61–68.

Jolanta, O. 2010. Consequences of sleep deprivation. *Int J Occup Med Environ Health.* 23:95–114.

Kagawa, D., Jokura, H., Ochiai, R., Tokimitsu, I., Tsubone, H. 2003. The sedative effects and mechanism of action of cedrol inhalation with behavioral pharmacological evaluation. *Planta Med.* 69:637–641.

Kato, K., Hirai, K., Nishiyama, K., et al. 2005. Neurochemical properties of ramelteon (TAK-375), a selective MT1/MT2 receptor agonist. *Neuropharmacology.* 48:301–310.

Kim, C.J., Kwak, T.Y., Bae, M.H., Shin, H.K., Choi, B.T. 2022. Therapeutic potential of active components from *Acorus gramineus* and *Acorus tatarinowii* in neurological disorders and their application in Korean medicine. *J Pharmacopuncture.* 25:326–343

Ko, L.W., Su, C.H., Yang, M.H., Liu, S.Y., Su, T.P. 2021. A pilot study on essential oil aroma stimulation for enhancing slow-wave EEG in sleeping brain. *Sci Rep.* 11:1078.

Koyama, S., and Heinbockel T. 2020. The effects of essential oils and terpenes in relation to their routes of intake and application. *Int J Mol Sci.* 21:1558.

Lie, J.D., Tu, K.N., Shen, D.D., Wong, B.M. 2015. Pharmacological treatment of insomnia. *P T.* 40:759–771.

Lillehei, A.S., and Halcon, L.L. 2014. A systematic review of the effect of inhaled essential oils on sleep. *J Altern Complement Med.* 20:441–451.

Lizarraga-Valderrama, L.R. 2021. Effects of essential oils on central nervous system: Focus on mental health. *Phytother. Res.* 35:657–679.

Lockie, A. 2006. *Encyclopedia of Homeopathy*. DK Publishing, New York, NY, USA.

Manor, R., Kumarnsit, E., Samerphob, N., Rujiralai, T., Puangpairote, T., Cheaha, D. 2021. Characterization of pharmaco-EEG fingerprint and sleep-wake profiles of *Lavandula angustifolia* Mill. essential oil inhalation and diazepam administration in rats. *J Ethnopharmacol*. 276:114193.

Masuo, Y., Satou, T., Takemoto, H., Koike, K. 2021. Smell and stress response in the brain: Review of the connection between chemistry and neuropharmacology. *Molecules*. 26:2571.

Monti, J.M. 2011. Serotonin control of sleep-wake behavior. *Sleep Med Rev*. 15:269–281.

Morin, C.M., Jarrin, D.C. 2022. Epidemiology of insomnia: Prevalence, course, risk factors, and public health burden. *Sleep Med Clin*. 17:173–191.

Nasiri Lari, Z., Hajimonfarednejad, M., Riasatian, M. et al. 2020. Efficacy of inhaled *Lavandula angustifolia* Mill.: Essential oil on sleep quality, quality of life and metabolic control in patients with diabetes mellitus type II and insomnia. *J Ethnopharmacol*. 251:112560.

National Association for Holistic Aromatherapy. 2016. What is aromatherapy? Retrieved from https://naha.org/explore-aromatherapy/about-aromatherapy/what-is-aromatherapy.

Nutt, D.J., and Stahl, S.M. 2010. Searching for perfect sleep: The continuing evolution of GABAA receptor modulators as hypnotics. *J Psychopharmacol*. 24:1601–1612.

Ohayon, M.M. 2002. Epidemiology of insomnia: What we know and what we still need to learn. *Sleep Med Rev*. 6:97e111.

Oliveira Júnior, R.G, Ferraz, C.A.A., Silva, J.C. et al. 2018. Neuropharmacological effects of essential oil from the leaves of *Croton conduplicatus* Kunth and possible mechanisms of action involved. *J Ethnopharmacol*. 221:65–76.

Önder, A. 2018. Chapter: 9. Coriander and Its Phytoconstituents for the Beneficial Effects. In *Potential of Essential Oils*. ed. Hany A. El-Shemy. In Tech Open, London, UK.

Oyemitan, I.A., Elusiyan, C.A., Akanmu, M.A., Olugbade, T.A. 2013. Hypnotic, anticonvulsant and anxiolytic effects of 1-nitro-2-phenylethane isolated from the essential oil of *Dennettia tripetala* in mice. *Phytomedicine*. 20:1315–1322.

Perricone, M., Arace, E., Corbo, M.R., Sinigaglia, M., Bevilacqua, A. 2015. Bioactivity of essential oils: A review on their interaction with food components. *Front Microbiol*. 6:76.

Perry, N., and Perry, E. 2006. Aromatherapy in the management of psychiatric disorders: Clinical and neuropharmacological perspectives. *CNS Drugs*. 20:257–280.

Ramsey, J.T., Shropshire, B.C., Nagy, T.R., Chambers, K.D., Li, Y., Korach, K.S. 2020. Essential oils and health. *Yale J Biol Med*. 93:291–305.

Reis, D., and Jones T. 2017. Aromatherapy: Using essential oils as a supportive therapy. *Clin J Oncol Nurs*. 21:16–19.

Ren, G., Zhong, Y., Ke, G. et al. 2019. The mechanism of compound Anshen essential oil in the treatment of insomnia was examined by network pharmacology. *Evid Based Complement Alternat Med*. 2019:9241403.

Riemann, D., Nissen, C., Palagini, L., Otte, A., Perlis, M.L., Spiegelhalder, K. 2015. The neurobiology, investigation, and treatment of chronic insomnia. *Lancet Neurol*. 14:547–558.

Sarris, J., and Byrne, G.J. 2011. A systematic review of insomnia and complementary medicine. *Sleep Med Rev*. 15:99e106.

Semyanov, A., Walker, M.C., Kullmann, D.M., Silver, R.A. 2004. Tonically active GABAA receptors: Modulating gain and maintaining the tone. *Trends Neurosci*. 27:262–269.

Setzer, W.N. 2009. Essential oils and anxiolytic aromatherapy. *Nat Prod Commun*. 4:1305–1316.

Sharifi-Rad, M., Berkay Yılmaz, Y., Antika, G. et al. 2021. Phytochemical constituents, biological activities, and health-promoting effects of the genus *Origanum*. *Phytother Res*. 35: 95–121.

Shi, M.M., Piao, J.H., Xu, X.L. et al. 2016. Chinese medicines with sedative-hypnotic effects and their active components. *Sleep Med Rev.* 29:108–118.

Shi, Y., Dong, J.W., Zhao, J.H. et al. 2014. Herbal insomnia medications that target GABAergic systems: A review of the psychopharmacological evidence. *Curr Neuropharmacol.* 12:289–302.

Siegel, J.M. 2004. The neurotransmitters of sleep. *J Clin Psychiatry.* 65(suppl 16):4–7.

Slattery, D.A. and Cryan, J.F. 2012. Using the rat forced swim test to assess antidepressant-like activity in rodents. *Nat. Protoc.* 7:1009–1014.

Soares, G.A.B.E., Bhattacharya, T., Chakrabarti, T., Tagde, P., Cavalu, S. 2021. Exploring pharmacological mechanisms of essential oils on the central nervous system. *Plants (Basel).* 11:21.

Stea, S., Beraudi, A., De Pasquale, D. 2014. Essential oils for complementary treatment of surgical patients: State of the art. *Evid Based Complement Alternat Med.* 2014:726341.

Suzana, U., Oliver, K., Miro, J., et al. 2010. Side effects of treatment with benzodiazepines. *Psychiatr Danub.* 22:90–93.

Szopa, A., Pajor, J., Klin, P. et al. 2020. *Artemisia absinthium* L.-Importance in the history of medicine, the latest advances in phytochemistry and therapeutical, cosmetological and culinary uses. *Plants (Basel).* 9:1063.

Tariq, S.H. and Pulisetty, S. 2008. Pharmacotherapy for insomnia. *Clin Geriatr Med.* 24:93.

Taylor, D.J., Lichstein, K.L., Durrence, H.H. 2003. Insomnia as a health risk factor. *Behav Sleep Med.* 1:227e47.

Twaij, B.M., and Hasan, M.N. 2022. Bioactive secondary metabolites from plant sources: Types, synthesis, and their therapeutic uses. *Int. J. Plant Biol. International Journal of Plant Biology.* 13:4–14.

Varkevisser, M., Van Dongen, H.P., Van Amsterdam, J.G., Kerkhof, G.A. 2007. Chronic insomnia and daytime functioning: An ambulatory assessment. *Behav Sleep Med.* 5:279e96.

Velasco-Rodríguez, R., Pérez-Hernández, M.G., Maturano-Melgoza, J.A. et al. 2019. The effect of aromatherapy with lavender (*Lavandula angustifolia*) on serum melatonin levels. *Complement Ther Med.* 47:102208.

Wang, Z.J., and Heinbockel, T. 2018. Essential oils and their constituents targeting the GABAergic system and sodium channels as treatment of neurological diseases. *Molecules.* 23:1061.

Winkler, A., Auer, C., Doering, B.K. et al. 2014. Drug treatment of primary insomnia: A meta-analysis of Polysomnographic randomized controlled trials. *CNS Drugs.* 28:799–816.

Xu, L., Li, X., Zhang, Y. et al. 2021. The effects of linalool acupoint application therapy on sleep regulation. *RSC Adv.* 11:5896–5902.

Xu, Y., Ma, L., Liu, F. et al. 2023. Lavender essential oil fractions alleviate sleep disorders induced by the combination of anxiety and caffeine in mice. *J Ethnopharmacol.* 302(Pt A):115868.

Yeung, W.F., Chung, K.F., Yung, K.P., Ng, T.H. 2015. Doxepin for insomnia: A systematic review of randomized placebo-controlled trials. *Sleep Med Rev.* 19:75–83.

Zhang, N., Zhang, L., Feng, L., Yao, L. 2016. The anxiolytic effect of essential oil of *Cananga odorata* exposure on mice and determination of its major active constituents. *Phytomedicine.* 23:1727–1734.

Zhong, Y., Zheng, Q., Hu, P. et al. 2019. Sedative and hypnotic effects of compound Anshen essential oil inhalation for insomnia. *BMC Complement Altern Med.* 19:306.

Zhong, Y., Zheng, Q., Hu, P. et al. 2021. Sedative and hypnotic effects of *Perilla frutescens* essential oil through GABAergic system pathway. *J Ethnopharmacol.* 279:113627.

# 7 Role of Egyptian Essential Oils in Health Care and Industry

*Hagar A. Sobhy, Ahmed E. Elissawy,*
*Omayma A. Eldahshan, and*
*Abdel Nasser B. Singab*

## 7.1 INTRODUCTION: BRIEF BACKGROUND ON ESSENTIAL OILS

Essential oils are polar and non-polar volatile compound mixtures prepared from plant parts; mainly herbs and spices from different families including *Asteraceae, Lamiaceae, Lauraceae, Cyperaceae, Piperaceae, Myrtaceae, Apiaceae, Apocynaceae, Solanaceae*, and *Zingerberaceae* by different means of extraction such as pressing and distillation. They protect the plants from pathogenic microorganisms, insect predators, and some herbivores. Besides, they can attract other insects that contribute to seed and pollen dispersion (Bakkali et al. 2008).

Essential oils are used as natural additives in food and food products owing to their antioxidant and antimicrobial activities. They possess a wide range of biological activities such as antimicrobial, antiseptic, analgesic, spasmolytic, carminative, diuretic, and hyperemic activities. They are widely used in perfumery, cosmetics industry, sanitary products, agriculture (bio-pesticide and repellent), and aromatherapy (Burt 2004; Sarkic et al. 2018).

Terpenoids and terpenes are the major components of essential oils, derived from the isoprene unit ($C_5H_8$). They are biosynthesized through mevalonate (MVA) pathway in the cytosol and methyl erythritol phosphate (MEP) pathway in the plastids yielding isopentenyl pyrophosphate (IPP) and dimethylallyl pyrophosphate (DMAPP) which are condensed to form monoterpenes. Terpenes are classified by the number of carbons as monoterpenes ($C_{10}H_{16}$), sesquiterpenes ($C_{15}H_{24}$), diterpenes ($C_{20}H_{32}$), triterpenes ($C_{30}H_{40}$), etc. Unique cyclase tends to form unique structures from terpenes which may be hydrocarbons, alcohols, aldehydes, ketones, ethers, or lactones. Sesquiterpenes have a wide variety of chemical structures owing to its longer chain of 15 carbons, increasing the number of possible cyclizations through the mevalonate pathway and so are diterpenes (Pavela and Benelli 2016). Only two or three components could represent almost 85% of the total mixture of the essential oil. These major components are attributed to the primary biological activities of the essential oil (Miguel 2010).

DOI: 10.1201/9781003389774-7

All parts of aromatic plants most probably contain volatile oils such as flowers including clove, lavender, and ylang ylang; leaves including thyme, eucalyptus, and savory; rhizomes including ginger; seeds including cardamom; fruits including fennel and anise; and wood and bark including cinnamon and sandalwood (Dhifi et al. 2016). Numerous extraction techniques can be used to extract essential oils from different parts of the aromatic plants such as hydro distillation and steam distillation being the oldest and simplest methods of extracting essential oils, cold pressing which is used for the peel of citrus fruits, crushing, hydrolysis, fermentation, and enfleurage which is used particularly for rose (Perricone et al. 2015). The classical method of hydro distillation and steam distillation is based on the use of the Clevenger apparatus which was discovered in 1928 and modified by Jakub Deryng in 1951 (Deryng 1951). Microwave and supercritical fluid assisted extractions are also modern methods used for extracting essential oils at the laboratory scale.

Egyptian perfumery was famous among the ancient worlds. In addition, the art of perfume preparation is assumed to be born in ancient Egypt (Fadel 2020). Aromatic plants and essential oils were widely used by ancient Egyptians for embalming to prevent body decay and bacterial growth. Furthermore, Egyptians used aromatic plants medicinally and spiritually. They practiced fumigation using smoldering plants during meditation, prayers, and healing particularly in the healing of women's reproductive disorders (Bird 2003). This chapter focuses on the different applications of essential oils from the Egyptian flora beginning in the old uses recorded in the medical papyri to the most recent applications in the pharmaceutical industry including their applications in the green chemistry and nanotechnology.

## 7.2 APPLICATIONS OF ESSENTIAL OILS FROM ANCIENT EGYPTIAN CIVILIZATION TO MODERN MEDICINE

The Egyptian civilization is one of the oldest and greatest civilizations in the history. Ancient Egypt lasted from 3300 to 525 BC when the dawn of modern medicine started including the use of different medicinal pharmacopias, dentistry, simple surgeries, and bone setting (Nunn 2002). Ancient Egyptians used perfumes and oils to give the body an agreeable odor. They produced perfumes from different herbs and plants such as balsam, iris, and iris root, whereas myrrh, lily, and frankincense were the most frequently used oils in ancient Egypt that were mixed with fruits, flowers, and herbs essences. Perfumes were made by three different techniques; the materials were ground, mixed, and then put on the heat (Fadel 2020). The medicinal use of essential oils against diseases and infections can be dated back as far as ancient Egypt. Ancient Egyptians widely cultivated those plants whose parts could be sources of essential oils. An Egyptian papyrus dated 2551–2528 BC proved the use of essential oils by ancient Egyptians for medical purpose. Ancient Egyptians used essential oils for beauty treatments, aromatherapy, and spiritual practice including mummification for its good preservation of mummies. They used to make mixtures of different herbal preparations such as cedar, grapes, aniseed, myrrh, and onion in perfumes and medicine (Baser et al. 2009). In 1922, 50 alabaster mason jars that were used in the storage of essential oils were found during the excavation of Tutankhamen's tomb (Sharangi 2021). It was said that ancient Egyptians strongly believed that spiritual transformation could be induced by inhalation of different fragrances. They used to extract essential oils from plants using the enfleurage technique through the infusion of plant material in a fatty substance following boiling, thus, the aroma evaporated and settled in the fat. The fats were either vegetable fat or animal fat that had been infused with the fragrance components of the flower, and when the fat became saturated with the fragrance, it was called "enfleurage pomade" (Bhadra and Parida 2021). Besides, there is evidence that they were aware of an oil extraction procedure through distillation (Gurib-Fakim 2006). Using essential oils as food preservatives can be dated back to ancient Egyptians (Abdel-Maksoud and El-Amin 2011). Moreover, ancient Egyptians used aromatic plants in embalming to prevent decay and stop any bacterial growth which is considerably attributed to their essential oils (Shuaib et al. 2016). Ancient Egyptians used fragrant oils and ointments all over themselves after daily ablutions. It is worth recalling that perfume and medicine were one and the same in ancient Egyptian civilization. The unguents were first used by priests who could be called the first perfumers and then the temple attendants and ancient people had been taught the skills. Moreover, the ancient Egyptian woman appreciated the value of perfumes to mask the body odors, fragrance hair, and scent homes and public meeting places (Tisserand 2017). On the other hand, ancient Egyptians believed that scents originated from gods in the first place (Tatomir 2016).

Essential oils have been studied for more than 60 years, but the increased interest in the rediscovery of natural remedies and the increased awareness regarding the use of synthetic drugs resulted in a growing interest in essential oils. Essential oils have a significant value in the global market such as cosmetics (skin creams, lotions, soaps, shampoos, etc.), perfumes, food (spices, additives, preservatives etc.), pharmaceutical (aromatherapy and medicinal supplements), and agricultural industries (Reddy 2019). The market value of essential oils varies according to their composition and purity. Essential oils have been reported to possess diverse biological activities. They are widely known for their powerful antioxidant, antimicrobial, anti-inflammatory, and antispasmodic activities. In addition, they can be used as local anesthetics. Recently, pharmaceutical companies and researchers have developed different means for impacting the effect of essential oils in pharmaceutical products. It was reported that gargles, mouth washes, and inhalation are the most effective methods for the external applications of essential oils. Essential oils are rarely used orally even though most of them have been proven to be safe for ingestion. In this respect, they are usually diluted with milk or soy milk if taken orally. The local applications of essential oils are generally safe, in spite of the fact that they have to be used cautiously because some oils, especially citrus oils, may cause skin reactions and irritations after exposure to sunlight (Chouhan et al. 2017). It is worth mentioning that the use of essential oils and the knowledge of their properties dates back to ancient Egyptian civilization. Many common essential oils of the ancient Egyptians are still in use today such as frankincense, myrrh, cedar, and coriander oils.

Some medical papyri dating back to 1850 BC proved the use of some species of genus *Artemisia* in the ancient Egyptian civilization (Elsharkawy et al. 2018). *Artemisia* species were grown in arid or desert zones of Egypt and have been used since ancient Egyptian civilization. Essential oils produced from *Artemisia* species such as *Artemisia sieberi*, *Artemisia judaica*, and *Artemisia monosperma* were found to possess significant antioxidant and antibacterial activities attributed to their richness of phytochemical components (Elsharkawy et al. 2018). Moreover, *Artemisia herba-alba*, *Artemisia judaica*, and *Artemisia monosperma* essential oils exhibited significant antimicrobial activity (Amin et al. 2019). Essential oil of *Artemisia annua* reported significant activity against the Gram-positive bacteria *Enterococcus hirae* and the fungi *Candida albicans* and *Saccharomyces cerevisiae* (Juteau et al. 2002).

Additionally, ancient Egyptians were already aware of the medical characteristics of *Nigella sativa* (black seeds) and essential oils which are still in use as spice and flavoring in bread, cheese, and other kinds of meals (Khalid and Shedeed 2016). *Nigella sativa* essential oils reported various biological properties such as antifungal, antibacterial, and antioxidant properties which gives this oil industrial and commercial importance to be used in food and non-food applications (Fawzy Ramadan 2015).

*Medemia argun* fruits were of a great significance in ancient Egypt and that was clear from the frequent occurrence of the fruits in the ancient tombs. It can be assumed that ancient Egyptians used it to preserve bodies or as a medicine for its possible antifungal and antibacterial activities that are attributed to the volatile constituents of its oil (Hamed et al. 2012).

Additionally, cedar oil was used in the mummifying process in ancient Egypt (Bhadra and Parida 2021). It was injected by ancient Egyptians inside the body cavities during the mummification process. It contains α-pinene, myrcene, limonene, terpinolene, and α-terpinene, which have major effects against fungi, bacteria, and insects, thereby protecting the mummies (Abdel-Maksoud and Elamin 2011). On the other hand, it was reported that cedar essential oil possesses remarkable antibiofilm activity against *Candida albicans*. It was also found that it has broad spectrum antimicrobial activity and insecticidal activity against insects that cause infectious diseases which would explain the reason of the use of cedar oil in the mummification process (Manoharan et al. 2017; Ramadass et al. 2015).

Furthermore, ancient Egyptians used oils and ointments to protect against high temperature. They used ingredients from rosemary together with other plants extracts such as thyme, cedar, chamomile, and myrrh (Ogden et al. 2000), whereas in modern medicine, *Rosmarini aetheroleum* (rosemary) essential oil is used in cosmetics to maintain skin homeostasis and prevent the appearance of some skin diseases. It is also used in cosmetic preparations as a fragrance. Rosemary derivatives are formulated in essential oils for aromatherapy, deodorants, shampoos, soaps, creams, eye contour, etc., for their antioxidant, antifungal, bactericidal, and anti-inflammatory activities (González-Minero et al. 2020; Diniz do Nascimento et al. 2020; Khan et al. 2017; Genena et al. 2008; Hussain et al. 2010).

Moreover, it was reported that ancient Egyptians used cinnamon (*Cinnamomum zeylanicum*) as beverage flavoring and to treat ailments as well (Vangalapati et al. 2012). Eventually, cinnamon oil would still be used today as an antifungal, antiviral, antibacterial, antiseptic, astringent, aphrodisiac, germicide, and digestive aid.

Myrrh oil (*Commiphora molmol*) was also used in the ancient times to make the skin young again and to embalm mummies as well (Young 2017). It contains α-pinene, sesquiterpene hydrocarbons, δ-elemene, β-bourbonene, furanosesquiterpenes, and germacrene-type compounds which are used to kill and repel pests. Ancient Egyptians referred to myrrh as "the tears of Horus". The "Papyrus Ebers" recorded the use of myrrh in embalming, mummification, wound healing, and bleeding control. More recently, myrrh continued to be used for sore throat, gum and gingival problems, gastrointestinal tract disorders, asthma, sinusitis, cough, wound/skin ailments, and traumatic injuries (Nomicos 2007).

In addition, rose petals mixed with fats formed into cones were used by ancient Egyptians and placed on their heads to eventually melt and perfume their bodies. Egyptians also used frankincense in the mummification process to stuff their body cavities. Consequently, several clinical studies have shown the anti-inflammatory, anti-arthritis, anti-proliferative, antimicrobial, and analgesic activities of frankincense (Noroozi et al. 2018). Besides, spikenard was one of the luxury perfumes in ancient Egypt (Fite et al. 2016).

It is noteworthy that pine oil containing $\beta$-thujene, $\alpha$-pinene, $\beta$-pinene, and bornyl acetate was used in the mummification process for its antifungal and antibacterial effects against Gram-positive and Gram-negative bacteria, and cassia oil was used in mummification for its antimicrobial, antiseptic, and antifungal effects (Abdel-Maksoud and El-Amin 2011).

*Matricaria chamomilla* (chamomile) essential oil, a universal remedy by the ancient Egyptians, reported several biological activities such as immunostimulant, analgesic, antimicrobial, antidiabetic, cytotoxic, astringent, antioxidant, and anti-inflammatory activities; they also used it for massage. These biological activities are attributed to its major volatile components, bisabolol and chamazulene (Nazir et al. 2022). Chamomile oil is either taken as a tea or used as aromatherapy to relieve insomnia (Sharangi 2021).

The essential oil extracted from Egyptian *Salvia officinalis* (common sage), that is considered sacred by the ancient Egyptians, was found to possess anti-urease activity and might provide antibacterial benefits as a co-adjuvant in the treatment of urease-producing bacterial infections or as a dietary supplement (Hassan et al. 2019).

*Mentha piperita* (peppermint) has a history of use as a part of herbal medicine dating back to the ancient Egyptians. Its essential oil is used topically for muscle pain, nerve pain, and itching relief. It was also found that it could minimize digestive tract mucosal irritation and heartburn and treat irritable bowel syndrome as well. The major components of peppermint oil, menthol and menthone, are most probably responsible for the therapeutic properties of peppermint essential oil (Sabzghabaee et al. 2011; Nazir et al. 2022).

*Pimpinella anisum* (anise) is one of the most important medicinal plants in Egypt. It has been known and cultivated as a spice fruit since the time of ancient Egypt. Ancient Egyptians used it for its pharmaceutical properties, such as analgesic against toothache and as a diuretic (Lotfy et al. 2022). Accordingly, its essential oil has been used in food and pharmaceutical industries for its biological activities as diuretic, appetite stimulant, and anti-insomnia. The major compound of anise essential oil is anethole (Tabanca et al. 2006; Nazir et al. 2022).

*Lavandula officinalis* (lavender) essential oil was used by the ancient Egyptians as a part of the mummification process (Sasannejad et al. 2012). In modern medicine, it was found that it is effective in relieving anxiety and insomnia owing to its sedative action. Linalool and linalyl acetate are the major components identified in the essential oil of lavender (Woronuk et al. 2011; Zuzarte et al. 2011).

Since ancient Egyptian times, *Anethum graveolens* (dill) has been used as a condiment and also used for medicinal purposes (Jana and Shekhawat 2010). More recently, its essential oil reported antispasmodic activity. It was found to reduce the bronchial secretions in lung infections as well (Nazir et al. 2022).

*Allium sativum* (garlic) was used by the ancient Egyptians for medicinal purposes. Garlic bulbs were found in Tutankhamun's tomb most likely to protect the king during the journey of the afterlife. Images of garlic have been found in ancient Egyptian burial chambers and Sumerian clay tablets dating back to 2600–2100 BC. Moreover, it was believed that large supplies of garlic were given to the construction workers of the great pyramid of Cheops to give them strength and protect them from illness. Additionally, crushed garlic protected the ancient Egyptians from mouth abscesses when applied to their teeth (Aviello et al. 2009). In recent times, the essential oil of garlic was found to reduce blood pressure, protect the cardiovascular system, and possess antimicrobial activity (Nazir et al. 2022).

Furthermore, the oldest archeological indications for the use of *Foeniculum vulgare* (fennel) by humans are from the ancient Egyptian Middle Kingdom, from the twenty-second to the eighteenth century BC (Afifi et al. 2021). In modern medicine, its essential oil reported hepatoprotective activities owing to its constituents of d-limonene and β-myrcene. Additionally, it has been found to help in gastrointestinal disorders such as chronic colitis and dyspepsia. It also helps in bronchial disorders by inducing the contraction of respiratory tract muscles and causing expectoration of mucus and bacteria to the tracheal tract (Ostad et al. 2001; Özbek et al. 2003).

In ancient Egypt, *Ocimum basilicum* (basil) was mixed with the essence of myrrh and incense in mummification process. Owing to its aromatic fragrances, it was used as an offering to their gods as well (Azzazy 2019). However, the essential oil extracted from its leaves reported strong antimicrobial activity against two Gram-positive bacteria, *Staphylococcus aureus* and *Bacillus subtilis*, two Gram-negative bacteria, *Escherichia coli* and *Pseudomonas aeruginosa*, and one yeast, *Candida albicans*; this activity might be attributed to the high contents of (E)-methyl cinnamate, methyl eugenol, eugenol, and other oxygenated compounds in it (Chenni et al. 2016). It also reported hypolipidemic, antioxidant, and digestive stimulant properties (Sharangi 2021).

The aforementioned aromatic plants and herbs such as black seeds, rosemary, peppermint, common sage, anise, lavender, dill, fennel, and basil are native to ancient Egypt with numerous applications in traditional medicine. Following their widespread successes in ancient Egypt for their multitude of medicinal uses, they were introduced to the Egyptian market as therapeutic remedies for modern-day illness through pharmaceutical industries.

## 7.3   ESSENTIAL OILS AND GREEN CHEMISTRY

Green chemistry has had a huge effect on research. Green chemistry can be defined as a set of twelve principles that reduce the use or the generation of hazardous substances (Anastas et al. 1998). The prominence of green chemistry has increased along with the increase in the global awareness of climate change and fossil fuel depletion (Tundo et al. 2018). Since essential oils have always been a part of people's daily lives as flavors, perfumes or even drugs, terpenes have been widely used in chemistry and the synthesis of natural and non-natural molecules with different applications (Touaibia et al. 2019).

Solvents are crucial for pharmaceutical, food nutraceutical, chemical, and cosmetics industries. The petrochemical industry usually provides the most commonly used solvents. Owing to the price volatility of petroleum, and the risk of the decrease in the world reserve, it has become necessary to focus on more sustainable alternatives. Green chemistry has had a positive influence on using and discovering alternative solvents according to green chemistry principles (Touaibia et al. 2019). Terpenes as bio-based solvents could be used as green solvents and good economic and ecological alternatives to petroleum.

For example, it has been found that limonene, the major constituent of citrus fruit essential oil, could be used to extract oil from rice bran instead of hexane (Mamidipally et al. 2004). Limonene was also found to be a suitable toluene substitute for moisture determination in food products (Veillet et al. 2010).

Furthermore, it was reported that the yield obtained when α-pinene, one of the major constituents found in pine essential oil, used for the extraction of sunflower, soya, peanuts, and olive oils, was better than the yield obtained by hexane (Bertouche et al. 2013). Moreover, pinene was used as an alternative to toluene for moisture determination of coriander, caraway, onion, olive, garlic, carrot, and oregano; and the results showed that the processing time of pinene was shorter than that of toluene with lower energy consumption. Additionally, it was used as a solvent in varnishes and dyes, an additive in perfumes, and for masking odor in some industrial products (Bertouche et al. 2012).

A cis-rich pinane, a stable terpene derived from the pine tree, was tested in the extraction of carotenoids from carrot, oil from rapeseeds, and aromas from caraway seed in comparison to hexane and showed comparable results (Yara-Varón et al. 2016).

Para-menthane, a saturated monocyclic terpenoid derived from eucalyptus essential oil and obtained by catalytic hydrogenation, was used for the solubilization of beta-carotene, carvone, linalool, limonene, and estragole and the results were similar to that of hexane. It was also used for the extraction of colza seed oil and the results were comparable to that of hexane (Touaibia et al. 2019).

It was also reported that the major constituents of essential oils from Egyptian flora can be used as synthons for green chemistry in the synthesis of basic or fine chemicals. The volatile fraction of some essential oils from Egyptian flora such as lemon oil, pine oil, clove oil, orange peel oil, peppermint oil, carrot seed oil, and lavender oil contains phenolic-origin or terpenoid compounds with different unsaturated levels. These compounds contain functional or asymmetric carbon groups which can be used as starting materials for functional modification and building blocks in the synthesis of industrial chemical products (Li et al. 2014).

## 7.4  ESSENTIAL OILS AND NANOTECHNOLOGY

Currently there is a considerable interest in the encapsulation of essential oils to decrease their volatility, regulate the rate of drug release, and enhance their biological activity. Many delivery systems loaded with essential oils have been reported to be effective, such as polymer-based and lipid-based nanoparticles.

Nanostructured lipid-based carriers loaded with eucalyptus oil reported good compatibility, bio adhesion, physicochemical properties, and good wound healing activity (Tanha et al. 2017). Furthermore, the nano-encapsulation of thymol resulted in enhanced antimicrobial activity (Li et al. 2012). It was reported that eucalyptus and rosemary essential oils, when loaded in lipid nanoparticles, resulted in medical devices with improved wound healing activities (Saporito et al. 2018). Additionally, it was reported that rosemary essential oil coated with nanoparticles possessed a significant antibiofilm activity against *C. albicans* and *C. tropicalis* (Chifiriuc et al. 2012).

In other studies, it was reported that nanoemulsion applications for essential oil encapsulation improved the bioavailability and solubilization of essential oils. Although essential oils have poor water solubility, they are used to improve the solubility of some poorly water-soluble drugs through making up the inner phase of oil in water nanoemulsions (Barradas et al. 2015). Various essential oils have been reported to be used in the development of nanoemulsions with proven biological activities. Thyme and rosemary essential oils nanoemulsions were prepared and investigated, they showed significant antibacterial activity against *Escherichia coli* and good stability over two months at ambient temperature which makes them interesting to be used in pharmaceutical and drug delivery systems (Moradi and Barati 2019).

Essential oils have also been used for the fabrication of metallic nanoparticles which is an easy single-step eco-friendly approach free of toxic chemicals and suitable for therapeutic applications. The active functional groups (C=C, −CH2, −CH3, −O-H, C-H, C=O, C-O-C, CH3-C-CH3, C-O, and −C-N) of terpenoids in essential oils are involved in the synthesis of metallic nanoparticles. For example, *Mentha piperita* essential oil was used in the synthesis of nanogold particles which showed good antifungal activity and were tested with different characterization methods (Thanighaiarassu et al. 2014). *Nigella sativa* essential oil coated gold spherical nanoparticles with the particle size 15 to 28 nm effectively controlled the growth and biofilm formation of Gram-positive *S. aureus* and Gram-negative *Vibrio harveyi*. Moreover, they showed good anticancer activity against human lung cancer cells (Manju et al. 2016). Rosemary essential oil was also successfully used as a green reducing agent in the synthesis of silver spherical nanoparticles possessing 29 nm (González-Rivera et al. 2017). In addition, a green, simple, and effective technique was developed for the synthesis of silver spherical nanoparticles using orange peel essential oil (Veisi et al. 2019).

## 7.5 CONCLUSION AND FUTURE PROSPECTS

Essential oils from the Egyptian flora represent an important part of the Egyptian civilization and traditional medicine. The use of some essential oils from Egyptian flora as alternative pharmaceutical agents has attracted considerable interest in modern medicine. In addition, the applications of some of these essential oils and their constituents in green chemistry and nanotechnology has garnered much interest in recent years. However, there is still a need for more rational research on the applications, safety, and toxicity of theses efficient essential oils for the manufacturing of novel, safe, and effective natural pharmaceutical remedies.

## REFERENCES

Abdel-Maksoud, Gomaa, and Abdel-Rahman El-Amin. 2011. "A review on the materials used during the mummification process in ancient Egypt." *Mediterranean Archaeology & Archaeometry* 11 (2).

Afifi, Sherif M, Amira El-Mahis, Andreas G. Heiss, and Mohamed A. Farag. 2021. "Gas chromatography-mass spectrometry-based classification of 12 fennel (Foeniculum vulgare Miller) varieties based on their aroma profiles and estragole levels as analyzed using chemometric tools." *ACS Omega* 6 (8):5775–5785. doi: 10.1021/acsomega.0c06188.

Amin, Sahar M, Hossam M Hassan, Abd El-Nasser G El Gendy, et al. 2019. "Comparative chemical study and antimicrobial activity of essential oils of three Artemisia species from Egypt and Saudi Arabia." *Flavour and Fragrance Journal* 34 (6):450–459.

Anastas, Paul T, and John C Warner. 1998. "Principles of green chemistry." *Green Chemistry: Theory and Practice* 29.

Aviello, G., L. Abenavoli, F. Borrelli, et al. 2009. "Garlic: empiricism or science?" *Nat Prod Commun* 4 (12):1785–1796.

Azzazy, Mohamed. 2019. "Micromorphology of pollen grains, trichomes of sweet basil, Egypt." 5:427–433. doi: 10.31031/ACAM.2019.05.000604.

Bakkali, F., S. Averbeck, D. Averbeck, and M. Idaomar. 2008. "Biological effects of essential oils: A review." *Food and Chemical Toxicology* 46 (2):446–475. doi: https://doi.org/10.1016/j.fct.2007.09.106.

Barradas, Thaís Nogueira, Vânia Emerich Bucco de Campos, Juliana Perdiz Senna, et al. 2015. "Development and characterization of promising o/w nanoemulsions containing sweet fennel essential oil and non-ionic sufactants." *Colloids and Surfaces A: Physicochemical and Engineering Aspects* 480:214–221. doi: https://doi.org/10.1016/j.colsurfa.2014.12.001.

Baser, K Husnu Can, and Gerhard Buchbauer. 2009. *Handbook of Essential Oils: Science, Technology, and Applications*: CRC press.

Bertouche, Sadjia, Valérie Tomao, Amina Hellal, Chahrazed Boutekedjiret, and Farid Chemat. 2013. "First approach on edible oil determination in oilseeds products using alpha-pinene." *Journal of Essential Oil Research* 25 (6):439–443.

Bertouche, Sadjia, Valérie Tomao, Karine Ruiz, et al. 2012. "First approach on moisture determination in food products using alpha-pinene as an alternative solvent for Dean-Stark distillation." *Food Chemistry* 134 (1):602–605.

Bhadra, Preetha, and Sagarika Parida. 2021. *Aromatherapy and Its Benefits*: Renu Publisher.

Bird, Stephanie Rose. 2003. "African aromatherapy: Past, present and future applications." *International Journal of Aromatherapy* 13 (4):185–195. doi: https://doi.org/10.1016/S0962-4562(03)00117-6.

Burt, Sara. 2004. "Essential oils: Their antibacterial properties and potential applications in foods: A review." *International Journal of Food Microbiology* 94 (3):223–253.

Chenni, Mohammed, Douniazad El Abed, Njara Rakotomanomana, Xavier Fernandez, and Farid Chemat. 2016. "Comparative study of essential oils extracted from Egyptian basil leaves (Ocimum basilicum L.) using hydro-distillation and solvent-free microwave extraction." *Molecules* 21 (1):113.

Chifiriuc, Carmen, Valentina Grumezescu, Alexandru Mihai Grumezescu, et al. 2012. "Hybrid magnetite nanoparticles/Rosmarinus officinalis essential oil nanobiosystem with antibiofilm activity." *Nanoscale Research Letters* 7 (1):209. doi: 10.1186/1556-276X-7-209.

Chouhan, Sonam, Kanika Sharma, and Sanjay Guleria. 2017. "Antimicrobial activity of some essential oils-present status and future perspectives." *Medicines* 4 (3):58.

Deryng, J. 1951. "Nowy aparat do oznaczanie olejków w materiale roślinnym." *Acta Pol. Pharm* 8:121–136.

Dhifi, Wissal, Sana Bellili, Sabrine Jazi, Nada Bahloul, and Wissem Mnif. 2016. "Essential oils' chemical characterization and investigation of some biological activities: A critical review." *Medicines* 3 (4):25.

Diniz do Nascimento, Lidiane, Angelo Antônio Barbosa de Moraes, Kauê Santana da Costa, et al. 2020. "Bioactive natural compounds and antioxidant activity of essential oils from spice plants: New findings and potential applications." *Biomolecules* 10 (7):988.

Elsharkawy, Eman Ramadan, Abdelaziz Ed-dra, Suliman Alghanem, and Emad Mohamed Abdallah. 2018. "Comparative studies of chemical compostion, antimicrobial and antioxidant activity of essential oil of some species from genus artemisia." *Journal of Natural Remedies* 18 (1):10–20. doi: 10.18311/jnr/2018/20052.

Fadel, Doaa Ragab. 2020. "History of the perfume industry in Greco-Roman Egypt." *International Journal of History and Cultural Studies* 6 (4):26–45. doi: 10.20431/2454-7654.0604003.

Fawzy Ramadan, Mohamed. 2015. "Nutritional value and applications of Nigella sativa essential oil: A mini review." *Journal of Essential Oil Research* 27 (4):271–275. doi: 10.1080/10412905.2015.1045564.

Fite, Vannoy Gentles, Michele Gentles McDaniel, and Vannoy Lin Reynolds. 2016. *Essential Oils for Healing: Over 400 All-Natural Recipes for Everyday Ailments*: St. Martin's Griffin.

Genena, Aziza Kamal, Haiko Hense, Artur Smânia Junior, and Simone Machado de Souza. 2008. "Rosemary (Rosmarinus officinalis): A study of the composition, antioxidant and antimicrobial activities of extracts obtained with supercritical carbon dioxide." *Food Science and Technology* 28:463–469.

González-Minero, Francisco José, Luis Bravo-Díaz, and Antonio Ayala-Gómez. 2020. "Rosmarinus officinalis L. (Rosemary): An ancient plant with uses in personal health-care and cosmetics." *Cosmetics* 7 (4):77.

González-Rivera, José, Celia Duce, Vincenzo Ierardi, et al. 2017. "Fast and eco-friendly microwave-assisted synthesis of silver nanoparticles using rosemary essential oil as renewable reducing agent." *Chemistry Select* 2 (6):2131–2138. doi: https://doi.org/10.1002/slct.201700244.

Gurib-Fakim, Ameenah. 2006. "Medicinal plants: Traditions of yesterday and drugs of tomorrow." *Molecular Aspects of Medicine* 27 (1):1–93. doi: https://doi.org/10.1016/j.mam.2005.07.008.

Hamed, Arafa I, Michele Leonardi, Anna Stochmal, Wieslaw Oleszek, and Luisa Pistelli. 2012. "GC-MS analysis of aroma of Medemia argun (Mama-n-Khanen or Mama-n-Xanin), an ancient Egyptian fruit palm." *Natural Product Communications* 7 (5):1934578X1200700523.

Hassan, Sherif TS, Emil Švajdlenka, Kannan RR Rengasamy, Radka Melichárková, and Shunmugiah Karutha Pandian. 2019. "The metabolic profile of essential oils and assessment of anti-urease activity by ESI-mass spectrometry of Salvia officinalis L." *South African Journal of Botany* 120:175–178.

Hussain, Abdullah Ijaz, Farooq Anwar, Shahzad Ali Shahid Chatha, et al. 2010. "Rosmarinus officinalis essential oil: Antiproliferative, antioxidant and antibacterial activities." *Brazilian Journal of Microbiology* 41:1070–1078.

Jana, S., and G. S. Shekhawat. 2010. "Anethum graveolens: An indian traditional medicinal herb and spice." *Pharmacogn Rev* 4 (8):179–184. doi: 10.4103/0973–7847.70915.

Juteau, Fabien, Veronique Masotti, Jean Marie Bessiere, Michel Dherbomez, and Josette Viano. 2002. "Antibacterial and antioxidant activities of Artemisia annua essential oil." *Fitoterapia* 73 (6):532–535.

Khalid, A. K, and M. R Shedeed. 2016. "GC-MS analyses of black cumin essential oil produces with sodium chloride." *International Food Research Journal* 23 (2):832.

Khan, Barkat Ali, Naveed Akhtar, Bouzid Menaa, et al. 2017. "Relative free radicals scavenging and enzymatic activities of hippophae rhamnoides and cassia fistula extracts: Importance for cosmetic, food and medicinal applications." *Cosmetics* 4 (1):3.

Li, Kang-Kang, Shou-Wei Yin, Xiao-Quan Yang, Chuan-He Tang, and Zi-Hao Wei. 2012. "Fabrication and characterization of novel antimicrobial films derived from thymol-loaded zein-sodium caseinate (SC) nanoparticles." *Journal of Agricultural and Food Chemistry* 60 (46):11592–11600. doi: 10.1021/jf302752v.

Li, Ying, Anne-Sylvie Fabiano-Tixier, and Farid Chemat. 2014. *Essential Oils as Reagents in Green Chemistry*. Vol. 1: Springer.

Lotfy, Shereen, Mohamed Ahmed, Rasha Saad, Fatma Abd El-Aleem, and Hoda Fadel. 2022. "Effects of ultrasonic and microwave pretreatments on the extraction yield, chemical composition and antioxidant activity of hydrodistilled essential oil from anise (Pimpinella anisum L.)." *Egyptian Journal of Chemistry* 65 (11):455–465. doi: 10.21608/ejchem.2022.125713.5584.

Mamidipally, Pavan K, and Sean X Liu. 2004. "First approach on rice bran oil extraction using limonene." *European Journal of Lipid Science and Technology* 106 (2):122–125.

Manju, Sivalingam, Balasubramanian Malaikozhundan, Sekar Vijayakumar, et al. 2016. "Antibacterial, antibiofilm and cytotoxic effects of Nigella sativa essential oil coated gold nanoparticles." *Microbial Pathogenesis* 91:129–135. doi: https://doi.org/10.1016/j.micpath.2015.11.021.

Manoharan, Ranjith Kumar, Jin-Hyung Lee, and Jintae Lee. 2017. "Antibiofilm and antihyphal activities of cedar leaf essential oil, camphor, and fenchone derivatives against Candida albicans." *Frontiers in Microbiology* 8. doi: 10.3389/fmicb.2017.01476.

Miguel, M. G. 2010. "Antioxidant activity of medicinal and aromatic plants.: A review." *Flavour and Fragrance Journal* 25 (5):291–312. doi: https://doi.org/10.1002/ffj.1961.

Moradi, S., and A. Barati. 2019. "Essential oils nanoemulsions: Preparation, characterization and study of antibacterial activity against escherichia coli." *International Journal of Nanoscience and Nanotechnology* 15 (3):199–210.

Nazir, Ishrat, and Sajad Ahmad Gangoo. 2022. "Pharmaceutical and therapeutic potentials of essential oils." In *Essential Oils-Advances in Extractions and Biological Applications*: IntechOpen.

Nomicos, Effie Y. H. 2007. "Myrrh: Medical marvel or myth of the magi?" *Holistic Nursing Practice* 21 (6).

Noroozi, S., H. Khadem Haghighian, M. Abbasi, M. Javadi, and S. Goodarzi. 2018. "A review of the therapeutic effects of frankincense." *Journal of Inflammatory Diseases* 22 (1):70–81. doi: 10.29252/qums.22.1.81.

Nunn, John F. 2002. *Ancient Egyptian Medicine*: University of Oklahoma Press.

Ogden, Jack, PT Nicholson, and I Shaw. 2000. *Ancient Egyptian Materials and Technology*: Cambridge University Press.

Ostad, S. N, M Soodi, M Shariffzadeh, N Khorshidi, and H Marzban. 2001. "The effect of fennel essential oil on uterine contraction as a model for dysmenorrhea, pharmacology and toxicology study." *Journal of Ethnopharmacology* 76 (3):299–304.

Özbek, H, S Uğraş, H Dülger, et al. 2003. "Hepatoprotective effect of foeniculum vulgare essential oil." *Fitoterapia* 74 (3):317–319.

Pavela, Roman, and Giovanni Benelli. 2016. "Essential oils as ecofriendly biopesticides? Challenges and constraints." *Trends in Plant Science* 21 (12):1000–1007.

Perricone, Marianne, Ersilia Arace, Maria R Corbo, Milena Sinigaglia, and Antonio Bevilacqua. 2015. "Bioactivity of essential oils: A review on their interaction with food components." *Frontiers in Microbiology* 6:76.

Ramadass, Manjula, and Padma Thiagarajan. 2015. "Importance and applications of cedar oil." *Research Journal of Pharmacy and Technology* 8:1714. doi: 10.5958/0974–360X.2 015.00308.X.

Reddy, Desam Nagarjuna. 2019. "Essential oils extracted from medicinal plants and their applications." In *Natural Bio-Active Compounds*, 237–283: Springer.

Sabzghabaee, Ali Mohammad, Firouzeh Nili, Alireza Ghannadi, Nastaran Eizadi-Mood, and Maryam Anvari. 2011. "Role of menthol in treatment of candidial napkin dermatitis." *World Journal of Pediatrics* 7 (2):167–170.

Saporito, F., G. Sandri, M. C. Bonferoni, et al. 2018. "Essential oil-loaded lipid nanoparticles for wound healing." *Int J Nanomedicine* 13:175–186. doi: 10.2147/ijn.s152529.

Sarkic, Asja, and Iris Stappen. 2018. "Essential oils and their single compounds in cosmetics: A critical review." *Cosmetics* 5 (1):11.

Sasannejad, P., M. Saeedi, A. Shoeibi, et al. 2012. "Lavender essential oil in the treatment of migraine headache: A placebo-controlled clinical trial." *European Neurology* 67 (5):288–291. doi: 10.1159/000335249.

Sharangi, Amit. 2021. *Aromatic Plants: The Technology, Human Welfare and Beyond*: Nova Publisher.

Shuaib, Ahmad, Adhav Rohit, and Mantry Piyush. 2016. "A review article on essential oils." *Journal of Medicinal Plants Studies* 4 (3):237–240.

Tabanca, Nurhayat, Betul Demirci, Temel Ozek, et al. 2006. "Gas chromatographic-mass spectrometric analysis of essential oils from Pimpinella species gathered from Central and Northern Turkey." *Journal of Chromatography A* 1117 (2):194–205.

Tanha, Shima, Morteza Rafiee-Tehrani, Mohamad Abdollahi, et al. 2017. "G-CSF loaded nanofiber/nanoparticle composite coated with collagen promotes wound healing in vivo." *Journal of Biomedical Materials Research Part A* 105 (10):2830–2842.

Tatomir, Renata. 2016. "To cause 'to make divine' through smoke: Ancient Egyptian incense and perfume.: An inter-and transdisciplinary re-evaluation of aromatic biotic materials used by the ancient Egyptians." *Moesica et Christiana-Studies in Honor of Professor Alexandru Barnea. Editura Istros. Braila*:665–78.

Thanighaiarassu, R. R, P Sivamai, R Devika, and Balwin Nambikkairaj. 2014. "Green synthesis of gold nanoparticles characterization by using plant essential oil Menthapiperita and their antifungal activity against human pathogenic fungi." *J. Nanomed. Nanotechnol* 5 (5).

Tisserand, Maggie. 2017. *Essential Oils for Lovers: How to Use Aromatherapy to Revitalize Your Sex Life*: Harper Thorsons.

Touaibia, Mohamed, Chahrazed Boutekedjiret, Sandrine Perino, and Farid Chemat. 2019. "Natural terpenes as building blocks for green chemistry." In Li Y, Chemat F, eds *Plant Based "Green Chemistry 2.0"*, 171–195: Springer.

Tundo, Pietro, and Elena Griguol. 2018. "Green chemistry for sustainable development." *Chemistry International* 40 (1):18–24. doi:10.1515/ci-2018–0105.

Vangalapati, Meena, N Sree Satya, D Surya Prakash, and Sumanjali Avanigadda. 2012. "A review on pharmacological activities and clinical effects of cinnamon species." *Research Journal of Pharmaceutical, Biological and Chemical Sciences* 3 (1):653–663.

Veillet, Sébastien, Valérie Tomao, Karine Ruiz, and Farid Chemat. 2010. "Green procedure using limonene in the Dean-Stark apparatus for moisture determination in food products." *Analytica Chimica Acta* 674 (1):49–52.

Veisi, Hojat, Nahid Dadres, Pourya Mohammadi, and Saba Hemmati. 2019. "Green synthesis of silver nanoparticles based on oil-water interface method with essential oil of orange peel and its application as nanocatalyst for A3 coupling." *Materials Science and Engineering: C* 105:110031. doi: https://doi.org/10.1016/j.msec.2019.110031.

Woronuk, Grant, Zerihun Demissie, Mark Rheault, and Soheil Mahmoud. 2011. "Biosynthesis and therapeutic properties of Lavandula essential oil constituents." *Planta Medica* 77 (01):7–15.

Yara-Varón, Edinson, A Selka, Anne-Sylvie Fabiano-Tixier, et al. 2016. "Solvent from forestry biomass: Pinane a stable terpene derived from pine tree byproducts to substitute n-hexane for the extraction of bioactive compounds." *Green Chemistry* 18 (24):6596–6608.

Young, Kac. 2017. *The Healing Art of Essential Oils: A Guide to 50 Oils for Remedy, Ritual, and Everyday Use*: Llewellyn Worldwide.

Zuzarte, Mónica, Maria José Gonçalves, Carlos Cavaleiro, et al. 2011. "Chemical composition and antifungal activity of the essential oils of Lavandula viridis L'Her." *Journal of Medical Microbiology* 60 (5):612–618.

# 8 Aromatherapy
## An Integrative Therapy of Essential Oils

*Sharada Nalla, Upendarrao Golla,*
*Sujatha Palatheeya, and Eswar Kumar Aouta*

## 8.1 INTRODUCTION

Aromatherapy is an alternative and integrative therapy which includes the usage of essential oils for medicinal and therapeutic purposes. Aromatherapy is simple to use and doesn't require any special instruments but produces positive effects even when used for a short time period. Aromatherapy includes the usage of various essential oils from flowers, fruits, roots, stems, seeds, and leaves of different plants, which absorb into the body through skin or mucus membranes and produce beneficial effects in different physiological and psychological disorders. These benefits can be achieved with inhalation, bathing or massage of essential oils (Park et al. 2012). Some studies suggest that essential oils enhance physical and psychological well-being by absorbing through skin and olfactory systems, resulting in immediate reduction in pain as well as changing in physiological parameters like blood pressure, pulse, brain activity, skin temperature, etc. (Lakhan et al. 2016). This grabs the attention to aromatherapy. Aromatherapy is most beneficial in reducing pain, anxiety, depression in different conditions like cancer therapy induced symptoms, labour-related anxiety and depression, etc. Because of its low cost and minimal or no side effects, aromatherapy is becoming the most common and complimentary treatment for many conditions. This chapter aims to provide the various applications of aromatherapy.

## 8.2 APPLICATIONS OF AROMATHERAPY

### 8.2.1 AROMATHERAPY IN MIGRAINE

Migraines are considered a major threat to human life because they affect the quality of life and health due to high pain intensity, high prevalence and attack rate. In the present era, migraine are treated by drug therapy, but because of its complex pathophysiology, the therapeutic effect is limited and varied from person to person and because of its side effects there is an increasing demand for alternative therapy. Aromatherapy is the most comfortable and pleasant all-natural therapy with efficient and rapid effect against migraine symptoms. Application of essential oils for

DOI: 10.1201/9781003389774-8

migraines has been evidenced in traditional Chinese medicine (Yuan et al. 2021). Migraines can be treated by using different essential oils from different plants: chamomile, *Angelicae dahuricae* Radix, Chuanxiong rhizome, etc. Some of them produce relief from nausea, vomiting, photophobia and other symptoms. This effect is different in different people with different doses (Niazi et al. 2017; Sasannejad et al. 2012; Yuan et al. 2021). Essential oils from *Lavandula angustifolia* Mill (dried flower heads and aerial foliage) (Sasannejad et al. 2012), garlic (bulb) (Marschollek et al. 2017), *Mentha piperita* L. (flowering aerial parts and leaves) (de Groot and Schmidt 2016), *Illicium verum* Hook.f. (fruit) (Mosaffa-Jahromi et al. 2016), *Rosa damascena* Herrm. (petals) (Niazi et al. 2017), *Vitis vinifera* L. (seed) (Woodman et al. 2022) and *Ocimum basilicum* L. (aerial part) (Ahmadifard et al. 2020) are also used to treat migraines.

### 8.2.2 Aromatherapy in Menstrual Pain

Menstrual pain is not actually a disease but it makes women uncomfortable periodically in the menstrual cycle. Aromatherapy is an effective alternative therapy to alleviate menstrual cramps and pain. A mixture of lavender, clary sage, rose and marjoram essential oils are beneficial in reducing menstrual cramps by different modes of applications like inhalation, massaging, etc. (Han et al. 2001, 2006; Marzouk et al. 2013).

### 8.2.3 Aromatherapy in Labour Pain

Pain during labour is an unavoidable reality that is associated with anxiety. It is mainly due to uterine muscle contraction and cervical dilation (Gholipour Baradari et al. 2017). If labour pain is inadequately managed then it is associated with many negative physiological and psychological complications during the delivery (Tabatabaeichehr and Mortazavi 2020). Therefore, pain should be managed either by pharmacological approach or non-pharmacological approach or both. Nowadays non-pharmacological approaches like acupuncture, massage therapy, acupressure, other relaxation techniques and aromatherapy are the most commonly used methods to reduce the pain sensation during labour because of their simplicity of use, low risk and cost effectiveness. Aromatherapy with lavender oil is more significant to reduce the pain and anxiety in labour (Seraji and Vakilian 2011). Some studies confirmed that rose essential oil inhalation reduces the pain intensity (Hamdamian et al. 2018). Jasmine extract massage shows significant reduction in pain severity (Joseph and Fernandes 2013). Essential oil of geranium (Rashidi Fakari et al. 2015), chamomile essential oil (Heidaryfard et al. 2015), essential oil of peppermint (Ozgoli et al. 2016), orange essential oil (Rashidi-Fakari et al. 2015) and clove essential oil (Han and Parker 2017) are reported for their significant efficacy in reducing labour pain with different route of administrations.

### 8.2.4 Aromatherapy in Anxiety

When a person is facing stressful or threatening situations, there is often a feeling of fear called anxiety. A number of factors leads to onset of anxiety and its serious consequences. Present available pharmacological approaches for the reduction or management of anxiety have many side effects, so alternative therapy has more attention for the management of anxiety without side effects. Aromatherapy is one of the best and most common therapies for alleviating anxiety in different conditions. For this, various essential oils like lavender, rose, citrus, orange and chamomile were reported to have a significant effect in reducing anxiety either through inhalation or massage (Gong et al. 2020).

### 8.2.5 AROMATHERAPY IN CANCER

Nowadays, cancer is a challenging health problem in the world. Mortality due to cancer is increasing day by day. Among all the types, lung and breast cancer are the most fatal types. Cancer produces so many physical and psychological complications, and with the current available pharmacological therapy, the patient suffers more with these effects along with the side effects of current medicines and radiation therapy, leading to decrease in the quality of life of cancer patient (Bartholomew et al. 2019). By considering the low risk, low cost and less or no complications, aromatherapy is the best and most common therapy to relieve the cancer patient from all the symptoms and also to reduce the side effects of other therapies when used as a complimentary therapy (Schnipper et al. 2015). Many studies reported that the aromatherapy shows a good recovery from all the complications of cancer. Farahani et al. reviewed several studies which showed that usage of aromatherapy with lavender essential oil by inhalation improves the physical complications (pain, nausea and vomiting, immune system, sleep quality, vital signs and others) and psychological complications (anxiety, depression, quality of life and other psychological complications) of cancer chemotherapy (Farahani et al. 2019).

### 8.2.6 AROMATHERAPY IN INSOMNIA

Sleep is considered as an important aid to recover from illness and in maintenance of health and strength for well-being of a person. Lack of sleep results in drowsiness, dizziness, nervousness, fatigue, instability and various attention disorders (Seo and Sohng 2011). So adequate sleep is essential for overall well-being. Insomnia is a sleep disorder that results in sleeplessness. The current available drug therapies have many side effects; insomnia can be improved by aromatherapy without side effects. Lavender, peppermint, bergamot, chamomile, clary sage, rosewood, lemon, marjoram, eucalyptus and rosemary oils are studied for their effect in insomnia. These results show that most of these essential oils have improved sleep and well-being but additional research is required to analyze the effect of aromatherapy in insomnia (Hwang and Shin 2015).

### 8.2.7 AROMATHERAPY IN WOMEN'S HEALTH

Women's health problems like premenstrual syndrome (PMS), vaginal infections, cystitis, infertility and menopausal symptoms may be treated with aromatherapy. Women experience relief by massaging on the abdomen or chest as needed with essential oils like neroli, ylang ylang or clary sage in PMS; stress and tension symptoms will be benefitted (Tillett and Ames 2010). For menstrual cramps, essential oils like roman chamomile, peppermint, black pepper, rosemary, sweet marjoram and ylang ylang are used for relief.

In dysmenorrhea, essential oils like Roman chamomile, angelica, clary sage and yarrow produce beneficial effects by massaging into the abdomen and lower back as needed, or they may also be added to a bath with carrier oil or Epsom salts. Women with recurrent cystitis will benefit from vaginal usage of tea tree and palmarosa and for abdominal usage of juniper and pine (Burns et al. 2000).

Aromatherapy is also beneficial in pregnancy to relieve stress and fatigue and to provide relaxation and emotional comfort and support. The most common routes of administration in pregnancy are dermal applications, massage and inhalation. Essential oils with high amounts of phenols, phenylpropanoids and ketones are mostly considered toxic and best avoided (Tiran 2000).

## 8.3　SUMMARY

Using essential oils for the treatment and management of different conditions like migraine, menstrual pain, labour pain, anxiety, cancers, insomnia and other women's health abnormalities is effective with lack of adverse effects and avoids the overusage of pharmaceuticals. Combining aromatherapy with other complimentary therapies like acupressure or massage will provide more effectiveness and contribute to the acceptance of these therapies.

## REFERENCES

Ahmadifard M, Yarahmadi S, Ardalan A, Ebrahimzadeh F, Bahrami P, Sheikhi E. The efficacy of topical basil essential oil on relieving migraine headaches: A randomized triple-blind study. Complementary Medicine Research. 2020; 27(5): 310–318.

Bartholomew AJ, Dervishaj OA, Sosin M, Kerivan LT, Tung SS, Caragacianu DL, Willey SC, Tousimis EA. Neoadjuvant chemotherapy and nipple-sparing mastectomy: Timing and postoperative complications. Annals of Surgical Oncology. 2019; 26(9): 2768–2772.

Burns E, Blamey C, Ersser SJ, Lloyd AJ, Barnetson L. The use of aromatherapy in intrapartum midwifery practice an observational study. Complementary Therapies in Nursing and Midwifery. 2000; 6(1): 33–34.

de Groot A, Schmidt E. Essential oils, part V: Peppermint oil, lavender oil, and lemongrass oil. Dermatitis. 2016; 27:325–332.

Farahani MA, Afsargharehbagh R, Marandi F, Moradi M, Hashemi SM, Moghadam MP, Balouchi A. Effect of aromatherapy on cancer complications: A systematic review. Complementary Therapies in Medicine. 2019; 47: 102169. doi: 10.1016/j.ctim.2019.08.003

Gholipour Baradari A, Firouzian A, Hasanzadeh Kiabi F, Emami Zeydi A, Khademloo M, Nazari Z, Sanagou M, Ghobadi M, Fooladi E. Bolus administration of intravenous lidocaine reduces pain after an elective caesarean section: Findings from a randomised, double-blind, placebo-controlled trial. Journal of Obstetrics and Gynaecology. 2017; 37(5): 566–570.

Gong M, Dong H, Tang Y, Huang W, Lu F. Effects of aromatherapy on anxiety: A meta-analysis of randomized controlled trials. Journal of Affective Disorders. 2020; 274: 1028–1040.

Hamdamian S, Nazarpour S, Simbar M, Hajian S, Mojab F, Talebi A. Effects of aromather-
    apy with Rosa damascena on nulliparous women's pain and anxiety of labor during first
    stage of labor. Journal of Integrative Medicine. 2018; 16(2): 120–125.
Han SH, Hur MH, Buckle J, Choi J, Lee MS. Effect of aromatherapy on symptoms of dys-
    menorrhea in college students: A randomized placebo-controlled clinical trial. Journal
    of Alternative and Complementary Medicine (New York, N.Y.). 2006; 12(6): 535–541.
Han SH, Ro YJ, Hur, MH. Effects of aromatherapy on menstrual cramps and dysmenorrhea in
    college student woman: A blind randomized clinical trial. Journal of Korean Academy
    of Adult Nursing. 2001; 13(3): 420–430. https://www.koreamed.org/SearchBasic.
    php?RID=2291155
Han X, Parker TL. Anti-inflammatory activity of clove (Eugenia caryophyllata) essential oil
    in human dermal fibroblasts. Pharmaceutical Biology. 2017; 55(1): 1619–1622.
Heidaryfard S, Amir Ali Akbari S, Mojab F, Shakeri N. Effect of Matricaria camomilla
    aroma on severity of first stage labor pain. Journal of Clinical Nursing and Midwifery.
    2015; 4(3): 23–31.
Hwang E, Shin S. The effects of aromatherapy on sleep improvement: A systematic literature
    review and meta-analysis. The Journal of Alternative and Complementary Medicine.
    2015; 21(2): 61–68.
Joseph RM, Fernandes P. Effectiveness of jasmine oil massage on reduction of labor pain
    among primigravida mothers. Journal of Health and Allied Sciences NU. 2013; 3(4):
    104–107. doi: 10.1055/s-0040-1703713
Lakhan SE, Sheafer H, Tepper D. The effectiveness of aromatherapy in reducing pain: A sys-
    tematic review and meta-analysis. Pain Research and Treatment. 2016; 2016: 8158693.
Marschollek C, Karimzadeh F, Jafarian M, Ahmadi M, Mohajeri SM, Rahimi S, Speckmann
    EJ, Gorji A. Effects of garlic extract on spreading depression: In vitro and in vivo inves-
    tigations. Nutritional Neuroscience. 2017; 20(2): 127–134.
Marzouk TM, El-Nemer AM, Baraka HN. The effect of aromatherapy abdominal massage
    on alleviating menstrual pain in nursing students: A prospective randomized cross-
    over study. Evidence-Based Complementary and Alternative Medicine. 2013; 2013:
    742421.
Mosaffa-Jahromi M, Lankarani KB, Pasalar M, Afsharypuor S, Tamaddon AM. Efficacy and
    safety of enteric coated capsules of anise oil to treat irritable bowel syndrome. Journal
    of Ethnopharmacology. 2016; 194: 937–946.
Niazi M, Hashempur MH, Taghizadeh M, Heydari M, Shariat A. Efficacy of topical Rose
    (Rosa damascena Mill.) oil for migraine headache: A randomized double-blinded
    placebo-controlled cross-over trial. Complementary Therapies in Medicine. 2017; 34:
    35–41.
Ozgoli G, Torkashvand S, Salehi Moghaddam F, Borumandnia N, Mojab F, Minooee S.
    Comparison of peppermint and clove essential oil aroma on pain intensity and anxiety
    at first stage of labor. The Iranian Journal of Obstetrics, Gynecology and Infertility.
    2016; 19(21): 1–11.
Park S, Park K-S, Ko Y-J, Lee B-Y, Yang HS, Park H-J, Woo Y-H, Lee J-Y, Park D-H. The
    effect of aroma inhalation therapy on fatigue and sleep in nurse shift workers. Journal
    of East-West Nursing Research. 2012; 18(2): 66–73.
Rashidi Fakari F, Tabatabaeichehr M, Kamali H, Rashidi Fakari F, Naseri M. Effect of inha-
    lation of aroma of geranium essence on anxiety and physiological parameters during
    first stage of labor in nulliparous women: A randomized clinical trial. Journal of Caring
    Sciences. 2015; 4(2): 135–141.
Rashidi-Fakari F, Tabatabaeichehr M, Mortazavi H. The effect of aromatherapy by essential
    oil of orange on anxiety during labor: A randomized clinical trial. Iranian Journal of
    Nursing and Midwifery Research. 2015; 20(6): 661–664.

Sasannejad P, Saeedi M, Shoeibi A, Gorji A, Abbasi M, Foroughipour M. Lavender essential oil in the treatment of migraine headache: A placebo-controlled clinical trial. European Neurology. 2012; 67(5): 288–291.

Schnipper LE, Davidson NE, Wollins DS, Tyne C, Blayney DW, Blum D, Dicker AP, Ganz PA, Hoverman JR, Langdon R, Lyman GH, Meropol NJ, Mulvey T, Newcomer L, Peppercorn J, Polite B, Raghavan D, Rossi G, Saltz L, Schrag D, Smith TJ, Yu PP, Hudis CA, Schilsky RL, American Society of Clinical Oncology. American Society of Clinical Oncology statement: A conceptual framework to assess the value of cancer treatment options. Journal of Clinical Oncology: Official Journal of the American Society of Clinical Oncology. 2015; 33(23): 2563–2577.

Seo HS, Sohng KY. The effect of footbaths on sleep and fatigue in older Korean adults. Journal of Korean Academy of Fundamentals of Nursing. 2011; 18(4): 488–496.

Seraji A, Vakilian K. The comparison between the effects of aromatherapy with lavender and breathing techniques on the reduction of labor pain. Complementary Medicine Journal CMJA. 2011; 1(1): 34–41. http://cmja.arakmu.ac.ir/article-1-63-en.html

Tabatabaeichehr M, Mortazavi H. The effectiveness of aromatherapy in the management of labor pain and anxiety: A systematic review. Ethiopian Journal of Health Sciences. 2020; 30(3): 449–458.

Tillett J, Ames D. The uses of aromatherapy in women's health. The Journal of Perinatal & Neonatal Nursing. 2010; 24(3): 238–245.

Tiran D. Clinical Aromatherapy for Pregnancy and Childbirth. 2nd ed. Edinburgh: Churchill Livingstone; 2000.

Woodman SE, Antonopoulos SR, Durham PL. Inhibition of nociception in a preclinical episodic migraine model by dietary supplementation of grape seed extract involves activation of endocannabinoid receptors. Frontiers in Pain Research (Lausanne, Switzerland). 2022; 3: 809352.

Yuan R, Zhang D, Yang J, Wu Z, Luo C, Han L, Yang F, Lin J, Yang M. Review of aromatherapy essential oils and their mechanism of action against migraines. Journal of Ethnopharmacology. 2021; 265: 113326.

# 9 Pharmacological Applications of Brazilian Aromatic Species
## Aniba Rosaeodora Ducke, Casearia Sylvestris Sw., Spilanthes Acmella Var. Oleracea (L.), and Xylopia Aromatica (Lam.) Mart

*Sachin P. Bhatt, Popat Mohite, Abhijeet Puri, Sudarshan Singh, Bhupendra G. Prajapati, Shruti Shiromwar, and Vijay R. Chidrawar*

## 9.1 INTRODUCTION

Natural compounds, particularly plant metabolites, have emerged as a vital source of medicine for people over the years. Yet, there has been a lot of scope for research on aromatic plants containing essential oils (EOs). EOs are among the several natural products that scientists have focused on due to their potent bioactive properties. They are a combination of volatile compounds, primarily mono- and sesquiterpenoids, benzenoids, and phenylpropanoids, among others. The chemical makeup of EOs, together with their antioxidant and antibacterial characteristics, influence a variety of physiological processes in both plant and human beings, using positive traits like pathogen growth suppression and free radical scavenging activity. Due to microbial resistance, conventional antimicrobials represent lower efficacy and a high incidence of negative effects on human health; due to this there has been a surge in interest in the study of EOs. Recent investigations show EOs possess broad array of medical properties including antibacterial, antiviral, antioxidant, anticancer, and hepatoprotective properties (Raut and Karuppayil, 2014).

Brazil has the most diverse plant life on the globe, with about 55,000 species of higher plants spread throughout several environments (Engelke, 2003). Brazil is also home to a sundry array of aromatic species, many of which have been used in

DOI: 10.1201/9781003389774-9

traditional medicine for centuries. Both biotic and non-biotic factors influence the EO-bearing aromatic plants to adapt to the varied environmental conditions. These plants contain a wide variety of bioactive compounds that have been studied for their therapeutic potential. Brazil has a diverse climate, which has a significant impact on the growth and development of aromatic plants. Different species of aromatic plants have varying tolerances to diverse environmental conditions, so the climate can positively affect their growth, yield, and quality. Over the past 25 years, several pre-clinical and clinical studies have been conducted by Brazilian researchers on EOs obtained from plants in various regions of Brazil. EOs extracted from aromatic plants have been screened for various pharmacological actions including anti-inflammatory, antiviral, immunomodulatory, anticancer, antioxidant, cardioprotective, and antidiabetic activities, as a skin penetration enhancer agent, in aromatherapy, and in massage therapy (Raut and Karuppayil, 2014).

EOs bear antioxidant capabilities that are commonly found in aromatic plants. Both the crude EOs and isolated components, which are both effective to tackle lipid oxidation, exhibit these qualities. The phytoconstituents responsible for the antioxidant activity are β-phellandrene, linalool, β-caryophyllene, and γ-eudesmol. A single volatile component in the chemical makeup of EOs or the synergistic interaction between numerous constituents can be attributed to their antioxidant capacity (Ferreira et al., 2022). The hunt for naturally occurring bioactive substances with antibacterial properties has grown. Therapeutic agents can be found in abundance in natural assets and their derivatives. Because EOs are made up of mixes of volatile components with antibacterial qualities, they have caught the attention of researchers in recent years (Silva et al., 2021). In Brazil, plants found in the Amazonian flora are sources of EOs, some of which have been studied for their antibacterial properties. The various phytoconstituents responsible for the antimicrobial activity against human pathogens include terpenes, sesquiterpene hydrocarbons, oxygenated sesquiterpenes, and *trans*-nerolidol (Scalvenzi et al., 2017). Further, EOs can be used solely or in combination with conventional antibiotics to avoid bacterial resistance and synergistic effect. Since most anticancer medications come from natural sources, the hunt for novel phyto-therapeutics with anticancer (tumor) potential is crucial. EOs from Amazonian plant species have demonstrated favorable cytotoxic activity. Various plant phytoconstituents were screened for cytotoxic activity by using a variety of mammalian cell lines. The chief chemical constituents responsible for the cytotoxic activity are α-bisabolol, β-eudesmol, α-eudesmol, γ-eudesmol, guaiol, caryophyllene oxide, β-bisabolene, terpenoids, sesquiterpenoids, germacrene, germacrene B, epi-β-bisabolol, and curzerene (Jerônimo et al., 2021). Moreover, Brazilian flora contain a variety of important phytoconstituents in the form of EOs which have shown significant protective effects in *in vivo* and *in vitro* models against cardiovascular complications; these phytoconstituents include thymoquinone, cinnamaldehyde, cinnamic acid, α-bisabolol, carvacrol, eugenol, limonene, linalool, α-terpineol, and 1,8-cineole (de Andrade et al., 2017). Among the infectious diseases, viral diseases included, hepatitis, respiratory syncytial virus, and COVID-19 are considered more challenging to treat due to their complex pathophysiology and rapid spread. In the search for antiviral drugs, the EOs were screened from the Brazilian species. A variety of plant species has shown antiviral activity due to the presence of

(*E*)-α-atlantone; 14-hydroxy-α-muurolene; allo-aromadendrene epoxide; amorpha-4,9-dien-2-ol; aristochene; azulenol; germacrene A; guaia-6,9-diene; hedycaryol; humulene epoxide II; α-amorphene; α-cadinene; α-calacorene, and α-muurolene (Amparo et al., 2021). Several studies show that EOs of Brazilian plants possess anti-diabetic activity due to the occurrence of diverse chemical compositions including eugenol, α-pinene, *C. cyminum* 6,10,14- Trimethyl-2-pentadecanone, hexadecanoic acid, methyl ester, hexadecanoic acid, 8,11- octadecadienoic acid, methyl ester, and 9,12,15-octadecatrien-1-ol (Chaudhry et al., 2020). Increasingly, EOs are becoming popular as a component of many topical formulations due to their penetration-enhancing activity. EOs interacts with the skin stratum corneum and increase the penetrability of many lipophilic and hydrophilic drugs. Popular EOs such as clove oil, angelica oil, chuanxiong oil, Cyperus oil, cinnamon oil, and eucalyptus oil are currently used in many topical formulations. The essential phytoconstituents present in many Brazilian species responsible for their penetration enhancement activity are ligustilide, trans-cinnamaldehyde, eugenol, cyperene, dehydrofukinone, and α-cyperone (Chen et al., 2015). In this chapter a brief on pharmacological and clinical application of Brazilian aromatic species including *Aniba rosaeodora* Ducke, *Casearia sylvestris* Sw., *Spilanthes acmella* var. *oleracea* (L.), and *Xylopia aromatica* (Lam.) Mart relating to EOs has been emphasized.

## ANIBA ROSAEODORA DUCKE

The *Aniba rosaeodora*, or Aniba, is a popular flowering plant (*Lauraceae*) that grows up to 30 meters tall and has yellow-brown bark (Maia et al., 2007). The commercial production of rosewood essential oil, utilized extensively in perfumery, began in the Brazilian interior state of Pará about 1930 (Amusant et al., 2016). Though the aroma may be enjoyed from the entire tree, only the trunk wood is taken and hydro-distilled to produce rosewood oil. This species serves several uses in the Amazon, such as a medicine for treating epileptic seizures, a component in regional scents, and a decorative plant (Teles et al., 2020). EOs typically contain terpenes, allyl phenols, alcohols, acids, and esters (Pimentel et al., 2018). *A. rosaeodora* oil, whose primary component is the monoterpene alcohol linalool, is a colorless or light-yellow liquid with a woody floral aroma (Sampaio Lde et al., 2012). Although there have been reports of rosewood oil's potential medicinal qualities, the oil is primarily of interest to the taste and fragrance industries due to the several lucrative derivatives that can be derived from it. Because of its high linalool concentration, *A. rosaeodora* is used extensively (85%) in the perfumery and cosmetics industries worldwide (da Trindade et al., 2021). *A. rosaeodora* oil is used for various purposes, including as an analgesic, anticonvulsant, anti-depressant, antimicrobial, antiseptic, aphrodisiac, bactericidal, cellular stimulant, cephalic, stimulant, tissue regenerator, and sleep aid (Sarrazin et al., 2016).

Kizak et al. studied the effects of *A. rosaeodora oil*, a potential novel herbal anesthetic, on goldfish in comparison to camphor (*Cinnamomum camphora*) EO and the widely used chemical agent 2-phenoxyethanol (2-PE) (*Carassius auratus*) (Kizak et al., 2018). These herbal EOs and 2-PE were tested for their anesthetic efficacy on standard-sized goldfish. A series of anesthetic concentrations were tested on fish, and the least effective concentrations (LECs) were determined based on the depth of unconsciousness achieved and the speed with which the fish recovered. The findings demonstrated that *A. rosaeodora* EOs are a potent anesthetic requiring at least three times lower doses than 2-PE; hence, it can be a possible novel anesthetic for fish. It can be utilized as an efficient natural drug, with quick induction and recovery times. Sœur et al. tested rosewood *A. rosaeodora* EOs on human epidermoid cancer line A431, immortal HaCaT cells assumed to represent an early stage of skin carcinogenesis, transformed normal HEK001 keratinocytes, and primary normal NHEK keratinocytes. Selective cytotoxicity against A431 and HaCaT cells was seen when EO was applied in a narrow concentration range. Cytotoxicity from the same treatments was low in both HEK001 and NHEK cells. Specifically, in A431 and HaCaT cells, EOs produced mitochondrial membrane depolarization, ROS generation, and caspase-dependent cell death defined by the early hallmark of apoptosis, phosphatidylserine externalization. EO-induced cell death was linked to both intrinsic and extrinsic apoptotic mechanisms. Finding that EO selectively induces apoptosis in precancerous and cancerous skin cells demonstrates the essential oil's potential anticancer action (Sœur et al., 2011). De Almeida et al. reported that the LORR test and latency estimation were used to test whether rosewood oil had any sedative effects on mice. After receiving an intraperitoneal injection of rosewood oil, mice took differing times to lose their righting reflex. Pentobarbital, a barbiturate with 40 mg/kg, generated latency periods comparable to those seen with rosewood oil at 100 mg/kg. Surprisingly, pentobarbital and rosewood oil showed a significant enhancement when injected jointly. These findings show that rosewood oil may have other therapeutic applications. Rosewood oil dose-dependently enhanced the mice's sleeping duration. According to the most recent data, combining pentobarbital with rosewood oil led to much longer periods of sleep than either component used alone (de Almeida et al., 2009). Singh et al. investigated the encapsulation of *A. rosaeodora* essential oil with chitosan nano-emulsion; it aimed to improve its antifungal and aflatoxin B1 (AFB1) inhibitory activity. The encapsulation of EOs within chitosan nano-emulsion was tested for *in vitro* release. Complete growth suppression and AFB1 production inhibition of *Aspergillus flavus* (AFLHPSi-1) by AREO-CsNe were achieved at 0.8 and 0.6 µl/mL, respectively, which was significantly better than AREO (1.4 and 1.2 µl/mL, respectively). It also confirmed the unique anti-aflatoxigenic mechanism of AREO and AREO-CsNe by measuring their ability to significantly suppress methylglyoxal (AFB1 inducer) formation in AFLHPSi-1 cells. The $IC_{50}$ values for AREO-antioxidant CsNes activity against DPPH and ABTS free radicals were 3.792 and 1.706 µl/mL, respectively. AREO-CsNe also showed a high safety profile with an LD50 value of 9538.742 µl/kg body weight (*Setaria italica* seeds) from becoming contaminated with AFB1 and experiencing lipid peroxidation for an entire year without affecting the grain's flavor or texture (Singh et al., 2022). Ferreira et al. evaluated EO solutions (10–100 mg/L) for antioxidant activity using ABTS and DPPH tests and larvicidal efficacy against *Aedes aegypti* larvae, wherein larval mortality was assessed using the Reed-Muench technique and $LC_{50}$ values were calculated. When tested for toxicity, $LC_{50}$ values fell outside the hazardous range (582–282 mg/L) and were considered safe. The EOs were effective against larvicides ($LC_{50}$=41.07 mg/L) and had significant antioxidant properties. Based on the findings, it was concluded that the studied EOs contain chemicals with a superior larvicidal action compared to *Aedes aegypti*, which bodes well for its future clinical utility (Ferreira et al., 2020). Sarrazin et al. applied disk-diffusion and plate micro-dilution tests to measure the *in vitro* antibacterial capability against *Escherichia coli*, *Klebsiella pneumoniae*, *Staphylococcus aureus*, *Staphylococcus epidermidis*, *Enterococcus faecalis*, and *Streptococcus pyogenes*. There was significant activity of both oils against these pathogenic bacteria, with the inhibition zone values for *A. rosaeodora* oil ranging from 8.80.6 mm to 38.41.4 mm (MIC, 1.3 to 10.0 µl/mL) and those for *A. parviflora* oil ranging from 9.20.4 mm to 15.40.9 mm (MIC, 1.3 to 10.0 µl/mL). Linalool and its concentration in the oils are responsible for their potency and bactericidal effects. Water-based extracts showed no antibacterial activity in the same tests. This proves that rosewood oil has antibacterial properties and might be utilized in pharmaceuticals or as a food preservative to combat multidrug-resistant bacterial strains (Sarrazin et al., 2016).

## CASEARIA SYLVESTRIS Sw.

Brazilian traditional medicine uses a plant called *C. sylvestris* (*Flacourtiaceae*) to cure trauma. It is also known as "guac atonga," a native term from the Tupi-Guarani language that alludes to the traditional use of species by Brazil's indigenous people. The medicinal qualities of the peel, which is used to cure fever, herpes, diarrhea, and snake bites, are comparable to those of the plant extract made by boiling the herbs (Esteves et al., 2005).

Plant extracts' chemical makeup is extremely complicated and varied because it depends on the temperature and/or the type of soil. Thin layer chromatography analysis indicated the presence of phytochemical flavonoids, which give it its orange color, and other phenolic components. The main phytoconstituent in hydroalcoholic extracts of *C. sylvestris* (flavonoids and polyphenols) were identified by TLC and spectrophotometrically measured, and their capacity to inhibit neuromuscular activity are quantified (Camargo et al., 2010).

The predominant species are yeasts and Gram-positive bacteria that *C. sylvestris* has a good action potential against (da Silva et al., 2008). In folk medicine, this plant's leaves are frequently employed as a purgative, analgesic, anti-inflammatory, anti-ulcerogenic, antiviral, and antibacterial drug. The EOs of *C. sylvestris* demonstrated significant antibacterial effect against *E. coli*, *S. aureus*, and *S. setubal* (Espinosa et al., 2015). *C. sylvestris* is sold in plant mixes that are used to make infusions and tea with therapeutic properties. Additionally, it functions as an active component in herpes lotions. Bicyclogermacrene, a compound with poor antitumoral potential, was found to be the predominant component of the EOs isolated from *C. sylvestris* leaves. However, two sesquiterpenes with strong and well-documented cytotoxic activity, caryophyllene and humulene, make up a large portion of this essential oil (da Silva et al.). *C. sylvestris* leaf hydroethanolic or aqueous extracts are extensively used as topical anti-inflammatory and wound-healing medications in Brazil. In inflammation model organisms, the aqueous extract, hydroethanolic extract, and EOs from *C. sylvestris* leaves indicated significant anti-inflammatory efficacy. Chemotaxonomy states that the presence of distinctive, highly oxygenated tricyclic cis-clerodane diterpenes with two acyloxy groups on the tetrahydrofuran ring distinguishes the *Casearia* genus (Pierri et al., 2017). Brazilian traditional medicine frequently uses *C. sylvestris* to treat skin lesions and small ulcerations, which is consistent with the plant's recently identified antiulcer properties. In pre-clinical tests, an extract of *C. sylvestris* leaves protected the rat stomach mucosa without affecting the gastric pH (Xia et al., 2015). Given that pepsin is used as a molecular target to threaten gastric ulcers, *in vivo* studies have shown that *C. sylvestris* extracts have antiulcerogenic activity, and pepsin has traditionally been used to threaten gastric injuries, pharmacological activity may be related to inhibition of pepsin (Rovedder et al., 2016). It has been demonstrated that *C. sylvestris* contains substances that affect the action of the enzymes Na+/K+-ATPase and acetylcholinesterase, DNA, and phospholipase A2 (De Mattos et al., 2007). *C. sylvestris* improved outcomes in terms of the growth of skin healings (Heymanns et al., 2021). Both the promastigote and amastigote forms of *Leishmania amazonensis* were immune to *C. sylvestris*'s antileishmanial actions. The main component of *C. sylvestris*, E-caryophyllene, showed lower toxicity and improved efficacy against *L. amazonensis* amastigote forms, suggesting potential as a leishmaniasis treatment candidate (Moreira et al., 2019). Smaller doses of *C. sylvestris* extracts have an antiproliferative effect and may be helpful as a supplementary therapy to traditional cytotoxic chemotherapy, regardless of whether larger doses are cytotoxic. By interacting with proteins linked to cell cycle arrest at G1 and senescence, the chloroform fraction and aqueous extract of *C. sylvestris* restrict cell growth in living things (Felipe et al., 2014). The inflammatory response to second-degree burn repair in diabetic rats was controlled by *C. sylvestris* leaves, which benefitted fibroplasia and collagenases and provided a useful treatment option for burns in diabetes (Martelli et al., 2018). There are no signs of renal, hepatic, or hemotoxic toxicity, and its species also shows preventative behavior against severe stomach lesions (Neto et al., 2020). Anti-inflammatory, anti-plasmodial, and antiulcer qualities are among its wide spectrum of pharmacological and cytotoxic abilities (Ribeiro et al., 2019).

## *Spilanthes acmella* Var. *Oleracea* (L.)

*Spilanthes acmella* var. oleracea (*Compositae*) is a class of naturally occurring bioactive compounds that usually act as important plant growth regulators (Nakatani and Nagashima, 1992). It is a native tropical plant that evolved in South America and Asia (Dias et al., 2012). The secondary metabolites of biological importance found in *S. acmella* L. are primarily phenolic acids and glycosylated flavonoids (Bellumori et al., 2022). Although this plant's roots contain less alkylamide than its aerial parts, they actually include twice as much total phenols (Bellumori et al., 2022). According to reports, the plant's flower head and roots are a rich source of active ingredients. The plant also contains triterpenoids (Dubey et al., 2013). Spilanthol, undeca-2E,7Z,9E-trienoic acid isobutylamide, undeca-2E-en-8,10-diyonic acid isobutylamide, 2E-N-(2-methylbutyl)-2-undecene-8,10-diynamide, and 7Z-N-isobutyl-2 are a few of the secondary metabolites of *Spilanthes* (Nascimento et al., 2020).

*S. acmella* extracts have been found to exhibit antibacterial, antioxidant, larvicidal, diuretic, analgesic, and mosquitocidal effects. It is extensively used as an appetite stimulant and to treat anemia and toothaches in addition to being widely utilized in cooking (Uthpala and Navaratne, 2021). A dose-dependent zone of inhibition was reported for EOs in a previous study (Dubey et al., 2013). The antioxidant activity of methanol extracts from the stem and leaves of *S. acmella* using DPPH and superoxide radical scavenging experiments demonstrated that the methanol extract had good superoxide radical scavenging activity, compared with the leaves of *S. acmella* (Joseph et al., 2013). Few instances of this genus exhibiting antiviral activity have been well documented (Paulraj et al., 2013). It has been demonstrated that many different chemical groups, including certain fatty acids and amides, facilitate skin penetration. Additionally, a great deal of study has been done on hybrid enhancers of transdermal penetration composed of two potent enhancer groups. Phytoconstituent identified azone (1-dodecylazacycloheptan-2-one) is made up of a cyclic amide (pyrrolidone) and a lengthy fatty acid chain (C12) (Sharma and Arumugam, 2021). The analgesic effect of spilanthol has been connected to an increase in GABA release in the temporal cerebral region of the brain, whereas echinacea alkylamides work on voltage-gated sodium channels in this part of the brain (Boonen et al., 2010b). It's possible that the plant extract's flavonoids lower prostaglandins like prostaglandin-PGE2 and prostaglandin-PGF2, which are known to play a role in pain perception (Prachayasittikul et al., 2013). When used as an extraction solvent, dichloromethane has been found to be more efficient than methanol or aqueous medium at preventing the growth of mycelial cells and sporulation in *Aspergillus* species (Sharma and Arumugam, 2021). The ability of dried *S. acmella* flowers to reduce inflammation has been demonstrated using the lipopolysaccharide-activated murine macrophage model (Rondanelli et al., 2020). In this biological model, nitric oxide (NO), which is utilized to mediate inflammation, is produced by macrophages with assistance from COX-2 and iNOS. The mRNAs in charge of iNOS and COX-2 are not allowed to express themselves when spilanthol is present (Wu et al., 2008). Well-known herbal enterprises create preparations with *Spilanthes* for use as dietary supplements and medical supplies. *S. acmella* extract is prepared using a patented technique by the French business Gattefossé SAS for use in cosmetic anti-wrinkle cream (Sharma and Arumugam, 2021). *S. acmella* was first introduced as a traditional remedy for toothache pain (Boonen et al., 2010a). The potent alkylamide-like spilanthol, one of *S. acmella*'s active components, is responsible for the drug's well-known anesthetic action (Ratnasooriya et al., 2004). It has been discovered that *Spilanthes* extracts are utilized in mouthwashes, mouth fresheners, and pharmaceuticals for treating periodontitis, pyrrhea, and items that reduce discomfort and gum swelling (Ong et al., 2011). *S. acmella* has received much financial value as a medicinal plant, horticultural ornamental plant, and food flavoring (Jansen, 1985). One of the earliest descriptions of the species's flavor was found in Lamarck's *Encyclopédie*, which described the plant's flavor as peppery but unattractive. The raw leaves can be added to soups and meats (Jansen, 1985), steamed as a vegetable, or used as a potent salad seasoning in India and the United States (Bailey, 1949). A recent study examined at the plants used by locals to treat tuberculosis in five towns in Brazil's Amazonas region, which has a substantial incidence of the disease and resistant forms of *Mycobacterium tuberculosis* (Storey and Salem, 1997). Since *Spilanthes acmella* flowers are strong diuretics with effects similar to those of furosemide and are known to significantly raise urine sodium ions (Na+) and potassium ions (K+) levels, they are employed to create the diuretic action (Ratnasooriya et al., 2004). In the current study, two African medicinal plants, *Aframomum melegueta* and *Spilanthes acmella*, were investigated for their ability to treat obesity. In many nations, medicinal plants have been utilized as dietary supplements to help people regulate and control their body weight (Yoshikawa et al., 2002).

## XYLOPIA AROMATICA (LAM.) MART

In the late nineteenth century, people began using the leaves and fruits of the underused species *X. aromatica* as food (Oliveira et al., 2018). Brazil is a hotspot for the search for biologically active compounds from plants such as *X. aromatica* (Lam.) due to its rich biodiversity. However, local Brazilian plants that are useful are not fully utilized (Brandão et al., 2011). The *X. aromatica* (Lam.) Mart. species, which belongs to the *Annonaceae* family, has a wide distribution in Brazil and is one of the 38 species that make up 50% of the Cerrado's vegetation. It is also found in Florentine regions (Yusuf et al., 2018). The findings of quantitative analysis measurements are in line with the components found in plants, such as flavonoids and phenolic acids. The leaves of the plant *O. cordata* contained 6.2 g/100 g of total phenolics compared to 3.2 g/100 g of flavonoids (Oliveira et al., 2018). Chromatography examination discovered the presence of several phytochemicals including gallic acid and quercetin in the crude aqueous extract of plant material from intermedia leaves (Simoni et al., 1996). It can be seen that the main ingredients included limonene, -pinene, -pinene, bicyclogermacrene, (E)-caryophyllene, and germacrene D. (Shakri et al., 2020). Out of all the oils, the species *X. aromatica* supplied the most, accounting for around 99.8% of them (Fournier et al., 1993). Monoterpene hydrocarbons, oxygenated, sesquiterpene hydrocarbons, and oxygenated sesquiterpenes predominated as the main group constituents of the essential oils in the plant *Xylopia* (Burkill, 1985). Esters, aldehydes, ketones, and phenylpropanoids are also found (Martins et al., 1995). In the genus *Xylopia*, alkaloids (Bouba A et al., 2010) and phenolic compounds have also been discovered (Maldini et al., 2011). All herpes viruses were actively inhibited by aromatic plant species. The greatest VII values against SuHV-1 were found in an aromatic extract (Silva Junior et al., 2009). According to several studies, quercetin enhanced the benefits against the inflammatory response associated with obesity, including a reduction in insulin sensitivity, monocytes, and systemic inflammation (Al-Fayez et al., 2006). In the current study, it was shown that CEXA increased liver inflammation, hepatic steatosis, insulin sensitivity, oral glucose tolerance, and inflammatory responses (Okuno et al., 1998). Polyphenols, particularly flavonoids, are the main components in plant extracts of *X. aromatica* with anti-inflammatory and antioxidant properties (Talhouk et al., 2007). The *X. aromatica* flower was found to have an inhibitory bacterial effect against several bacteria strains, including *S. aureus* (minimum inhibitory concentration 400 g/mL), *S. pyogenes* (ATCC 12345) (minimum inhibitory concentration 200 g/mL), and *P. aeruginosa* strains. This EO's antifungal efficacy versus *Candida* strains was only moderately effective when tested (Nascimento et al., 2018). The significant antibacterial action of the essential oils from spices may be explained by the fact that the leaves of *X. aromatica* have a greater concentration of oxygenated sesquiterpenes (70%) than the flowers (51%) (Dorman and Deans, 2000). By testing the oil's minimum inhibitory concentration against several bacteria and *Candida albicans*, the fungistatic properties of the substance were ascertained (Fournier et al., 1993). The stem bark oil of *X. aromatica* had a MIC of 5 mg/mL against *Mycobacterium smegmatis* (Fournier et al., 1994). There is currently a lot of interest in the use of functional foods, nutritional supplements, and dietary aids in the treatment of obesity and related metabolic diseases. However, many herbal medicines are widely used in the treatment of obesity, and those plants allow easy metabolism of the fats and lipids (de Oliveira, 2012). In lab trials, *X. aethiopica* fruits were given to animal models, and they demonstrated improved glucose and lipid metabolism as well as acting on metabolic dysfunction, which is usually associated with obesity (Ezekwesili et al., 2010). South and Central America, as well as some Caribbean islands, are where *X. aromatica* (Lam.) Mart. (pepemato, sembe) is found. It is used to treat malaria effectively in the Colombian region, and it also has antiprotozoal effects (Blair et al., 1991).

## 9.2   CONCLUSIONS

Brazil is home to a rich biodiversity, including numerous aromatic plant species that have been traditionally used in Brazilian folk medicine for their medicinal properties. Many of these species have been investigated for their pharmacological potential in clinical applications. Moreover, the future fortification of EOs within nanostructure materials expected to play a pivotal role in treatment of several infectious diseases due to their excellent antibacterial efficacy. Among them in this chapter the therapeutic potential of EOs obtained from *Aniba rosaeodora* Ducke, *Casearia sylvestris* Sw., *Spilanthes acmella* var. *oleracea* (L.), and *Xylopia aromatica* (Lam.) Mart were elaborated, which are just a few examples of Brazilian aromatic species. Many more species are currently being studied for their therapeutic potential, and their use in traditional medicine to inspire new research into natural remedies.

## REFERENCES

Al-Fayez, M., Cai, H., Tunstall, R., Steward, W. P. & Gescher, A. J. 2006. Differential modulation of cyclooxygenase-mediated prostaglandin production by the putative cancer chemopreventive flavonoids tricin, apigenin and quercetin. *Cancer Chemotherapy and Pharmacology*, 58, 816–825.

Amparo, T. R., Seibert, J. B., Silveira, B. M., Costa, F. S. F., Almeida, T. C., Braga, S. F. P., da Silva, G. N., dos Santos, O. D. H. & de Souza, G. H. B. 2021. Brazilian essential oils as source for the discovery of new anti-covid-19 drug: A review guided by in silico study. *Phytochemistry Review*, 20, 1013–1032.

Amusant, N., Beauchène, J., Digeon, A. & Chaix, G. 2016. Essential oil yield in rosewood (*Aniba rosaeodora* ducke): Initial application of rapid prediction by near infrared spectroscopy based on wood spectra. *Journal of Near Infrared Spectroscopy*, 24, 507–515.

Bailey, L. H. 1949. *Manual of cultivated plants: Most commonly grown in the continental United States and Canada*. The Macmillan Company, New York.

Bellumori, M., Zonfrillo, B., Maggini, V., Bogani, P., Gallo, E., Firenzuoli, F., Mulinacci, N. & Innocenti, M. 2022. Acmella oleracea (l.) Rk jansen: Alkylamides and phenolic compounds in aerial parts and roots of in vitro seedlings. *Journal of Pharmaceutical and Biomedical Analysis*, 220, 114991.

Blair, S., Correa, A., Madrigal, B., Zuluaga, C. & Franco, H. 1991. Plantas antimaláricas, una revisión bibliográfica. *Medellin: universidad de antioquia*, 214.

Boonen, J., Baert, B., Burvenich, C., Blondeel, P., de Saeger, S. & de Spiegeleer, B. 2010a. Lc-ms profiling of n-alkylamides in Spilanthes acmella extract and the transmucosal behaviour of its main bio-active spilanthol. *Journal of Pharmaceutical and Biomedical Analysis*, 53, 243–249.

Boonen, J., Baert, B., Roche, N., Burvenich, C. & de Spiegeleer, B. 2010b. Transdermal behaviour of the n-alkylamide spilanthol (affinin) from Spilanthes acmella (compositae) extracts. *Journal of Ethnopharmacology*, 127, 77–84.

Bouba A., Njintang, Y., Scher, J. & Mbofung, C. 2010. Phenolic compounds and radical scavenging potential of twenty cameroonian spices. *Agriculture and Biology Journal of North America*, 1, 213–224.

Brandão, M. G., Grael, C. F. & Fagg, C. W. 2011. European naturalists and medicinal plants of brazil. *Biological Diversity and Sustainable Resources Use*, 101, 120.

Burkill, H. 1985. The useful plants of West Africa. *Royal Botanical Gardens, Kew*, 1, 319.

Camargo, T., Nazato, V., Silva, M., Cogo, J., Groppo, F. & Oshima-Franco, Y. 2010. Bothrops jararacussu venom-induced neuromuscular blockade inhibited by Casearia gossypiosperma briquet hydroalcoholic extract. *Journal of Venomous Animals and Toxins Including Tropical Diseases*, 16, 432–441.

Chaudhry, Z. R., Shakir, S., Rasheed, S., Rashid, E., Rafique, S. & Rasheed, F. 2020. Glucose-lowering and weight improving effect of Syzygium aromaticum (clove) extract on diabetic rats. *Pakistan Journal of Medical & Health Sciences*, 14(2), 1589–1591.

Chen, J., Jiang, Q. D., Wu, Y. M., Liu, P., Yao, J. H., Lu, Q., Zhang, H. & Duan, J. A. 2015. Potential of essential oils as penetration enhancers for transdermal administration of ibuprofen to treat dysmenorrhoea. *Molecules*, 20, 18219–18236.

da Silva, S. L., Chaar, J. D. S., Damico, D. C., Figueiredo, P. D. M. & Yano, T. 2008. Antimicrobial activity of ethanol extract from leaves of casearia sylvestris. *Pharmaceutical Biology*, 46, 347–351.

da Trindade, R. C. S., Xavier, J. K. A. M., Setzer, W. N., Maia, J. G. S. & da Silva, J. K. R. 2021. Chemical diversity and therapeutic effects of essential oils of aniba species from the amazon: A review. *Plants*, 10, 1854.

de Almeida, R. N., Araújo, D. A. M., Gonçalves, J. C. R., Montenegro, F. C., de Sousa, D. P., Leite, J. R., Mattei, R., Benedito, M. A. C., de Carvalho, J. G. B., Cruz, J. S. & Maia, J. G. S. 2009. Rosewood oil induces sedation and inhibits compound action potential in rodents. *Journal of Ethnopharmacology*, 124, 440–443.

de Andrade, T. U., Brasil, G. A., Endringer, D. C., da Nóbrega, F. R. & de Sousa, D. P. 2017. Cardiovascular activity of the chemical constituents of essential oils. *Molecules*, 22.

de Mattos, E., Frederico, M., Colle, T., de Pieri, D., Peters, R. & Piovezan, A. 2007. Evaluation of antinociceptive activity of Casearia sylvestris and possible mechanism of action. *Journal of Ethnopharmacology*, 112, 1–6.

de Oliveira, V. B. 2012. Potencial dos frutos de xylopia aromatica (lam.) Mart. (Annonaceae) no tratamento de alterações metabólicas, induzidas por dieta em camundongos balb/c. Universidade Federal de Minas Gerais, 1–135. http://hdl.handle.net/1843/BUOS-8U4G2N

Dias, A., Santos, P., Seabra, I., Júnior, R., Braga, M. & de Sousa, H. 2012. Spilanthol from Spilanthes acmella flowers, leaves and stems obtained by selective supercritical carbon dioxide extraction. *The Journal of Supercritical Fluids*, 61, 62–70.

Dorman, H. D. & Deans, S. G. 2000. Antimicrobial agents from plants: Antibacterial activity of plant volatile oils. *Journal of Applied Microbiology*, 88, 308–316.

Dubey, S., Maity, S., Singh, M., Saraf, S. A. & Saha, S. 2013. Phytochemistry, pharmacology and toxicology of Spilanthes acmella: A review. *Advances in Pharmacological and Pharmaceutical Sciences*, 2013.

Engelke, F. 2003. Fitoterápicos e legislaçao. *Jornal brasileiro de fitomedicina*, 1, 10–15.

Espinosa, J., Medeiros, L. F., Souza, A. D., Güntzel, A. R. D. C., Rücker, B., Casali, E. A., Ethur, E. M., Wink, M. R. & Torres, I. L. D. S. 2015. Ethanolic extract of Casearia sylvestris sw exhibits in vitro antioxidant and antimicrobial activities and in vivo hypolipidemic effect in rats. *Revista brasileira de plantas medicinais*, 17, 305–315.

Esteves, I., Souza, I. R., Rodrigues, M., Cardoso, L. G. V., Santos, L. S., Sertie, J. A. A., Perazzo, F. F., Lima, L. M., Schneedorf, J. M. & Bastos, J. K. 2005. Gastric antiulcer and anti-inflammatory activities of the essential oil from Casearia sylvestris sw. *Journal of Ethnopharmacology*, 101, 191–196.

Ezekwesili, C., Nwodo, O., Eneh, F. & Ogbunugafor, H. 2010. Investigation of the chemical composition and biological activity of Xylopia aethiopica dunal (annonacae). *African Journal of Biotechnology*, 9, 7352–7356.

Felipe, K. B., Kviecinski, M. R., da Silva, F. O., Bücker, N. F., Farias, M. S., Castro, L. S. E. P. W., de Souza Grinevicius, V. M. A., Motta, N. S., Correia, J. F. G. & Rossi, M. H. 2014. Inhibition of tumor proliferation associated with cell cycle arrest caused by extract and fraction from Casearia sylvestris (Salicaceae). *Journal of Ethnopharmacology*, 155, 1492–1499.

Ferreira, A. M., Mouchrek Filho, V. E., Mafra, N. S. C., Sales, E. H., Júnior, P. S. S. & Everton, G. O. 2020. Constituintes químicos, toxicidade, potencial antioxidante e atividade larvicida frente a larvas de aedes aegypti do óleo essencial de *Aniba rosaeodora* ducke. *Research, Society and Development*, 9, e520985663.

Ferreira, O. O., Cruz, J. N., de Moraes Â, A. B., de Jesus Pereira Franco, C., Lima, R. R., Anjos, T. O. D., Siqueira, G. M., Nascimento, L. D. D., Cascaes, M. M., de Oliveira, M. S. & Andrade, E. H. A. 2022. Essential oil of the plants growing in the Brazilian Amazon: Chemical composition, antioxidants, and biological applications. *Molecules*, 27.

Fournier, G., Hadjiakhoondi, A., Charles, B., Fourniat, J., Leboeuf, M. & Cave, A. 1994. Chemical and biological studios of Xylopia aromatica stem bark and leaf oils. *Planta Medica*, 60, 283–284.

Fournier, G., Hadjiakhoondi, A., Leboeuf, M., Cavé, A., Fourniat, J. & Charles, B. 1993. Chemical and biological studies of Xylopia longifolia a. Dc. Essential oils. *Journal of Essential Oil Research*, 5, 403–410.

Heymanns, A. C., Albano, M. N., d Silveira, M. R., Muller, S. D., Petronilho, F. C., Gainski, L. D., Cargnin-Ferreira, E. & Piovezan, A. P. 2021. Macroscopic, biochemical and hystological evaluation of topical anti-inflammatory activity of Casearia sylvestris (Flacourtiaceae) in mice. *Journal of ethnopharmacology*, 264, 113139.

Jansen, R. K. 1985. The systematics of Acmella (Asteraceae-heliantheae). *Systematic Botany Monographs*, 1–115.

Jerônimo, L. B., da Costa, J. S., Pinto, L. C., Montenegro, R. C., Setzer, W. N., Mourão, R. H. V., da Silva, J. K. R., Maia, J. G. S. & Figueiredo, P. L. B. 2021. Antioxidant and cytotoxic activities of Myrtaceae essential oils rich in terpenoids from Brazil. *Natural Product Communications*, 16, 1934578x21996156.

Joseph, B., George, J. & Mv, J. 2013. The role of Acemella oleracea in medicine: A review. *World Journal of Pharmaceutical Res*earch, 2, 2781–2788.

Kizak, V., Can, E., Danabaş, D. & Can, Ş. S. 2018. Evaluation of anesthetic potential of rosewood (*Aniba rosaeodora*) oil as a new anesthetic agent for goldfish (*Carassius auratus*). *Aquaculture*, 493, 296–301.

Maia, J. G. S., Andrade, E. H. A., Couto, H. A. R., Silva, A. C. M. D., Marx, F. & Henke, C. 2007. Plant sources of Amazon rosewood oil. *Química nova*, 30, 1906–1910.

Maldini, M., Montoro, P. & Pizza, C. 2011. Phenolic compounds from byrsonima crassifolia l. Bark: Phytochemical investigation and quantitative analysis by lc-esi ms/ms. *Journal of Pharmaceutical and Biomedical Analysis*, 56, 1–6.

Martelli, A., Theodoro, V., Gaspi, F. O., Amaral, M. E., Dalia, R. A., Aro, A. A., Esquisatto, M. A., Mendonça, F. A., Andrade, T. A. & Santos, G. M. 2018. *Casearia sylvestris* improved cutaneous burn repair in diabetic rats. *Journal of Pharmacy and Pharmacology*, 6, 551–562.

Martins, D., Alvarenga, M., Roque, N. F. & Felício, J. 1995. Diterpenes and alkaloids from Brazilian Xylopia species. *Química nova*, 18, 14–16.

Moreira, R. R. D., Santos, A. G. D., Carvalho, F. A., Perego, C. H., Crevelin, E. J., Crotti, A. E. M., Cogo, J., Cardoso, M. L. C. & Nakamura, C. V. 2019. Antileishmanial activity of Melampodium divaricatum and Casearia sylvestris essential oils on Leishmania amazonensis. *Revista do instituto de medicina tropical de são paulo*, 61.

Nakatani, N. & Nagashima, M. 1992. Pungent alkamides from Spilanthes acmella l. var. Oleracea clarke. *Bioscience, Biotechnology, and Biochemistry*, 56, 759–762.

Nascimento, L. E. S., Arriola, N. D. A., da Silva, L. A. L., Faqueti, L. G., Sandjo, L. P., de Araújo, C. E. S., Biavatti, M. W., Barcelos-Oliveira, J. L. & Amboni, R. D. D. M. C. 2020. Phytochemical profile of different anatomical parts of jambu (Acmella oleracea (l.) Rk jansen): A comparison between hydroponic and conventional cultivation using pca and cluster analysis. *Food Chemistry*, 332, 127393.

Nascimento, M., Junqueira, J. G. M., Terezan, A. P., Severino, R. P., Silva, T. D. S., Martins, C. H. G., Severino, V. G., Cacuro, T. & Waldman, W. 2018. Chemical composition and antimicrobial activity of essential oils from Xylopia aromatica (Annonaceae) flowers and leaves. *Revista Virtual de Quimica*, 10, 1578–1590.

Neto, J. A. R., Tarôco, B. R. P., dos Santos, H. B., Thomé, R. G., Wolfram, E. & de A Ribeiro, R. I. M. 2020. Using the plants of Brazilian cerrado for wound healing: From traditional use to scientific approach. *Journal of Ethnopharmacology*, 260, 112547.

Okuno, A., Tamemoto, H., Tobe, K., Ueki, K., Mori, Y., Iwamoto, K., Umesono, K., Akanuma, Y., Fujiwara, T. & Horikoshi, H. 1998. Troglitazone increases the number of small adipocytes without the change of white adipose tissue mass in obese zucker rats. *The Journal of Clinical Investigation*, 101, 1354–1361.

Oliveira, V. B., Araújo, R. L., Eidenberger, T. & Brandão, M. G. 2018. Chemical composition and inhibitory activities on dipeptidyl peptidase iv and pancreatic lipase of two underutilized species from the Brazilian Savannah: Oxalis cordata a. St.-hil. and Aylopia aromatica (lam.) Mart. *Food Research International*, 105, 989–995.

Ong, H. M., Mohamad, A. S., Makhtar, N. A., Khalid, M. H., Khalid, S., Perimal, E. K., Mastuki, S. N., Zakaria, Z. A., Lajis, N. & Israf, D. A. 2011. Antinociceptive activity of methanolic extract of Acmella uliginosa (sw.) Cass. *Journal of Ethnopharmacology*, 133, 227–233.

Paulraj, J., Govindarajan, R. & Palpu, P. 2013. The genus spilanthes ethnopharmacology, phytochemistry, and pharmacological properties: A review. *Advances in Pharmacological Sciences*, 2013.

Pierri, E. G., Castro, R. C., Vizioli, E. O., Ferreira, C. M., Cavalheiro, A. J., Tininis, A. G., Chin, C. M. & Santos, A. G. 2017. Anti-inflammatory action of ethanolic extract and clerodane diterpenes from Casearia sylvestris. *Revista brasileira de farmacognosia*, 27, 495–501.

Pimentel, R. B. Q., Souza, D. P., Albuquerque, P. M., Fernandes, A. V., Santos, A. S., Duvoisin, S. & Gonçalves, J. F. C. 2018. Variability and antifungal activity of volatile compounds from *Aniba rosaeodora* ducke, harvested from central amazonia in two different seasons. *Industrial Crops and Products*, 123, 1–9.

Prachayasittikul, V., Prachayasittikul, S., Ruchirawat, S. & Prachayasittikul, V. 2013. High therapeutic potential of Spilanthes acmella: A review. *Excli Journal*, 12, 291.

Ratnasooriya, W., Pieris, K., Samaratunga, U. & Jayakody, J. 2004. Diuretic activity of Spilanthes acmella flowers in rats. *Journal of Ethnopharmacology*, 91, 317–320.

Raut, J. S. & Karuppayil, S. M. 2014. A status review on the medicinal properties of essential oils. *Industrial Crops and Products*, 62, 250–264.

Ribeiro, S. M., Fratucelli, É. D., Bueno, P. C., de Castro, M. K. V., Francisco, A. A., Cavalheiro, A. J. & Klein, M. I. 2019. Antimicrobial and antibiofilm activities of Casearia sylvestris extracts from distinct Brazilian biomes against Streptococcus mutans and Candida albicans. *BMC Complementary and Alternative Medicine*, 19, 1–16.

Rondanelli, M., Fossari, F., Vecchio, V., Braschi, V., Riva, A., Allegrini, P., Petrangolini, G., Iannello, G., Faliva, M. A. & Peroni, G. 2020. Acmella oleracea for pain management. *Fitoterapia*, 140, 104419.

Rovedder, A. P. M., Piazza, E. M., Thomas, P. A., Felker, R. M., Hummel, R. B. & Farias, J. A. D. 2016. Potential medicinal use of forest species of the deciduous seasonal forest from Atlantic forest biome, South Brazil. *Brazilian Archives of Biology and Technology*, 59.

Sampaio Lde, F., Maia, J. G., de Parijós, A. M., de Souza, R. Z. & Barata, L. E. 2012. Linalool from rosewood (Aniba rosaeodora ducke) oil inhibits adenylate cyclase in the retina, contributing to understanding its biological activity. *Phytotherapy Research*, 26, 73–77.

Sarrazin, S. L. F., Oliveira, R. B. D., Maia, J. G. S. & Mourão, R. H. V. 2016. Antibacterial activity of the rosewood (*Aniba rosaeodora* and *a. Parviflora*) linalool-rich oils from the Amazon. *European Journal of Medicinal Plants*, 12, 1–9.

Scalvenzi, L., Grandini, A., Spagnoletti, A., Tacchini, M., Neill, D., Ballesteros, J. L., Sacchetti, G. & Guerrini, A. 2017. Myrcia splendens (sw.) Dc. (syn. M. Fallax (rich.) Dc.)(Myrtaceae) essential oil from Amazonian Ecuador: A chemical characterization and bioactivity profile. *Molecules*, 22, 1163.

Shakri, N. M., Salleh, W. M. N. H. W. & Ali, N. A. M. 2020. Chemical composition and biological activities of the essential oils of genus Xylopia l. (Annonaceae): A review. *Rivista Italiana Delle Sostanze Grasse*, 97, 25–34.

Sharma, R. & Arumugam, N. 2021. N-alkylamides of spilanthes (syn: Acmella): Structure, purification, characterization, biological activities and applications: A review. *Future Foods*, 3, 100022.

Silva, S. G., de Oliveira, M. S., Cruz, J. N., da Costa, W. A., da Silva, S. H. M., Maia, A. A. B., de Sousa, R. L., Junior, R. N. C. & de Aguiar Andrade, E. H. 2021. Supercritical CO2 extraction to obtain Lippia thymoides Mart. & Schauer (Verbenaceae) essential oil rich in thymol and evaluation of its antimicrobial activity. *The Journal of Supercritical Fluids*, 168, 105064.

Silva Junior, I. E., Cechinel Filho, V., Zacchino, S. A., Lima, J. C. D. S. & Martins, D. T. D. O. 2009. Antimicrobial screening of some medicinal plants from Mato Grosso Cerrado. *Revista brasileira de farmacognosia*, 19, 242–248.

Simoni, I., Fernandes, M., Gonçalves, C., de Almeida, A., Costa, S. & Lins, A. 1996. A study on the antiviral characteristics of Persea americana extracts against Aujeszky's disease virus. *Biomedical Letters (United Kingdom)*, 54(215), 173–181.

Singh, B. K., Chaudhari, A. K., Das, S., Tiwari, S., Maurya, A., Singh, V. K. & Dubey, N. K. 2022. Chitosan encompassed Aniba rosaeodora essential oil as innovative green candidate for antifungal and antiaflatoxigenic activity in millets with emphasis on cellular and its mode of action. *Frontiers in Microbiology*, 13.

Sœur, J., Marrot, L., Perez, P., Iraqui, I., Kienda, G., Dardalhon, M., Meunier, J.-R., Averbeck, D. & Huang, M.-E. 2011. Selective cytotoxicity of *Aniba rosaeodora* essential oil towards epidermoid cancer cells through induction of apoptosis. *Mutation Research/ Genetic Toxicology and Environmental Mutagenesis*, 718, 24–32.

Storey, C. & Salem, J. I. 1997. Lay use of amazonian plants for the treatment of tuberculosis. *Acta amazonica*, 27, 175–182.

Talhouk, R., Karam, C., Fostok, S., EL-Jouni, W. & Barbour, E. 2007. Anti-inflammatory bioactivities in plant extracts. *Journal of Medicinal Food*, 10, 1–10.

Teles, A. M., Silva-Silva, J. V., Fernandes, J. M. P., Calabrese, K. D. S., Abreu-Silva, A. L., Marinho, S. C., Mouchrek, A. N., Filho, V. E. M. & Almeida-Souza, F. 2020. *Aniba rosaeodora* (var. Amazonica ducke) essential oil: Chemical composition, antibacterial, antioxidant and antitrypanosomal activity. *Antibiotics (Basel)*, 10.

Uthpala, T. & Navaratne, S. 2021. Acmella oleracea plant; Identification, applications and use as an emerging food source: Review. *Food Reviews International*, 37, 399–414.

Wu, L. C., Fan, N. C., Lin, M. H., Chu, I. R., Huang, S. J., Hu, C. Y. & Han, S. Y. 2008. Anti-inflammatory effect of spilanthol from Spilanthes acmella on murine macrophage by down-regulating lps-induced inflammatory mediators. *Journal of Agricultural and Food Chemistry*, 56, 2341–2349.

Xia, L., Guo, Q., Tu, P. & Chai, X. 2015. The genus casearia: A phytochemical and pharmacological overview. *Phytochemistry Reviews*, 14, 99–135.

Yoshikawa, M., Shimoda, H., Nishida, N., Takada, M. & Matsuda, H. 2002. Salacia reticulata and its polyphenolic constituents with lipase inhibitory and lipolytic activities have mild antiobesity effects in rats. *The Journal of Nutrition*, 132, 1819–1824.

Yusuf, A. A., Lawal, B., Yusuf, M. A., Adejoke, A. O., Raji, F. H. & Wenawo, D. L. 2018. Free radical scavenging, antimicrobial activities and effect of sub-acute exposure to Nigerian Xylopia aethiopica seed extract on liver and kidney functional indices of albino rat. *Iranian Journal of Toxicology*, 12, 51–58.

# 10 Pharmacological Aspects and Chemical Characterization of *Syzygium Aromaticum*
## *Current and Future Trends*

*Jigar Vyas, Nensi Raytthatha, and Bhupendra G. Prajapati*

## 10.1 INTRODUCTION TO CLOVE

Clove, i.e., *Syzygium aromaticum* from the *Myrtaceae* family, is a widely used spice that has been employed for decades as a natural preservative and for a wide range of medical purposes. It is native to Indonesia but is currently cultivated through-out several countries worldwide, including Brazil's Bahia state. It is a rich reservoir of phenol chemicals including eugenol acetate, eugenol, and gallic acid. In a fresh new plant, eugenol is the primary pharmacological compound found in clove, with quantities ranging from 9.3817 to 14.65 gm per 100 gm (Figure 10.1). Other common constituents are beta caryophyllene, methyl salicylate, pinene, vanillin, eugenyl acetate, and α-humulene. It has tremendous possibilities for medicinal, agricultural, and cosmetics use and for a variety of food commodities (Cortés-Rojas et al. 2014).

## 10.2 TECHNOLOGICAL ADVANCEMENTS FOR THE CHEMICAL CHARACTERIZATION OF *SYZYGIUM AROMATICUM*

Numerous techniques are employed for estimation of components of clove; the estimation methods are described further.

### 10.2.1 HPLC-UV DETECTION TECHNIQUE

A Rheodyne injecting valve with a 50-millilitre loop and an Ultraviolet-Visible (UV) detector were used in the HPLC system. Eugenol was analyzed using HPLC-UV at a 380-nanometre range. The stationary phase, i.e., HPLC column was 150 × 3-millimetre internal diameter and contained 5 mm Carbon-18 as packing material

DOI: 10.1201/9781003389774-10

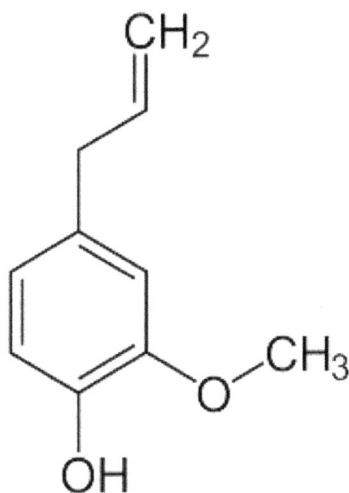

**FIGURE 10.1**   Structure of eugenol.

particles. A Chromatopac Model Co-R8A integration was adopted to character-ize the maxima. Then 0.62 L of acetonitrile was added to 0.38 L of Milli-Q water containing trifluoro-acetic acid (0.1 v/v%) to make the mobile phase. The speci-mens were eluted through the column at room temperature at a rate of 0.43 mL/min (Higashi and Fujii 2010).

## 10.2.2   FTIR Spectroscopy

FTIR spectrum was recorded using a Bruker Tensor II FTIR spectrometer equipped with the temperature-controlled single solitary diamond-attenuated total reflectance (SB-ATR) detector and a crystal-deuterated triglycine sulphate detector. The spec-trum was observed in the 4000–400 cm range (128 scans/sample or background). Using chloroform as a solvent, fluid specimens or physical blends were studied as a film on a NaCl salt plate. The KBr pellet process was employed to record the FTIR spectrum of powdered specimens (Rodríguez et al. 2018).

## 10.2.3   GC-MS Detection Technique

For the GC-MS analysis, a chromatograph was linked to a mass spectrometry detec-tor. The capillaries HP-5MS UI (cross-linkage with 5% phenyl methyl Silox) (30,000 mm × 0.25 mm, layer width 250 mm) have been used. The oven's heating was ele-vated from 40°C to 200°C at a pace of 6°C per minute. After that, the oven was run for 10 minutes at 280°C. The gas phase included helium, having a flow rate of 1.0 mL/min. The injectors and detectors reached temperatures approaching 250–255°C. It was performed with 1 μL of the sample (0.1% in absolute methanol) with scanning modes as well as spitless (Amelia et al. 2017).

### 10.2.4    LC-MS Detection Technique

The distilling residual then macerated in ethanol for 1 day, 3 times, with a sample ratio of 25% and 75%. Column chromatography using LH-20 with ethanol as the solvent was followed by silica chromatography with n-hexane-ethyl acetate 75% and 25% as the eluent. Analysis of LC-MS with auto-sampler. The specifications of the C-18 solvent system are 0.0046 m × 0.25 m. The eluents for separation were 0.110% formic acid in a water medium (solvent A), followed by acetonitrile (solvent B).

### 10.2.5    Nuclear Magnetic Resonance Spectroscopy (NMR)

[1]H NMR data were acquired at 22.85°C using a 500 MHz FT-NMR analyzer using a 5 mm probe. A typical [1]NMR pulsing programmer was used for data acquisition, with the corresponding input parameters: DQD acquisition mode, 6.50 µs pre-scan lag, 0.01 MHz spectrum width, 0.3 Hz FID resolution, 3.277 s acquisition time, 8 scans having a relaxing delay of 1.0 s to observe the findings. Specimens were tested with deuterated chloroform (CCl4) (Kemprai et al. 2019).

### 10.2.6    HPTLC Chromatographic Method

The chromatography was performed out on an aluminium plate (0.1 m × 0.1 m) treated using 0.2 mm silica gels 60 F254. The specimens were placed on the plates in 6 mm bands using a Camag Linomat 5 applicator as well as a 100 µl syringe. The application was constant at 150 mL/s, and the distance between 2 bands was 15 mm. The mobile phase was a 7:3 v/v mixture of e-toluene and ethyl acetate. The chromatogram run was 80 mm in length. Following the development, the plates were withdrawn and air-dried. TLC was used for densitometric scanning at 560 nm (Zanwar et al. 2022).

## 10.3    AN ASSESSMENT OF TOXICITY AND SAFETY ISSUES IN THE USAGE OF *SYZYGIUM AROMATICUM*

Overdoses have been characterized by the loss of consciousness and coma within hours after intake (10–30 mL). There is usually acidosis, respiratory depression, and severe hypoglycaemia, which necessitates ventilation and intravenous (IV) glucose. Liver damage occurs 12–24 hours after intake, with significant increases in blood aminotransferase concentrations with early coagulation difficulties (Mohamed Fawzy Ramadan 2022). When ingested in doses less than 1500 mg/kg, clove oil is usually regarded as a safe substance. On either side, the World Health Organization determined that the daily amount of clove permissible in humans is 2.5 mg/kg. It is readily absorbed if administered orally, reaching plasma and blood rapidly with typical half-lives of 14 and 18 hours, respectively.

The submandibular cell line of humans was employed to study the cytotoxic activity of clove oil, the generation of reactive oxygen species (ROS), and lower levels of γ-l-glutamyl-l-cysteinyl-glycine (GSH). The formation of benzyl radicals is thought to be the primary cause of eugenol's lower GSH, which has been linked to reactive oxygen species independent pathways. Eugenol has less cytotoxic properties than isoeugenol, and this property is dependent on dosage.

## 10.4 PHARMACOLOGICAL ASPECTS OF DIFFERENT *SYZYGIUM AROMATICUM*

Clove is a prominent therapeutic herb due to the substantial range of pharmacologic features consolidated from centuries of traditional usage and outlined in scientific texts. The main pharmacological aspects include those delineated in this section.

### 10.4.1 ANTIOXIDANT ASPECT

The hydroxyl position on the heterocyclic ring is responsible for eugenol's antioxidant activity. Phenolic compounds impede the oxidative pathway by electron transfer to free radicals and neutralizes them.

Three main key pathways of clove activity could underlie this interesting high antioxidant efficacy:

- *Hydrogen donation accompanied by dissociation of a group modified at the para-position*
- *Dimerization of 2 phenoxylated radicals forming the complex*
- *Formation of DPPH with an aryl radical*

It is well known for their functionality to neutralize free radicals, inhibit the formation of ROS and reactive nitrogen species (RNS), increase cytoantioxidant ability, and protect the functioning of proteins and microbial DNA. It may also help with the elimination of damaged fragments, repairing the oxidative damage, and the prevention of cancer-triggering mutations. It is the structure of eugenol which allows it to repair phenoxy ions and free radicals by absorbing provided $H_2$ atoms, which is responsible for its antioxidative property.

In contrast to standard antioxidant substances such as butylated hydroxytoluene, butylated hydroxyanisole, and vitamin E (a natural antioxidant), clove oil was discovered as an efficient antioxidant in multiple *in vitro* experiments. The clove essential oil scavenged a 2,2-diphenyl-1-picryl hydrazyl (DPPH) peroxide at doses lower than that of standard drugs which include BHT, BHA, and vitamin E. Abojid et al. demonstrated enhanced lipid metabolism, renal function, and overall antioxidant condition in clove-treated rats, suggesting that its preventive role in $H_2O_2$-induced cellular damage may well be attributable to bioactive substances present in essential oil or plant extract (Bakour et al. 2018).

Based on the findings of the research, clove can normalize overall amounts of oxidative stress indices (CAT, GSH, H202) in serum and skin, as well as decrease inflammation damages regulated by the NF-κB signalling structure. It can also control the AMPK signalling pathway's energy metabolism and reduce UV-B exposure by regulating Na+-K+ ATPase, which decreases oxidative stress and inflammation in mice, limiting epidermal damage and safeguarding the epidermis. Five active antioxidant components of clove (dihydroquercetin, rutin, ferulic acid, isoquercitrin, and quercitrin) aid in the avoidance of UV-B skin damage, making cloves an essential nutrient for sunscreen.

Sokamte et al. interpreted the strong antioxidant potential as a result of synergistic effects of eugenol and eugenyl acetate as well as the other minor components found in this essential oil. The extracts of clove might potentially be employed as dietary antioxidants (Selles et al. 2020). The storage or cooking durability of encapsulated and unencapsulated eugenol-rich clove preparations in soybean oil was investigated by Chatterjee and Bhattacharjee (2013). Entrapped clove powder produced by spray drying with maltodextrin and gum arabic as barrier elements might provide a controlled release of antioxidants.

## 10.4.2 ANTI-INFLAMMATORY EFFECT

Inflammation is characterized as a complex defensive response of the system towards potentially harmful stimuli such as microorganisms, with the biotic system's target aiming at toxic stimuli from the body while also boosting the treatment. The NF-B signalling pathway is important in the immunological response. By hindering the Raf/MEK/ERK phosphorylated pathways, eugenol may inhibit neutrophils from forming superoxide radicals. Moreover, it is known to suppress proinflammatory mediators such as tumour TNF-alpha, InterLeukins-6 and Interleukin-1, PGE2, inducible oxide nitrate synthase (iNOS), and interpretation of COX-2, leukotriene C4 as well as 5-lipoxygenase (5-LOX), and NF-B. Eugenol's anti-inflammatory property is related with inhibiting neutrophil/macrophage chemotaxis and obstructing the formation of proinflammatory neurotransmitters including LTs and PTGs. 5-LOX and COX-2 are blocked by eugenol so eugenol has the potential to act as an anti-inflammatory agent, allowing it to be a substitute for specific NSAIDs in a variety of conditions. Additionally, it could be used in the expansion of new interdisciplinary molecules to combat ailments associated with inflammation activities, such as cancer or osteoarthritis.

According to Banerjee et al., after 3 hours, similarly to diclofenac gel, eugenol possesses anti-inflammatory effects, promoting healing by 20%–60%. Eugenol-treated mice having developed lesions healed by more than 95% in the first 15 days. The data also revealed that eugenol-treated mice had healing of wounds comparable to neomycin-treated mice, which would be currently used to decrease inflammation and expedite the healing of wounds. As a result, it's essential to avoid both the chronic and the acute harmful consequences of synthesized medicines, especially if they are administered on a regular basis (Banerjee et al. 2020).

With the perspective of eugenol's significance, Barboza et al. investigated its anti-inflammatory and antioxidant characteristics, as well as its modes of action and therapeutic ability to heal inflammatory diseases *in vivo*/*in vitro* (Barboza et al. 2018). According to De Paula Porto et al., eugenol stimulates the dysregulation of TNF-α in LPS-activated macrophages, which is related to antigenotoxic action if DNA damage is caused by doxorubicin. Thus, this research suggests that such molecular mechanisms behind eugenol's anti-inflammatory effects are mediated via the control of inflammatory mediator production by macrophages (de Paula Porto et al. 2014).

The implications of eugenol on the inflammatory response have also been studied in dental tissue fibroblast and recovered molar teeth. Post-operative complications like alveolar osteitis, an inflamed disorder with prolonged recovery and chronic pain, can occur with permanent tooth extractions. In this regard, Martínez-Herrera et al. found that when fibroblasts were subjected to lipopolysaccharide, eugenol suppressed TNF-alpha expression as well as the NF-beta signalling pathway, but not IL-1, indicating its anti-inflammatory activity in bone problems. Interestingly, in the lack of preceding inflammation, eugenol also triggered modest inflammatory gene expression in fibroblasts (Martínez-Herrera et al. 2016).

### 10.4.3 Anti-Viral Aspect

Clove oil has antiviral activities against viruses like HSV types 1 and 2, influenza A viruses, and Ebola. According to the latest study, clove derivatives can reduce the activities of the West Nile virus, rendering them a beneficial treatment for flaviviruses including zika, dengue, and yellow fever. Eugenin, a component isolated from buds of clove, demonstrated antiviral activity against the HSV at a dosage of 10 g/ml. Eugenol may disrupt the highly contagious envelope of newly generated virions thus impeding viral replication at the outset; additionally with eugenol, viruses were deactivated directly, and intracellular and extracellular viruses were inhibited after replication. There is a synergism involving eugenol with acyclovir in the regulation of HSV *in vitro*. Topical treatment of eugenol was observed to prevent the growth of HSV-induced keratitis in mice models (Zhou et al. 2012). Eugenol demonstrated antiprotozoal action against Leishmania, a group of bacteria responsible for a broad spectrum of clinical manifestations; ovicidal activity against *H. contortus*, a parasite found in the gastrointestinal tract; and virucidal effectiveness towards HSV1 and HSV2 viruses. Eugenol may be a viable blocker of the initial process of HIV1 infection due to its capacity to decrease viral multiplication. Eugenol can also promote lymphocyte synthesis, which might explain how it has an anti-HIV1 impact (Aboubakr et al. 2016).

Clove oil has antiviral action against feline calicivirus, which is used to substitute human norovirus. As a consequence, employing clove oil in the procedure of rinsing vegetables and fruits removes the virus loading that might occur. Furthermore, the use of clove oil in cleansing wipes enables surface cleansing (Lane et al. 2019). Additionally, clove oil has been demonstrated to be more effective than moroxydine hydrochloride in increasing tomato plant resistance to tomato yellow leaf curl virus. All therapeutic applications of clove essential oil are depicted in Figure 10.2.

### 10.4.4 Anti-Fungal Aspect

Even after the discovery of several innovative antifungals which have greatly improved the therapies of invasive mycoses, new antifungals still confront obstacles

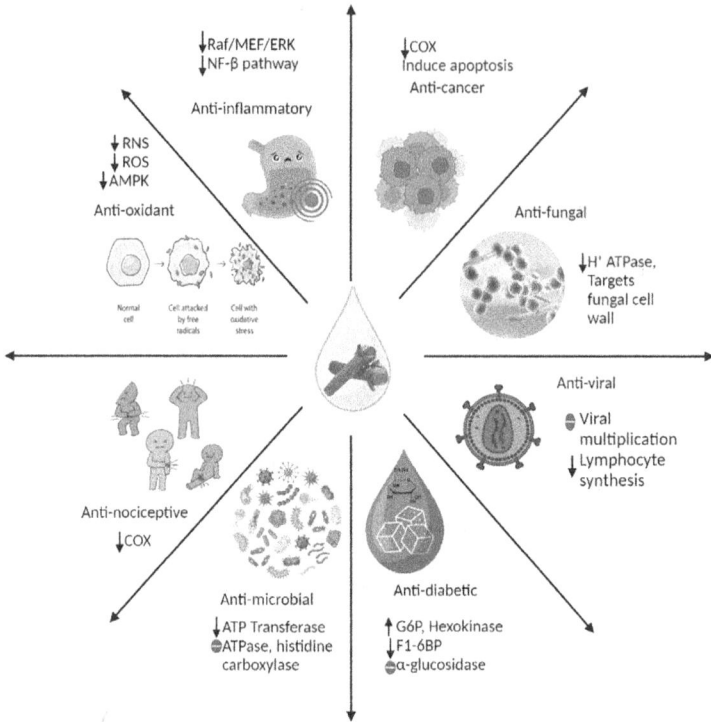

**FIGURE 10.2** Therapeutic applications of clove essential oil.

due to the toxic effects involved with long-term use; as a result, the development of new antifungal agents with better safety profiles is strongly influenced by the adverse effects of the current traditional antifungal drug as well as fungal resistance (Palaniappan and Holley 2010). Eugenol has demonstrated significant antifungal activity on *Candida albicans* preformed biofilms, adhering cells, continued biofilm formation, and cell morphogenesis. It is hypothesized that cell wall modification leads to eugenol's antifungal effectiveness on *S. cerevisiae*.

The fungicidal pathogenic actions of eugenol in *Candida albicans* are mostly attributable to membrane disruption as well as substantial reduction of the defense mechanism by free radical cascade mediated LPO, which results in membrane lesions. Interestingly, the inhibition of amino acid permeases adds to eugenol's inhibitory impact. The research showed eugenol inhibited the transportation of amino acid residues across the yeast cytoplasmic barrier via two permeases (Tat1p and Gap1p). Secondly, the synergistic antifungal activity of eugenol and cinnamaldehyde is caused by the inhibition of fungal cell wall formation along with cell wall degradation in fungal cells. The chromatography analyses revealed eugenol was the major component accountable for the antifungal activity produced through spore or micelle lysis. Devi et al. reported a comparable mode of action of membrane disruption and macromolecule deformation induced by eugenol (Yadav et al. 2015).

Noticeably, clove oil had significant fungicidal activity towards pathogenic fungus strains resistant to azoles, which has been related to the suppression of $H^+$ATPase functioning (Devi et al. 2010). Antigonorrheal efficacy also was reported in a number of multiresistant *N. gonorrhoeae* strains. Interestingly, eugenol was shown to be more effective than the synthetic antiseptics chlorhexidine, cetylpyridinium salt, and triclosan towards fluconazole-resistant *Candida dubliniensis*.

### 10.4.5 INSECTICIDAL ASPECT

Since the 1940s, researchers have been investigating the insecticidal effects of clove oil and its derivatives. The toxicity of clove oil differs among insects due to changes in insect sensitivity, variation in the content of eugenol, and other active components in the clove oil.

Clove oil has acaricidal effects. The results revealed that clove oil was particularly harmful to scabies mites. Acetyl eugenol and isoeugenol acted as a positive control acaricide, eradicating mites within 60 mins of contact. In comparison to typical scabies treatment, which includes the synthetic pesticide permethrin as well as the oral medication ivermectin, a natural choice like clove is much more highly desired. Clove oil killed mites at concentrations ranging between 1.56% to 25% clove oil in under 15 minutes, compared to mites killed by permethrin (Pasay et al. 2010).

Clove oil was discovered to be the most efficient termiticide for termite management. It was also efficient as a fumigant as well as a feeding deterrent, which made it ideal for managing grass and ornamental insect pests. A mixture of 50% clove oil, 50% geranium oil, or 50% thyme oil reduced biting. The best efficient mosquito repellents were thyme and clove oils, which gave 1.5 to 3.5 hrs of repellent activity in *A. aegypti* and *A. albimanus* (Devi et al. 2010).

### 10.4.6 ANTIDIABETIC ASPECT

Clove oil is a potent anti-diabetic bioactive compound. Because of its multiple pharmacological effects, clove oil has been proven in trials to be effective in healing a variety of metabolic ailments. Clove oil stimulates carbohydrate metabolic enzymes such as hexokinase and glucose-6-phosphate dehydrogenase. According to studies, the use of clove oil has a lowering effect on fructose-1,6-bisphosphatase, creatine kinase, blood urea nitrogen, and glucose-6-phosphatase (Srinivasan et al. 2014).

According to Anuj et al., clove oil primarily inhibits alpha-glucosidases after interfering with the production of enhanced glycation end products. Dietetic complex carbohydrates do not release absorbable monosaccharides in the presence of α-glycosidase inhibitors such as eugenol. By delaying glucose absorption into the bloodstream, the inhibitors limit any significant increase in meal-induced glucose levels in the blood (Nisar et al. 2021).

The activity of the enzymes involved in glucose metabolism was investigated by Srinivasan et al., by administering streptozotocin (40 mg/kg B.W.) to male rats to evaluate the effectiveness of clove oil. A 10 mg/kg of B.W. dose of clove oil significantly increased liver glucose and insulin in plasma, while decreasing glycosylated hemoglobin and blood sugar levels (Carvalho et al. 2018).

### 10.4.7  ANTI-MICROBIAL ASPECT

Clove has shown extensive microbial-inhibitory activity. The hydroxyl group in the para and meta positions of the primary chemical structure has been associated with antimicrobial activity. The chromatographic assessments indicated that eugenol was the major component implicated in the antimicrobial activity mediated via spores and micelle ruptures.

Certain functional groups can engage with the cytoplasm membrane of microbial cells. Clove can penetrate cellular membranes due to its lipid-soluble characteristics. When clove interacts with fatty acids, phospholipids, and polysaccharides, the cell membrane's integrity is disrupted, the components of the cells leak out, and the proton pump is disrupted, resulting in cell death.

### 10.4.8  ANTINOCICEPTIVE ASPECT

Since the 1300s, clove has been used as a painkiller for toothache, joint pain, and antispasmodic, with eugenol being the major component responsible for this effect. The evolved mechanism has been linked to the stimulation of calcium and chloride channels within ganglion cells. The voltage-dependent actions of eugenol in both calcium and sodium channels, as well as receptor located in the trigeminal ganglia, also contributed to clove's analgesic effect. Nuziel et al. reported found that eugenol had antinociceptive effect in the peripheral nervous system at dosages of 50, 75, and 100 mg/kg (Oliveira and Arruda 2021). Ethanol extracts of clove were found to possess anti-nociceptive as well as anti-inflammatory effects in *Rattus norvegicus* rats and mice, as assessed by acetic acid-induced contractions in the mice gut as well as formalin-stimulated hind paw edoema in *Rattus norvegicus* rats lending creditability to the plant's conventional use in painful and inflammatory conditions. The local anaesthetic effect of β-caryophyllene was able to significantly diminish electrically elicited contraction of the rat phrenic hemidiaphragm in a dose-dependent manner.

### 10.4.9  ANTI-TUMOUR ASPECT

Cancer often produces tumours through cellular build-up and uncontrollable cell proliferation. It is the second largest cause of mortality globally, accounting for 6 million deaths each year. Cell aggregation may emerge as a result of inflammation due to improper functioning of the signalling pathway (Oliveira and Arruda 2021). Chemotherapy is chiefly used to eradicate cancerous cells; however, it also induces the division of normal cells in hair follicles, bone marrow, and other tissues. So, chemoprotective biological agents such as clove oil are recommended for tumour treatment. These agents have no cytotoxic impact on healthy normal cells even at large doses. The US FDA has certified clove oil to be a non-mutagenic and non-carcinogenic agent. Clove oil has been shown to have anticancer activities against colon carcinoma, breast carcinoma, cervical carcinoma, lung carcinoma, and gastric carcinoma.

**TABLE 10.1**

**Effectiveness of Clove Oil against Different Types of Cancers**

| Type of Carcinoma | Mechanism of Action | Clinical Studies | References |
|---|---|---|---|
| Colon | Clove oil with cisplatin, doxorubicin, and cinnamaldehyde-like drugs synergistically boost the apoptotic and cytotoxic effects. | Petrocelli et al. identified cinnamaldehyde and eugenol as anticancer agents that specifically target modified colonic cells. Both cinnamaldehyde and eugenol induced death of cells, necrosis, and cell cycle deceleration in Caco-2 including SW-620 cells after 3 days of treatment, but not NCM-460 cells. | (Petrocelli et al. 2021) |
| Breast | Inhibits E2F1 as well as its downstream anti-apoptosis target and inhibits breast cancer-related gene mutations. | Abdullah et al. evaluated the possibility of using clove oil against MDA-MB-231 and SK-BR-3 carcinoma cells of the breast as an antitumor and antiproliferative agent. Clove oil treatment significantly reduces MMP2 and MMP9 expression while enhancing TIMP1 expression in both triple negative and HER2-positive breast carcinoma cells. It significantly increased the fraction of MDA-MB-231 and SK-BR-3 cells exhibiting death of cells and increased the expression of Caspase3, Caspase7, and Caspase9. | (Abdullah et al. 2018) |
| Cervical | Apoptosis is enhanced by cellular migration and suppression using clove oil at high concentrations. | Permatasari et al. investigated eugenol's effect on cellular migration, specifically in HeLa cells which were exposed to various concentrations of eugenol in scratched wellbores. Eugenol increases apoptosis in HeLa cells. It was cytotoxic to HeLa cells at doses that ranged from 50 to 200 μM. | (Happy Kurnia et al. 2021) |
| Lung | Clove oil decreases cyclo-oxygenase-2 (COX-2) activity, causes S-phase cellular phase arrest, and initiates apoptosis. | Choudhury et al. investigated drug-resistant and strongest cancerous cells identified as cancer stem cells by studying their regulator molecule β-catenin. A safe dose of eugenol was shown to cause death of cells while suppressing cell migration inside the lung tissues of cancer-treated mice while having no effect on healthy mice. | (Choudhury et al. 2021) |
| Gastric | Stops tumor progression, boosts pro-invasive and angiogenesis factors, and induces death of cells via the mitochondrial route via regulating B-cell leukemia/lymphoma-2 proteins. | Manikandan et al. investigated the chemoprotective effects of clove oil on N-methyl-N'-nitro-N-nitrosoguanidine induced gastric carcinoma on *Rattus norvegicus* rats. N-methyl-N'-nitro-N-nitrosoguanidine-treated rats acquired gastric carcinogenesis, evading death of cells and increasing pro-invasive and angiogenic elements. Clove oil treatment-induced death of cells through modulating B-cell leukemia/lymphoma-2 protein family proteins, apoptotic protease activating factor-1, cytochrome C, and caspase, while decreasing cell growth and thus causing cell death. | (Padhy et al. 2022) |

## 10.5 CLINICAL AND META-CLINICAL STUDIES DONE WITH *SYZYGIUM AROMATICUM* UTILIZING THEIR PHARMACEUTICAL APPLICATION

Clove has several applications, including dentistry, skincare, and anticancer.

- Dentistry: Clove oil was proven to be efficient in preventing tooth erosion, leading to the assumption that clove oil may prevent cavities just as fluorides. Many marketed formulations including gels, toothpastes, and creams are available for toothache, anti-inflammatory, and analgesic effects. Applying clove oil to a painful tooth may help ease pain. Clove oil has also been proven to reduce oral pain.
- Skincare: Clove is one spice that is rich in antioxidants and antimicrobial qualities. According to Ayurveda, clove oil is rich in therapeutic qualities and has some excellent skin benefits. This oil aids in the prevention and treatment of acne, as well as the reduction of redness, discomfort, blemishes, and scars. It aids in the removal of impurities from the pore, hence avoiding future outbursts. It also inhibits allergies and bacterial development in the skin, which aids in the appearance of healthy skin. To enhance the quality of skin, several formulations such as creams, oils, and gels are available.
- Cancer therapy: The researchers developed a clove oil-based emulsion to treat cancer, stating that the formulation has tremendous potential in the treatment of undifferentiated melanoma cells and can also bypass anti-microbial resistance. Clove essential oils have provided the way for the development of new alternatives to the drawbacks of synthetic medications.

## 10.6 CONCLUSION

The FDA considers *Syzygium aromaticum* to be relatively acceptable and is a precious spice that has been used for ages as a food preservative. Based on the scientific proofs, it is possible to infer that clove is a highly intriguing plant with significant pharmacological potential. It has shown numerous biological activities that have led to the development of several classes of medicine, and it has effectively replaced many synthetic drugs for treatment of various ailments.

## REFERENCES

Abdullah, Mashan L., et al. "Anti-Metastatic and Anti-Proliferative Activity of Eugenol against Triple Negative and HER2 Positive Breast Cancer Cells." *BMC Complementary and Alternative Medicine*, vol. 18, no. 1, Dec. 2018, https://doi.org/10.1186/s12906-018-2392-5.

Aboubakr, Hamada A., et al. "In Vitro Antiviral Activity of Clove and Ginger Aqueous Extracts against Feline Calicivirus, a Surrogate for Human Norovirus." *Journal of Food Protection*, vol. 79, no. 6, June 2016, pp. 1001–1012, https://doi.org/10.4315/0362-028x.jfp-15-593.

Amelia, B., et al. "GC-MS Analysis of Clove (Syzygium Aromaticum) Bud Essential Oil from Java and Manado." *AIP Conference Proceedings*, 2017, https://doi.org/10.1063/1.4991186.

Bakour, Meryem, et al. "The Antioxidant Content and Protective Effect of Argan Oil and *Syzygium aromaticum* Essential Oil in Hydrogen Peroxide-Induced Biochemical and Histological Changes." *International Journal of Molecular Sciences*, vol. 19, no. 2, Feb. 2018, p. 610, https://doi.org/10.3390/ijms19020610.

Banerjee, Kaushita, et al. "Anti-Inflammatory and Wound Healing Potential of a Clove Oil Emulsion." *Colloids and Surfaces: B, Biointerfaces*, vol. 193, Sept. 2020, p. 111102, https://doi.org/10.1016/j.colsurfb.2020.111102.

Barboza, Joice Nascimento, et al. "An Overview on the Anti-Inflammatory Potential and Antioxidant Profile of Eugenol." *Oxidative Medicine and Cellular Longevity*, vol. 2018, 2018, p. 3957262, https://doi.org/10.1155/2018/3957262.

Carvalho, M., et al. "In Vitro Antimicrobial Activities of Various Essential Oils against Pathogenic and Spoilage Microorganisms." *Journal of Food Quality and Hazards Conrol*, vol. 5, no. 2, June 2018, pp. 41–48, https://doi.org/10.29252/jfqhc.5.2.3.

Chatterjee, Dipan, and Paramita Bhattacharjee. "Comparative Evaluation of the Antioxidant Efficacy of Encapsulated and Un-Encapsulated Eugenol-Rich Clove Extracts in Soybean Oil: Shelf-Life and Frying Stability of Soybean Oil." *Journal of Food Engineering*, vol. 117, no. 4, Aug. 2013, pp. 545–550, https://doi.org/10.1016/j.jfoodeng.2012.11.016.

Choudhury, Pritha, et al. "Eugenol Emerges as an Elixir by Targeting β-Catenin, the Central Cancer Stem Cell Regulator in Lung Carcinogenesis: An in Vivo and in Vitro Rationale." *Food & Function*, vol. 12, no. 3, Feb. 2021, pp. 1063–1078, https://doi.org/10.1039/D0FO02105A.

Cortés-Rojas, Diego Francisco, et al. "Clove (Syzygium Aromaticum): A Precious Spice." *Asian Pacific Journal of Tropical Biomedicine*, vol. 4, no. 2, Feb. 2014, pp. 90–96, https://doi.org/10.1016/s2221-1691(14)60215-x.

de Paula Porto, Marilia, et al. "Citral and Eugenol Modulate DNA Damage and Pro-Inflammatory Mediator Genes in Murine Peritoneal Macrophages." *Molecular Biology Reports*, vol. 41, no. 11, Aug. 2014, pp. 7043–7051, https://doi.org/10.1007/s11033-014-3657-9.

Devi, K. Pandima, et al. "Eugenol (an Essential Oil of Clove) Acts as an Antibacterial Agent against Salmonella Typhi by Disrupting the Cellular Membrane." *Journal of Ethnopharmacology*, vol. 130, no. 1, July 2010, pp. 107–115, https://doi.org/10.1016/j.jep.2010.04.025.

Happy Kurnia, Permatasari, et al. "Eugenol Isolated from *Syzygium aromaticum* Inhibits HeLa Cancer Cell Migration by Altering Epithelial-Mesenchymal Transition Protein Regulators." *Journal of Applied Pharmaceutical Science*, vol. 11, no. 5, May 2021, https://doi.org/10.7324/japs.2021.110507.

Higashi, Yasuhiko, and Youichi Fujii. "HPLC-UV Analysis of Eugenol in Clove and Cinnamon Oils after Pre-Column Derivatization with 4-Fluoro-7-Nitro-2,1,3-Benzoxadiazole." *Journal of Liquid Chromatography & Related Technologies*, vol. 34, no. 1, Dec. 2010, pp. 18–25, https://doi.org/10.1080/10826076.2011.534689.

Kemprai, Phirose, et al. "*Piper Betleoides* C. DC.: Edible Source of Betel-Scented Sesquiterpene-Rich Essential Oil." *Flavour and Fragrance Journal*, vol. 35, no. 1, Oct. 2019, pp. 70–78, https://doi.org/10.1002/ffj.3537.

Lane, Thomas, et al. "The Natural Product Eugenol Is an Inhibitor of the Ebola Virus in Vitro." *Pharmaceutical Research*, vol. 36, no. 7, May 2019, p. 104, https://doi.org/10.1007/s11095-019-2629-0.

Martínez-Herrera, Andrea, et al. "Effect of 4-Allyl-1-Hydroxy-2-Methoxybenzene (Eugenol) on Inflammatory and Apoptosis Processes in Dental Pulp Fibroblasts." *Mediators of Inflammation*, vol. 2016, 2016, pp. 1–7, https://doi.org/10.1155/2016/9371403.

Mohamed Fawzy Ramadan. *Clove (Syzygium Aromaticum)*. Academic Press, 2022.

Nisar, Muhammad Farrukh, et al. "Pharmacological Properties and Health Benefits of Eugenol: A Comprehensive Review." *Oxidative Medicine and Cellular Longevity*, edited by Antonella Smeriglio, vol. 2021, Aug. 2021, pp. 1–14, https://doi.org/10.1155/2021/2497354.

Oliveira, Natália Sakuray, and Evilanna Lima Arruda. "Estudos in Silico Sobre as Atividades Anticancerígenas Do Eugenol Presente No Cravo Da Índia (Syzygium Aromaticum)." *Research, Society and Development*, vol. 10, no. 4, Apr. 2021, p. e27910414165, https://doi.org/10.33448/rsd-v10i4.14165.

Padhy, Ipsa, et al. "Molecular Mechanisms of Action of Eugenol in Cancer: Recent Trends and Advancement." *Life*, vol. 12, no. 11, Nov. 2022, p. 1795, https://doi.org/10.3390/life12111795.

Palaniappan, Kavitha, and Richard A. Holley. "Use of Natural Antimicrobials to Increase Antibiotic Susceptibility of Drug Resistant Bacteria." *International Journal of Food Microbiology*, vol. 140, no. 2–3, June 2010, pp. 164–168, https://doi.org/10.1016/j.ijfoodmicro.2010.04.001.

Pasay Cielo, Mounsey Kate, Stevenson Graeme, Davis Rohan, Arlian Larry, et al. "Acaricidal Activity of Eugenol Based Compounds against Scabies Mites." *PLoS One,* vol. 5, no.8, Aug. 2010, p. e12079, doi:10.1371/journal.pone.0012079.

Petrocelli, Giovannamaria, et al. "Molecules Present in Plant Essential Oils for Prevention and Treatment of Colorectal Cancer (CRC)." *Molecules*, vol. 26, no. 4, Feb. 2021, p. 885, https://doi.org/10.3390/molecules26040885.

Rodríguez, José Daniel Wicochea, et al. "Rapid Quantification of Clove (Syzygium Aromaticum) and Spearmint (Mentha Spicata) Essential Oils Encapsulated in a Complex Organic Matrix Using an ATR-FTIR Spectroscopic Method." *PLoS One*, edited by Christopher Michael Fellows, vol. 13, no. 11, Nov. 2018, p. e0207401, https://doi.org/10.1371/journal.pone.0207401.

Selles, Sidi Mohammed Ammar, et al. "Chemical Composition, In-Vitro Antibacterial and Antioxidant Activities of *Syzygium aromaticum* Essential Oil." *Journal of Food Measurement and Characterization*, vol. 14, no. 4, May 2020, pp. 2352–2358, doi:https://doi.org/10.1007/s11694-020-00482-5.

Srinivasan, Subramani, et al. "Ameliorating Effect of Eugenol on Hyperglycemia by Attenuating the Key Enzymes of Glucose Metabolism in Streptozotocin-Induced Diabetic Rats." *Molecular and Cellular Biochemistry*, vol. 385, nos. 1–2, 2014, pp. 159–169.

Yadav, Mukesh Kumar, et al. "Eugenol: A Phyto-Compound Effective against Methicillin-Resistant and Methicillin-Sensitive Staphylococcus Aureus Clinical Strain Biofilms." *PLoS One*, edited by Christophe Beloin, vol. 10, no. 3, Mar. 2015, p. e0119564, https://doi.org/10.1371/journal.pone.0119564.

Zanwar, Aarti S., et al. "Spectrophotometric Methods for the Analysis of Berberine Hydrochloride and Eugenol in Formulated Emulgel." *Journal of Natural Remedies*, vol. 22, no. 3, July 2022, pp. 440–448, https://doi.org/10.18311/jnr/2022/30166.

Zhou, Liman, et al. "Eugenol Inhibits Quorum Sensing at Sub-Inhibitory Concentrations." *Biotechnology Letters*, vol. 35, no. 4, Dec. 2012, pp. 631–637, https://doi.org/10.1007/s10529-012-1126-x.

# 11 Advanced Anticancer Application of *Thymus Zygis* Essential Oil (EOT)

*Jaya Rautela, Shivani Rawat, and Vikash Jakhmola*

## 11.1 INTRODUCTION

*Thymus zygis (Th. zygis)* is an aromatic plant which belongs to the genus *Thymus L.*, family *Lamiaceae*. *Th. zygis* has been used for a long time as a spice or drug and is immensely important economically. As spice it enhances the flavour of food and acts as a preservative. On the Iberian Peninsula, the genus *Thymus L.* is widely dispersed (Gonçalves et al. 2010; Schmidt et al. 2004). *Th. zygis* leaves and flowers are covered in glandular trichomes that secrete essential oil that is high in monoterpenes (Rota et al. 2008; Yakoubi et al. 2014). The synonyms of *Th. zygis* are Spanish thyme, which is indigenous to Portugal, Spain, Algeria, and Morocco (Anastasia et al. 2021); and 'erva-de-Santa-Maria' and 'Ziitra' which are regional names for *Th. zygis* (Zerkani et al. 2022). EOT is widely known for its bioactive properties, which include antimicrobial, antifungal, antiviral, insecticidal, and other characteristics. Nevertheless, recently, *Th. zygis*'s anticancer activity has also been thoroughly investigated (Cutillas et al. 2018; Viuda-Martos et al. 2010; Mosmann et al. 1983; Raudone et al. 2017; Vlaicu et al. 2022; Abeer et al. 2019).

## 11.2 CHEMICAL COMPONENTS OF THYME

Chromatographic combined with spectrometric study of the chemical composition of the EOT revealed 18 constituents, which accounted for 94% of the total portion of the EO (Table 11.1 and Figure 11.2). The main constituents were identified as thymol (43.17%), carvacrol (13.00%), and p-cymene (10.58%) (Figure 11.1) (Coimbra et al. 2022; Silva et al. 2020; Afonso et al. 2018; Radi et al. 2021).

Other miscellaneous components of EOT are sabinene, α-cadinol, trans-verbenol, α-terpineol, δ-2-carene, Z-ocimenone, β-pinene, α-terpinene-7-al, campholenal, α-phellandrene, bornyl acetate, thymol, δ-3-carene, ethylether carvacrol, 1,4-cineole, 1,8-cineole, nerol, geraniol, linalyl acetate, carvacrol, E-caryophyllene, β-humulene, ρ-cymene, o-cymene, D-germacrene, β-E-ocimene, β-Z-ocimene, δ-cadinene, D-4-ol de germacrene, γ-terpinene, allo-aromadendrene, trans-β-elemenone, carvone, cis-oxide de linalool, caryophyllene oxide, neral, geranial, metacymenene, bicyclogermacrene, and myrcene (Abdoul-Latif et al. 2021).

DOI: 10.1201/9781003389774-11

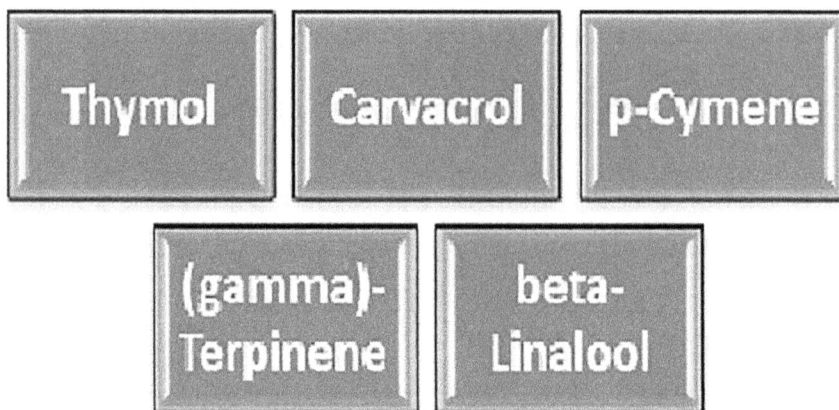

**FIGURE 11.1**    The most abundant phytoconstituents of EOT.

**TABLE 11.1**
**Phytochemical Constituents of EOT**

| S. No. | Phytoconstituents | Retention Time | Percentage |
|---|---|---|---|
| 1 | Thymol | 22.78 | 43.17 |
| 2 | Carvacrol | 22.99 | 13.00 |
| 3 | p-Cymene | 14.31 | 10.58 |
| 4 | γ-Terpinene | 15.50 | 8.04 |
| 5 | β-Linalool | 16.85 | 3.77 |
| 6 | β-Caryophyllene | 26.03 | 1.43 |
| 7 | α-Terpinene | 13.98 | 1.38 |
| 8 | β-Myrcene | 13.14 | 1.29 |
| 9 | Camphene | 11.50 | 1.19 |
| 10 | Trans-Sabinene hydrate | 15.71 | 1.14 |
| 11 | Camphor | 18.16 | 1.10 |
| 12 | α-Pinene | 10.98 | 1.01 |
| 13 | Trans-pinocarveol | 18.31 | 0.89 |
| 14 | α-Thujene | 10.75 | 0.73 |
| 15 | Caryophyllene oxide | 30.01 | 0.59 |
| 16 | Limonene | 14.42 | 0.56 |
| 17 | Borneol | 18.90 | 0.46 |
| 18 | 4-Terpineol | 19.21 | 0.46 |

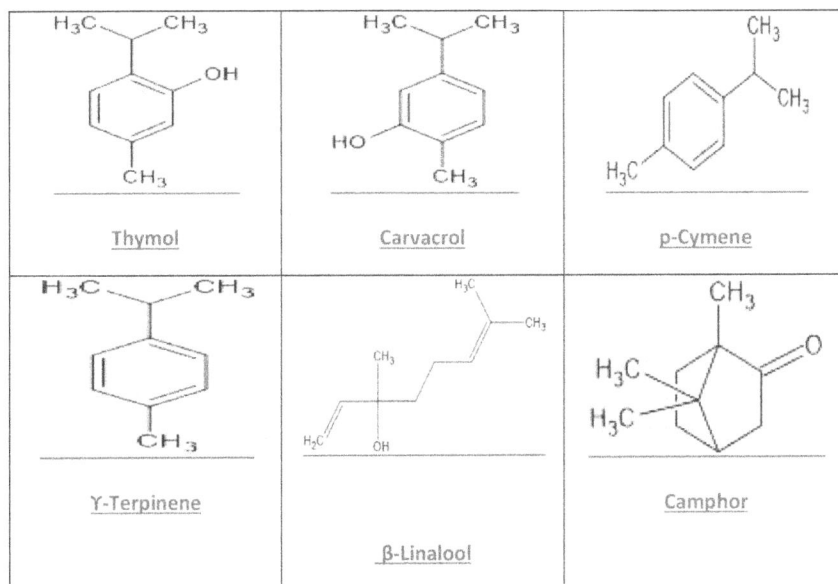

FIGURE 11.2   Chemical structures of phytoconstituents from EOT.

## 11.3   PHARMACOLOGICAL PROPERTIES OF EOT WITH SPECIAL REFERENCE OF ANTICANCER ACTIVITY

### 11.3.1   ANTICANCER ACTIVITY

Initially, inflammatory and oxidative disorders have been the focus of research into and use of essential oils. As a result of the EOT's reaction with oxygen species, which have been associated with the cause of oxidation and inflammation that can result in cancer, it is evident that the EOT can also engage as a cancer-preventive agent (Jackson and Loeb 2001). Thymol is a monoterpene; it serves as the primary ingredient of thyme essential oil and has anti-inflammatory, antibacterial, and antioxidant qualities. Thymol exhibits anti-tumour effects through a number of mechanisms, including apoptosis induction, induction of cell death (antiproliferative activity), and generation of subcellular ROS. Several studies have been conducted that demonstrate the potential of EOT as an anticancer agent (Luís et al. 2017).

In 2020, A.M. Silva and his colleagues used the alamarBlue™ assay to investigate cytotoxic and other effects of different extracts of *Th. zygis* on Caco-2 and HepG2 cell lines. Different *Th. zygis* extract concentrations (50, 100, 200, 500, and 750 g/mL) were treated with the cells for 24 or 48 hours. Cytotoxic assay results contrasted with control cells. Cell viability is decreased to values below 20% of control at doses more than 200 g/mL (both cell lines, both exposure times). However, the antiproliferative/cytotoxic effect has been tested against Caco-2 and HepG2 cells, with evidence showing that the AD extract had only slightly reduced cell viability at higher concentrations ($IC_{50} > 600$ µg/mL, 48 hours exposure), denoting very low toxicity, while the HE extract showed a high antiproliferative effect, especially at 48 hours exposure ($IC_{50}$ of 85.01 ± 15.10 µg/mL and 82.19 ± 2.46 µg/mL, for Caco-2 and HepG2, respectively) (Silva et al. 2020).

A.J. Delgado and his team evaluated the antioxidant, antimicrobial, and cytotoxic activities of EOs from *T. capitata* and *Thymus* species. The high antioxidant capacity has been observed with significant antimicrobial activity in both plants. For cytotoxicity, the minimum inhibitory concentration obtained in range from 0.1 to 0.01 µL/mL (Delgado-Adámez et al. 2017).

Vanessa Rodrigues and her colleagues investigate the anti-inflammatory activity of *Thymus zygis* L. subsp. sylvestris (Hoffmanns. & Link) Cout. oil and its constituents. The anti-inflammatory activity of *Th. zygis* subsp. sylvestris essential oil was examined in lipopolysaccharide (LPS)-induced nitric oxide (NO) generation by macrophages and microglia treated concurrently with LPS. At doses of up to 0.32 and 0.16 L/mL, respectively, our data showed a significant decrease in LPS-induced NO generation. The essential oil of *Th. zygis* and its principal components were tested for cell viability in the following cell lines: macrophages (RAW 264.7), microglia (BV2), keratinocytes (HaCaT), hepatocytes (HepG2), and alveolar epithelial (A549). A colorimetric assay using the MTT reduction was used to assess cell viability. At densities of $0.6 \times 10^6$, $0.3 \times 10^6$, $0.2 \times 10^6$, $0.2 \times 10^6$, and $0.2 \times 10^6$ cells/well, macrophages (RAW 264.7), microglia (BV2), keratinocytes (HaCaT), hepatocytes (HepG2), and alveolar epithelial cells (A549) were cultivated. Cells were grown in 48-well microplates with a final capacity of 600 L for 12 hours before being exposed to various concentrations of essential oil and its major compounds (600 L medium − control; 588 L media + 12 L each dilution of essential oil or major compound). The highest dose that can be employed without impacting cell viability in macrophages is 0.32 L/mL, and at this concentration, an inhibition of more than 30% was attained. In microglia, the highest safe dose of the oil is 0.16 L/mL, with inhibition more than 70% at this concentration (Rodrigues et al. 2019).

Because thymol is abundant in *Thymus zygis*, Elbe and his colleagues investigated the anti-cancer activity of thymol in particular. They investigated thymol's antiproliferative and apoptotic activities in prostate cancer (PC-3, DU145), breast cancer (MDA-MB-231), and lung cancer (KLN205) cell lines. At 24 hours, 48 hours, and 72 hours, the cancer cells were treated with various doses of thymol (100, 200, 400, 600, and 800 M). The MTT assay was used to measure cell viability, while the annexin V assay was used to determine apoptosis. Thymol was found to have a dose- and time-dependent cytotoxic effect in cancer cell lines PC-3, DU145, MDA-MB-231, and KLN205. Their findings showed that thymol had antiproliferative and apoptotic characteristics in lung, breast, and prostate cancer cell lines (Elbe et al. 2020).

Devasahayam Jaya Balan and his coworker conducted another research in 2020. The cytotoxic effect of thymol on A549 cells was evaluated using the MTT test. The stains DCF-DA, PI, and AO/EtBr were used to evaluate ROS generation, macromolecular damage, and apoptosis, respectively. Thymol's antiproliferative activity on A549 cells was discovered to be dosage- and time-dependent, with $IC_{50}$ values of 112 g/mL (745 M) at 24 h. The aforementioned research indicates that *Thymus zygis*, which contains thymol, may be a potent therapeutic agent for the treatment of several types of cancer (Balan et al. 2021).

## 11.3.2 ANTIPROLIFERATIVE MECHANISMS OF ACTION OF EOT

Resisting cell death, maintaining proliferative signals, and dodging growth suppressors are important characteristics of cancer (Vimalanathan and Hudson 2014). As a result, medicinal approaches that aim to cause apoptosis and cellular arrest are clearly significant. Both the internal (and mitochondria-dependent) and extrinsic (or death receptor-dependent) apoptosis mechanisms have been demonstrated to be induced by EOT.

Carvacrol, a phenolic monoterpenoid that is prevalent in the essential oils of oregano and thyme, was examined in another investigation to determine its mode of action. Carvacrol triggered apoptosis in MDA-MB-231 by permeabilizing the mitochondrial membrane, which led to the release of cytochrome C, the stimulation of caspases as seen by PARP cleavage, and DNA fragmentation (Arunasree et al. 2010). In MDA-MB-231 cells, preparations of frankincense from the *Boswellia sacra* tree caused PARP breakage and apoptosis with a better cancer cell specificity (Suhail et al. 2011). Citral has also been demonstrated to activate caspase and therefore induce apoptosis in a variety of cancer cell types, including glioblastoma and colorectal cancer (Dudai et al. 2005; Queiroz et al. 2014; Sheikh et al. 2017). Other studies have demonstrated that citral therapy can decrease the expression of stemness and prosurvival markers such as microtubule activity regulating kinase 4 (MARK4) and aldehyde dehydrogenase 1A3 (ALDH1A3) in cancer, respectively (Tomas et al. 2016; Naz et al. 2018). A crucial protein known as PKB (protein kinase B) is involved in cellular metabolism, transcription, cell cycle progression, and survival (Fayard et al. 2005). Non-small cell lung carcinoma cells, a cancer form with a high mortality rate, underwent cell cycle arrest and apoptosis when exposed to the vapour of plant-derived seed oil. The study found that apoptosis was caused by a significant decrease in the expression of the mTOR protein (mechanistic target of rapamycin) and a fall in PPDK1's phosphorylating capacity, which dephosphorylated PKB and started the caspase-dependent apoptosis pathway (Seal et al. 2012).

A monoterpenoid alcohol called gamma-terpineol was able to block the transcription of NFB in a variety of tumour cells, with NCI-H69 small cell lung carcinoma cell line having the largest inhibitory effect (Hassan et al. 2010).

## 11.4 EMERGING MEDICINAL STRATEGIES FOR EOT AND ITS PHYTOCONSTITUENTS: SYNERGIC EFFECT WITH SYNTHETIC MEDICATION

EOT demonstrates strong anticancer potential, but when combined with synthetic antibiotics, it has synergistic effects against a variety of microorganisms. An effective strategy for battling antimicrobial resistance against *S. aureus* is the combination of EOT with a synthetic antimicrobial agent. This is demonstrated in the review by Owen and Laird. In this regard, EOT exhibits encouraging outcomes (Owen and Laird 2018). The majority of the interactions between EOT and the antibiotics studied predominantly manifested as additive interactions; nevertheless, a number of these additive combinations restored antibiotic sensitivity in accordance with the Clinical and Laboratory Standards Institute's breakpoints (Clinical and Laboratory Standards Institute 2021). Additionally, EOT plus ampicillin, ciprofloxacin, or vancomycin combinations had additive or synergistic effects, according to the isobolograms. In actuality, as discussed by Langeveld et al., numerous research studies revealed interactions between thymol and various antibiotic classes among various microbes (Langeveld et al. 2014). It's possible that this connection relates to how thymol works. Thymol affected the integrity of the *S. aureus* cell membrane, as demonstrated by Wang et al. (2017).

The synergistic effect of EOT with antibiotics is proven by the investigations described in this section. This illustrates that possibly coupling EOT with anticancer medication can also enhance the anticancer activity of EOT, which may be explored further in the future.

## 11.5  CONCLUSION

EOT possesses a variety of anticancer characteristics and mechanisms that have been demonstrated. More focused therapy and greater specificity to cancer cells over non-cancer tissue might be possible with more *in vitro* and *in vivo* research to determine the most effective cytotoxic EOT combination composition. Additionally, the concentrations of already used conventional chemotherapy medications may be lowered when paired with EOT, which may also lessen chemotherapy-related toxicity. Furthermore, components of EOT may be modified synthetically to increase their overall efficacy. The ability of EOT and their constituents to have such diverse anticancer effects through working on numerous routes and cellular mechanisms is impressive, despite the fact that this is a fairly inexperienced and growing area of cancer research. However, additional research is necessary to increase our understanding of these pathways in order to advance the development of cell-specific and customized cancer therapies. Additionally, their novel treatment formulations, which contain these substances and include nanoparticles and microspheres, can be effective in cancer treatment. The extensive application of EOT in the healthcare industry is highly promising, although additional research is still necessary.

## REFERENCES

Abdoul-Latif FM, Ainane A, Mohamed J, Attahar W, Ouassil M, Ainane T. Essential oil of Thymus zygis: Chemical composition and biological valorization proposals. AMA, Agricultural Mechanization in Asia, Africa and Latin America. 2021;51:801–810.
Abeer M, Ahlam R, Marwa H. Impact of anise, clove, and thyme essential oils as feed supplements on the productive performance and digestion of barki ewes. Australian Journal of Basic and Applied Sciences. 2019 Jun; 13:1–3.

Afonso AF, Pereira OR, Válega M, Silva AM, Cardoso SM. Metabolites and biological activities of Thymus zygis, Thymus pulegioides, and Thymus fragrantissimus grown under organic cultivation. Molecules. 2018 Jun 22;23(7):1514.

Arunasree KM. Anti-proliferative effects of carvacrol on a human metastatic breast cancer cell line, MDA-MB 231. Phytomedicine. 2010;17(8–9):581–588.

Balan DJ, Rajavel T, Das M, Sathya S, Jeyakumar M, Devi KP. Thymol induces mitochondrial pathway-mediated apoptosis via ROS generation, macromolecular damage and SOD diminution in A549 cells. Pharmacological Reports. 2021 Feb;73(1):240–254.

Clinical and Laboratory Standards Institute (CLSI). Performance Standards for Antimicrobial Susceptibility Testing, Approved Standard, CLSI Document M100-S31, 31st ed.; CLSI: Wayne, PA, USA. 2021;31.

Coimbra A, Miguel S, Ribeiro M, Coutinho P, Silva L, Duarte AP, Ferreira S. Thymus zygis essential oil: Phytochemical characterization, bioactivity evaluation and synergistic effect with antibiotics against staphylococcus aureus. Antibiotics. 2022 Jan 24;11(2):146.

Cutillas AB, Carrasco A, Martinez-Gutierrez R, Tomas V, Tudela J. Thyme essential oils from Spain: Aromatic profile ascertained by GC–MS, and their antioxidant, antilipoxygenase and antimicrobial activities. Journal of Food and Drug Analysis. 2018 Apr 1;26(2):529–544.

Delgado-Adámez J, Garrido M, Bote ME, Fuentes-Pérez MC, Espino J, Martín-Vertedor D. Chemical composition and bioactivity of essential oils from flower and fruit of thymbra capitata and Thymus species. Journal of Food Science and Technology. 2017 Jun;54(7):1857–1865.

Dudai N, Weinstein Y, Krup M, Rabinski T, Ofr R. Citral is a new inducer of caspase-3 in tumor cell lines. Planta Medica. 2005;71(5):484–488.

Elbe H, Yigitturk G, Cavusoglu T, Uyanikgil Y, Ozturk F. Apoptotic effects of thymol, a novel monoterpene phenol, on different types of cancer. Bratislavske Lekarske Listy. 2020 Jan 1;121(2):122–128.

Fayard E, Tintignac LA, Baudry A, Hemmings BA. Protein kinase B/Akt at a glance. Journal of Cell Science. 2005;118(24):5675–5678.

Gonçalves MJ, Cruz MT, Cavaleiro C, Lopes MC, Salgueiro L. Chemical, antifungal and cytotoxic evaluation of the essential oil of Thymus zygis subsp. sylvestris. Industrial Crops and Products. 2010 Jul 1;32(1):70–75.

Hassan SB, Muhtasib H, Goransson H Larsson R. Alpha terpineol: A potential anti-cancer agent which acts through suppressing NF-B signalling. Anticancer Research. 2010; 30(6):1911–1919.

Jackson AL, Loeb LA. The contribution of endogenous sources of DNA damage to the multiple mutations in cancer. Mutation Research/Fundamental and Molecular Mechanisms of Mutagenesis. 2001 Jun 2;477(1–2):7–21.

Langeveld WT, Veldhuizen EJA, Burt SA, Synergy between essential oil components and antibiotics: A review. Critical Reviews in Microbiology. 2014;40:76–94.

Luís Â, Duarte AP, Pereira L, Domingues F. Chemical profiling and evaluation of antioxidant and anti-microbial properties of selected commercial essential oils: A comparative study. Medicines. 2017; 4:36.

Mosmann T. Rapid colorimetric assay for cellular growth and survival: Application to proliferation and cytotoxicity assays. Journal of Immunological Methods. 1983;65:55–63.

Naz F, Khan FI, Mohammad T et al. Investigation of molecular mechanism of recognition between citral and MARK4: A newer therapeutic approach to attenuate cancer cell progression. International Journal of Biological Macromolecules. 2018;107:2580–2589.

Owen L, Laird K. Synchronous application of antibiotics and essential oils: Dual mechanisms of action as a potential solution to antibiotic resistance. Critical Reviews in Microbiology. 2018 Jul 4;44(4):414–435.

Queiroz RM, Takiya CM, Guimaraes LP. Apoptosis inducing efects of Melissa officinalis L. essential oil in glioblastoma multiforme cells. Cancer Investigation. 2014;32(6):226–235.

Radi FZ, Bouhrim M, Mechchate H, Al-Zahrani M, Qurtam AA, Aleissa AM, Drioiche A, Handaq N, Zair T. Phytochemical analysis, antimicrobial and antioxidant properties of Thymus zygis L. and Thymus willdenowii Boiss. essential oils. Plants. 2021 Dec 22;11(1):15.

Raudone L, Zymone K, Raudonis R, Vainoriene R, Motiekaityte V, Janulis V. Phenological changes in triterpenic and phenolic composition of Thymus L. species. Industrial Crops and Products. 2017 Dec 15;109:445–451.

Rodrigues V, Cabral C, Evora L, Ferreira I, Cavaleiro C, Cruz MT, Salgueiro L. Chemical composition, anti-inflammatory activity and cytotoxicity of Thymus zygis L. subsp. sylvestris (Hoffmanns. & Link) Cout. essential oil and its main compounds. Arabian Journal of Chemistry. 2019 Dec 1;12(8):3236–3243.

Rota MC, Herrera A, Martínez RM, Sotomayor JA, Jordán MJ. Antimicrobial activity and chemical composition of Thymus vulgaris, Thymus zygis and Thymus hyemalis essential oils. Food Control. 2008 Jul 1;19(7):681–687.

Schmidt A, Bischof-Deichnik C, Stahl-Biskup E. Essential oil polymorphism of Thymus praecox subsp. arcticus on the British Isles. Biochemical Systematics and Ecology. 2004 Apr 1;32(4):409–421.

Seal S, Chatterjee P, Bhattacharya S et al. Vapor of volatile oils from litsea cubeba seed induces apoptosis and causes cell cycle arrest in lung cancer cells. PLoS One. 2012;7:10.

Sheikh BY, Sarker MMR, Kamarudin MNA, Mohan G. Antiproliferative and apoptosis inducing effects of citral via p53 and ROS-induced mitochondrial-mediated apoptosis in human colorectal HCT116 and HT29 cell lines. Biomedicine & Pharmacotherapy. 2017;96:834–846.

Silva AM, Martins-Gomes C, Souto EB, Schäfer J, Santos JA, Bunzel M, Nunes FM. Thymus zygis subsp. zygis an endemic Portuguese plant: Phytochemical profiling, antioxidant, anti-proliferative and anti-inflammatory activities. Antioxidants. 2020 Jun;9(6):482.

Suhail MM, Wu W, Cao A et al. Boswellia sacra essential oil induces tumor cell-specific apoptosis and suppresses tumor aggressiveness in cultured human breast cancer cells. BMC Complementary and Alternative Medicine. 2011;11:129.

Tomas ML, Antueno Rde, Coyle KM et al. Citral reduces breast tumor growth by inhibiting the cancer stem cell marker ALDH1A3. Molecular Oncology. 2016;10(9):1485–1496.

Vimalanathan S, Hudson J. Anti-influenza virus activity of essential oils and vapors. American Journal of Essential Oils and Natural Products. 2014;2(1):47–53.

Viuda-Martos M, ElGendy A El-NGS, Sendra E, Fernández-López J, ElRazik KA, Omer EA, Pérez-Alvarez JA. Chemical composition and antioxidant and anti-listeria activities of essentials oils obtained from some Egyptian plants. Journal of Agricultural and Food Chemistry. 2010;58:9063–9070.

Vlaicu PA, Untea AE, Turcu RP, Saracila M, Panaite TD, Cornescu GM. Nutritional composition and bioactive compounds of basil, thyme and sage plant additives and their functionality on broiler thigh meat quality. Foods. 2022 Apr 12;11(8):1105.

Wang LH, Zhang ZH, Zeng XA, Gong DM, Wang MS. Combination of microbiological, spectroscopic and molecular docking techniques to study the antibacterial mechanism of thymol against staphylococcus aureus: Membrane damage and genomic DNA binding. Analytical and Bioanalytical Chemistry. 2017;409:1615–1625.

Yakoubi S, Cherrat A, Diouri M, Hilali FE, Zair T. Chemical composition and antibacterial activity of Thymus zygis subsp. gracilis (Boiss.) R. Morales essential oils from Morocco. Mediterranean Journal of Chemistry. 2014 Apr 1;3(1):746–758.

Zerkani H, Kharchoufa L, Tagnaout I, Fakchich J, Bouhrim M, Amalich S, Addi M, Hano C, Cruz-Martins N, Bouharroud R, Zair T. Chemical composition and bioinsecticidal effects of Thymus zygis L., Salvia officinalis L. and Mentha suaveolens Ehrh. Essential Oils on Medfly Ceratitis capitata and Tomato Leaf Miner Tuta absoluta. Plants. 2022 Nov 14;11(22):3084.

# 12 Cinnamon Oil
## An Insight into Pharmacological and Pharmaceutical Potential

*Madhavi Patel and Bhupendra G. Prajapati*

## 12.1 INTRODUCTION TO ESSENTIAL OILS AND THEIR HEALTH BENEFITS

Essential oils, also known as volatile or ethereal oils, are known for their several powerful medicinal benefits from ancient times and this trend is continuing even today. They evaporate on exposure to the environment and contain mixtures of highly odorous aromatic compounds, stored in special secretory structures of plants (Sangwan et al., 2001; Hamid et al., 2011). For many years, essential oils have been utilized as flavours and perfumes and for healing the mind and body in many traditional medicinal systems. Distillation, expression and solvent extraction are common traditional extraction methods, whereas supercritical fluid extraction and phytonic process are used in modern days (Surburg and Panten, 2006). They are major agronomically based products and their world production and utilization are rapidly growing. On the medicinal front, they are proven as antibacterial, antiseptic, carminative, antiviral, antifungal, antioxidant, anticancer, insect repellent, anti-inflammatory, etc. They are preferred for aromatherapy for physical and psychological wellbeing (Tanu and Harpreet, 2016).

## 12.2 INTRODUCTION TO CINNAMON

Around 250 species of cinnamon genera have been identified throughout the world (Barceloux, 2008). The word cinnamon is derived from a Greek word that means sweet wood. Bark, leaves, roots, and fruits of the cinnamon tree are used, but most often the bark of different cinnamon species is a widely used popular spice and as a medicinal herb worldwide (Vangalapati et al., 2012). The oil of cinnamon is mostly extracted from bark or leaves. The rich composition of phytoconstituents in cinnamon are responsible for the wide range of its biological actions. In Ayurveda, an Indian system of medicine, its medicinal properties have been mentioned for over 6,000 years (Rao and Gan, 2014).

DOI: 10.1201/9781003389774-12

## 12.2.1 Cinnamon Species

Out of 250 known aromatic species of the genus *Cinnamomum* (family: *Lauraceae*), *Cinnamomum zeylanicum* Blume (also known as Ceylon cinnamon) and *Cinnamomum cassia* J. Presl are widely used and economical species (Muhammed and Dewettinck, 2017). Ceylon cinnamon, called true cinnamon, is indigenous to Sri Lanka, the leading supplier of pure cinnamon worldwide (Ghodki and Goswami, 2016). The cinnamon tree is large, tropical and evergreen, 10–14 m tall. After 3 years, they are coppiced annually to harvest the bark from the young branches which are brown and smooth. The bark of cinnamon is papery and possesses a yellowish brown colour (Pathirana, 2007).

## 12.2.2 Cultivation and Harvesting

Seed or vegetative propagation (stem cuttings) are used for cultivation of Ceylon cinnamon. They are first raised in nursery beds for the initial 4 to 6 months before transplanting to field. Aftercare operations like manuring, soil conservation, and weed and pest management are performed. After 3 to 4 years of plantation, the commercial production can be started and can last up to 35 to 40 years of plants' lifespan. Initial plant treatment is of utmost importance to produce good quality straight shoots (Azad et al., 2019). When the bark turns brown after 3 years, the first harvest can be done and the subsequent harvesting can be performed from shoots after around 1.5 years. Conventionally, when the young leaves turn light green, that stage is considered the right time to peel the bark. The stems are coppiced and a few stems are left to make the bush grow further. Top portions of the branches are removed and processed for leaf oil distillation. The bark is then scraped and sticks are rubbed to loosen the bark from the hardwood. The small quills are fitted inside the bigger quills and the edges are trimmed as required. Drying is performed indoors for 4 to 7 days. After drying, they are graded based on the uniformity, thickness and colour (Wijesekera and Chichester, 1978).

## 12.2.3 Preparation for Market with Emphasis on Oil Extraction

Cinnamon oil, usually extracted from its bark and leaf, became high-value added products on the market. Both traditional and advanced extraction methods are employed for cinnamon oil preparation. The distillation and solvent extraction are conventional methods whereas supercritical fluid extraction, ultrasound extraction, microwave extraction, microdistillation, etc., are the modern methods for oil extraction. Conventional methods suffer from few drawbacks whereas the advanced techniques like supercritical fluid extraction possess large versatility. However, due to high cost investment, supercritical fluid technique is not adopted widely. After its extraction, the oil is analyzed traditionally for its chemical and physical composition using chromatography and spectroscopy (Doughari, 2012; Ravindran et al., 2003).

### 12.2.4 PHYTOCHEMICALS

Terpenoids are a major category of phytochemicals found in cinnamon. However, variability in the amounts and types of chemicals present in cinnamon are different according to the species of cinnamon. Volatile oil extracted from *C. zeylanicum* bark and leaf yield 0.93% to 3% and 1.5% to 4.7% respectively. Major essential oil compounds present in it are cinnamaldehyde (49%–97%), eugenol, cinnamic acid, α-pinene, β-caryophyllene, cinnamyl acetate, myrcene, limonene, 1,8-cineole, benzaldehyde, linalool and cinnamyl acetate. Leaf and bark also contain oleoresin chemicals (Muhammed and Dewettinck, 2017; Jayaprakasha and Rao, 2011). Furthermore, the presence of coumarin, catechins and mucilage are reported in cinnamon (Tanaka et al., 2008). Some of the important constituent structures of the oil are displayed in Figure 12.1.

### 12.2.5 USES OF CINNAMON

Since ancient times, cinnamon has been the preferred spice and flavouring agent, used widely in food and confectionaries. Literature suggests its use in *vata roga* diseases, piles, oral cavity disease, worm infection and heart issues (Anonymous, 2001). Cinnamon oil and cinnamaldehyde are reported as antimicrobial, antioxidant, antifungal and antidiabetic. Therapeutically, the drug is proven as an anticancer, anti-inflammatory, anti-hyperlipidaemic, and insect repellent, in neurological and heart diseases and an anticoagulant (Rao and Gan, 2014).

### 12.2.6 TOXICITY OF CINNAMON

Cinnamon oil is generally recognized as a safe substance, so does not have any quantitative boundaries to use. Oil is reported to have an acute oral $LD_{50}$ 2650 mg/kg in rats that is equivalent to 258 to 324 mg for a 60 kg adult (Tisserand and Young, 2013; Opdyke, 1979).

## 12.3 BIOLOGICAL APPLICATIONS OF CINNAMON OIL

Cinnamon and its constituents possess a wide range of therapeutic benefits. It is important to note that the oil exerts therapeutic benefits due to its potent phytocomponents.

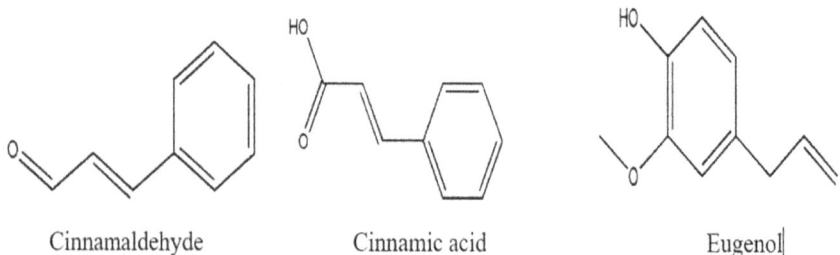

Cinnamaldehyde          Cinnamic acid          Eugenol

**FIGURE 12.1** Some phytoconstituents of cinnamon.

The details about biological activities exerted by cinnamon oil and/or its constituent cinnamaldehyde are depicted in this section.

## 12.3.1 ANTIBACTERIAL ACTIVITY

The major category of volatile oils is known for exerting an antibacterial effect. Various studies reported several antimicrobial activities of cinnamon oil and cinnamon (Matan et al., 2006; Abdollahzadeh et al. 2014). Oil of cinnamon, extract and major phytochemicals like cinnamaldehyde and eugenol are found active against both Gram-positive and Gram-negative bacteria. Cinnamon oil demonstrated strong antibacterial activity against *Salmonella enterica*, *Bacillus subtilis*, *Staphylococcus aureus*, *Micrococcus luteus*, *Escherichia coli*, *Listeria monocytogenes*, *Pseudomonas aeruginosa*, *Enterobacter cloacae*, *Klebsiella pneumonia*, *Alcaligenes faecalis* and *Serratia marcescens* (Friedman et al., 2004; Chao et al., 2000). Incorporation of cinnamaldehyde in biofilm revealed negative effects on many uropathogenic *E. coli*, on *Candida* species, *Salmonella* species and *P. aeruginosa* (Niu and Gilbert, 2004; Khan and Ahmad, 2012; Zhang et al., 2014; Kim et al., 2015). Cinnamaldehyde is also found to be effective on *Streptococcus pneumonia*, *S. aureus*, *Haemophilus influenza* like gastrointestinal tract and respiratory pathogens (Inouye et al., 2001).

Alteration of the cell membrane and its lipid profile, ATPase inhibition, inhibition of cell division and membrane porins, inhibition of biofilm formation and antiquorum sensing effect are core mechanisms exerted by cinnamon oil and its major constituents to demonstrate antibacterial effect (Vasconcelos et al., 2018).

## 12.3.2 ANTIDIABETIC AND DIABETIC NEUROPATHY

Cinnamon oil, when tested on rats at the dosage of 25, 50 and 100 mg/kg b.w., led to a noticeable decrease in fasting blood glucose of diabetic animals. There was a decline in total cholesterol, blood urea nitrogen, serum triglyceride and plasma C-peptide observed with concomitant elevation of HDL. They have also observed increased immunoreactivity of β-cells and improved glucose tolerance (Ping et al., 2010). Similar studies reported at the various dosage levels to track the antidiabetic effects of oil on animals (Budiastuti et al., 2020). Encapsulated cinnamon oil in STZ-induced diabetic rats at the dose of 200 or 400 mg/kg b.w. demonstrated improved glucose and insulin levels, lipid profile, amylase, GSH and SOD along with favourable histological changes in the pancreas and liver (Mohammed et al., 2020). A human study of cinnamon oil reported improvement in fasting blood glucose and insulin levels at 400 mg/day but pharmacokinetic data revealed low bioavailability of oil (Stevens, 2020). The major constituent of cinnamon oil, cinnamaldehyde, was also evaluated by several studies as was the oil. Cinnamaldehyde at 20 mg/kg b.w. in diabetic rats increased glucose uptake via GLUT4 receptors, improved lipid profile and glucose tolerance (Anand et al., 2010; Zhao et al., 2021). *In vitro* effects of cinnamaldehyde on HEK293 and 3T3-L1 led induced expression of PPAR genes and target mRNA expression, thereby contributing to insulin sensitivity (Li et al., 2015).

STZ-induced diabetic rats, when treated with cinnamaldehyde, exhibited decreased blood glucose, IL-2 and TNF-α with amelioration of neurochemical and behavioural deficits (Jawale et al., 2016).

### 12.3.3  ANTIOXIDANT

Cinnamon essential oil and its actives exerted good antioxidant effect suggesting extensive usage of cinnamon in food and herbal medicines (Przygodzka et al., 2014). Cinnamaldehyde, when tested for inhibitory effect on nitric oxide production, showed 81.5% inhibitory effect at 1 µg/µl (Lee et al., 2002). Singh et al. (2007) studied antioxidant effects of leaf and bark cinnamon oil along with other constituents by DPPH and hydroxyl radical scavenging effect; bark volatile oil exhibited 79.6% scavenging effect.

### 12.3.4  CARDIOVASCULAR HEALTH

The major constituent cinnamaldehyde, when tested for cardiovascular health, demonstrated a mainly protective effect on heart. It was found to prevent ischemic injury via good antioxidant effect, exerted hypotensive effect, prevent cardiac hypertrophy via blocking extracellular signal-regulated kinase signalling pathway, promote vasorelaxation via decreasing calcium influx and release, inhibit platelet aggregation and decrease hyperlipidaemia, hyperglycaemia and hypertension (Das et al., 2022).

### 12.3.5  ANTICANCER

Cinnamon essential oil was tested for head and neck cancer where it has exhibited significant anticancer activity against HNSCC (head and neck squamous cell carcinoma) cells *in vitro*, where the suppression of epidermal growth factor receptor tyrosine kinase (EGFR-TK) has resulted in anticancer potential of the oil (Yang et al., 2015). It has been reported as a promising agent for stomach cancer and melanoma. Cinnamaldehyde and eugenol are commonly employed as nutraceuticals for colon and liver cancer. Also, they have demonstrated good effect against leukaemia and lymphoma (Goel and Mishra, 2020).

### 12.3.6  NEUROLOGICAL DISEASE

Effect of cinnamon oil on deltamethrin-induced neurotoxicity was evaluated in albino rats. Cinnamon oil at 0.5 mg/kg b.w. significantly improved behavioural and antioxidant capacity of the brain along with an increase in acetylcholine esterase activity. It has reduced the serum corticosterone, serotonin and malonaldehyde (MDA) levels in the brain. Gene expression study revealed down regulation of iNOS and CYP1A1 depicting prevention of neurotoxicity by the oil (Ahmed et al., 2021). Cinnamaldehyde is reported to ameliorate cerebral ischemia-induced brain injury where inhibition of neuroinflammation was observed via attenuation of iNOS, NFκB signalling and COX-2 expression (Chen et al., 2016). Effects of cinnamaldehyde in Alzheimer's disease depends on the amount of its metabolites and the interaction with blood–brain barrier. Cinnamon oil, when studied in Parkinson's disease, can potentially delay the progression of neurodisorders (Dolgacheva et al., 2019).

## 12.3.7 ANTI-INFLAMMATORY ACTIVITY

Leaf essential oil inhibited pro IL-1β protein expression at 60 μg/ml in murine macrophages. It has inhibited IL-1β and IL-6 production *in vitro* suggesting good anti-inflammatory action (Chao et al., 2005). Similarly, the effect of volatile oil on nitric oxide production in macrophages was evaluated. Cinnamaldehyde, being the major responsible component of cinnamon oil, strongly inhibited nitric oxide production at $IC_{50}$ value 9.7–15.5μg/ml (Tung et al., 2010). Cinnamon bark essential oil demonstrated promising anti-inflammatory effect on human dermal fibroblast suggesting its very good application in chronic inflammation (Han and Parker, 2017).

## 12.3.8 COSMETIC APPLICATIONS

Essential oil of cinnamon demonstrated its positive place in a wide range of cosmetics and oral care products. It might be attributed to the oil's antiseptic and antimicrobial activity. Antiacne concealer containing cinnamon oil demonstrated very good effect against *Propionibacterium acnes* with 5 mg/ml inhibitory concentration (Veerasophon et al., 2020).

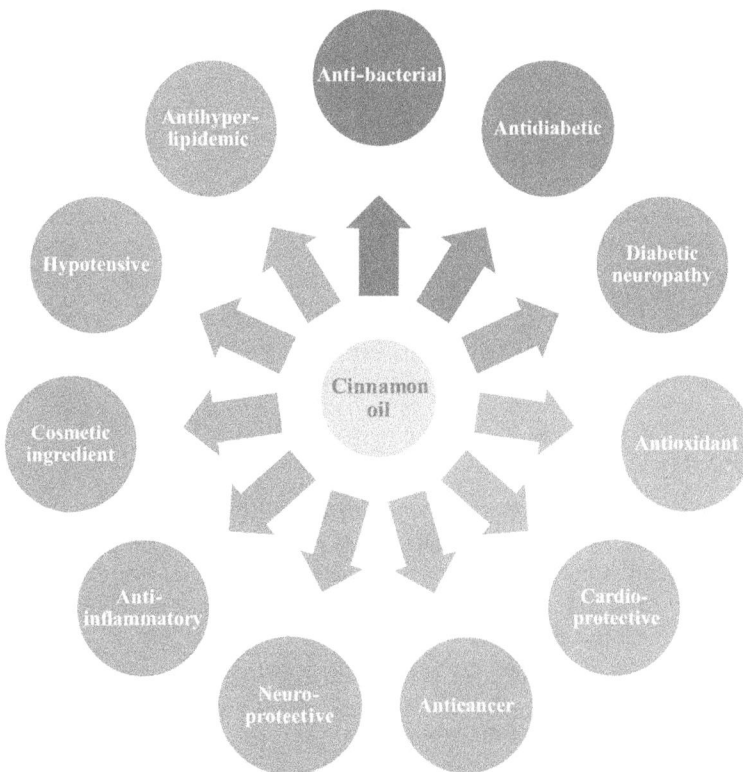

FIGURE 12.2   Health benefits of cinnamon oil.

### 12.3.9 Other Miscellaneous Applications

Cinnamon oil components were proven to activate brown adipose tissue in the body where mitochondria numbers and thermogenic protein expression were increased, suggesting its effect on hypothermia (Li et al., 2021).

Cinnamon oil, when tested in mice, demonstrated significant protection against genotoxicity, oxidative stress and reproductive troubles induced by titanium nanoparticles (Salman et al., 2021). In mouthwash preparations, it is employed as an antimicrobial substance.

Cinnamon is also incorporated in many preparations for utilization as insecticidal, acaricidal, nematocidal and repellent property (Kim et al., 2004; Park et al., 2005; Prajapati et al., 2005).

## 12.4   CINNAMON OIL IN/AS PHARMACEUTICALS

Cinnamon oil is a very attractive ingredient not only in food but also in cosmetic and in pharmaceutical industries where it found vast application. Cinnamon oil, due to its antioxidant activity, can be incorporated as a food preservative. Also, antimicrobial and antiseptic effects of cinnamon oil lead to formulation of many cosmetic preparations to cure skin issues. Cinnamon oil incorporation in various conventional and nano dosage forms for different applications are mentioned in Table 12.1. A few patents on cinnamon oil are mentioned in Table 12.2.

## 12.5   FUTURE PROSPECTS

Plenty of literature available on pharmacological potential and pharmaceutical application of cinnamon oil confirmed major interests of researchers in the oil. Many activities and mechanisms of its biological effects have been well established in *in vitro* and *in vivo* animal studies along with a few clinical study reports. However, systemic clinical trials and establishment of efficacy of cinnamon, its oil and its phytoactives are the need of the hour. Using advanced cultivation techniques with all required care can boost quality production of this important spice.

## 12.6   CONCLUSION

Cinnamon, its different parts and the volatile oil extracted from cinnamon have found their potent use in food, flavouring and health problems since ancient times. Volatile oil components such as cinnamaldehyde and eugenol were identified and isolated from cinnamon as major phytochemicals. Different traditional and modern extraction methods are employed for essential oil extraction. The oil and the phytoconstituents present in it demonstrate a wide range of biological effects ranging from antibacterial, antidiabetic to anticancer with good bioavailability. Various research documented encapsulation of oil, emulsion or gel preparation and nanoparticle formulation using cinnamon oil or cinnamaldehyde for enhancing its therapeutic potential. Increasing trade of cinnamon worldwide has proven the special potential of this medicinal herb and its products.

## TABLE 12.1
### Conventional and Nano Dosage Forms of Cinnamon Oil

| Formulation | Core Ingredient/s | Application | Reference |
|---|---|---|---|
| Nanocream | Cinnamon leaf oil 2% | Topical | Zainol et al., 2015 |
| Nanostructures (Nanoemulsion and nanocapsules) | Cinnamon oil 5% | To control *Rhipicephalus microplus* ticks on cattle | Dos Santos et al., 2017 |
| Microemulsion for sustained release | Cinnamon essential oil | Insecticide | Shi et al., 2022 |
| Microencapsulated oil | Cinnamon essential oil minimum inhibitory concentration – 220.5 to 440.5 μg/mL | Antidermatophytic effect | Makimori et al., 2020 |
| Nanoemulsion | Cinnamon oil and usnic acid blend | Skin carcinogenicity | Mukerjee et al., 2019 |
| Nano/microstructured hybrid composite particles | Cinnamon oil | Antibiotic alternative for foodborne pathogens | Yostawonkul et al., 2021 |
| Erythromycin loaded transethosomes cinnamon oil based emulgel | Erythromycin and cinnamon oil | Antimicrobial activity | Abdallah et al., 2023 |
| Nanoemulgel | Cinnamon oil | Antifungal, antibacterial and analgesic effects on oral microbiota | Hosny et al., 2021 |
| Nanoformulation | Maltodextrin and cinnamon essential oil | Protective effect against titanium nanoparticles-induced oxidative stress, genotoxicity and reproductive disturbances in male mice | Salman et al., 2021 |
| Sanitizer gel | Cinnamon oil | Antibacterial activity | Diviyagahage et al., 2021 |

**TABLE 12.2**
**Patents Available for Cinnamon Oil**

| Patent No. | Title | Country | Year | Specifications |
|---|---|---|---|---|
| KR1020210092052 | Composition for inhibiting oral biofilm formation comprising nano-emulsified cinnamon oil as active component | Republic of Korea | 2022 | The composition was prepared for dental caries and periodontal disease. |
| CN102697852 | Hydrochloric acid cicletanine and cinnamon oil nanoemulsion antihypertensive drug | China | 2022 | Antihypertensive nanoemulsion contains 1%–20% of cinnamon oil as one of the ingredients. |
| CN114632061 | Cinnamon oil nano emulsion stabilized by natural oil-based nonionic surfactant and preparation method thereof | China | 2022 | 5% to 10% of cinnamon oil, along with other ingredients |
| IN201941033087 | Cinnamon oil mediated gold nanoparticles and its dental applications | India | 2021 | Exerted antimicrobial activity against dental pathogen |
| IN201811028254 | A method of formulation of cinnamon oil nanoemulsion for antibacterial efficacy | India | 2020 | Nanoemulsion |
| CN111616344 | Preparation method for cinnamon essential oil and cellulose nano-microsphere suspension | China | 2020 | Nano-microspheres of particle size of 200–400 nm |
| KR102016009747 | Manufacturing method of multilayered nano-capsule encapsulating unsaturated fatty acids and cinnamon oil | Republic of Korea | 2018 | Nano-emulsion with encapsulated cinnamon oil |
| CN103653179 | Cinnamon essential oil nano lipidosome and preparation method thereof | China | 2014 | Cinnamon essential oil, soybean lecithin, cholesterol, vitamin E and a surfactant |
| CN102166257 | Oil-in-water type cinnamon oil nanoemulsion oral liquid | China | 2011 | 0.1% to 8% of cinnamon oil |

# REFERENCES

Abdallah, M.H., Elghamry, H.A., Khalifa, N.E., Khojali, W.M., Khafagy, E.S., Shawky, S., El-Horany, H.E.S. and El-Housiny, S. 2023. Development and optimization of erythromycin loaded transethosomes cinnamon oil based emulgel for antimicrobial efficiency. *Gels* 9(2), 137.

Abdollahzadeh, E., Rezaei, M. and Hosseini, H. 2014. Antibacterial activity of plant essential oils and extracts: The role of thyme essential oil, nisin, and their combination to control Listeria monocytogenes inoculated in minced fish meat. *Food Control* 35(1), 177–183.

Ahmed, W.M., Abdel-Azeem, N.M., Ibrahim, M.A., Helmy, N.A. and Radi, A.M. 2021. Neuromodulatory effect of cinnamon oil on behavioural disturbance, CYP1A1, iNOStranscripts and neurochemical alterations induced by deltamethrin in rat brain. *Ecotoxicology and Environmental Safety* 209, 11820.

Anand, P., Murali, K.Y., Tandon, V., Murthy, P.S. and Chandra, R. 2010. Insulinotropic effect of cinnamaldehyde on transcriptional regulation of pyruvate kinase, phosphoenolpyruvate carboxykinase, and GLUT4 translocation in experimental diabetic rats. *Chemico-Biological Interactions* 186(1), 72–81.

Anonymous 2001. The ayurvedic pharmacopoeia of India. Part I, Vol. I, Edn. 1, Ministry of Health and Family Welfare Government of India Department of Ayurveda, Yoga: Naturopathy, Unani, Siddha & Homeopathy (AYUSH), New Delhi. 151–152.

Azad, R., Jayasekara, L., Ranawaka, R.A., Senanayake, G., Kumara, K.W., Pushpakumara, D.K. and Geekiyanage, S. 2019. Development of a core collection for Sri Lankan cinnamon germplasm based on morphological characterization using an eco-geographic survey. *Australian Journal of Crop Science* 13(9), 1473–1485.

Barceloux, D.G. 2008. Cinnamon (Cinnamomum Species). In Medical Toxicology of Natural Substances: Foods, Fungi, Medicinal Herbs, Toxic Plants, and Venomous Animals. Hoboken, New Jersey: John Wiley & Sons, Inc. 39–43.

Budiastuti, B., Safitri, Y., Plumeriastuti, H., Srianto, P., Effendi, M. and Helmi, M. 2020. Effect of cinnamon (Cinnamomum burmannii) bark oil on testicular histopathology in streptozotocin induced diabetic wistar male rats. *Journal of Global Pharma Technology* 12, 901–907.

Chao, L.K., Hua, K.F., Hsu, H.Y., Cheng, S.S., Liu, J.Y. and Chang, S.T. 2005. Study on the antiinflammatory activity of essential oil from leaves of Cinnamomum osmophloeum. *Journal of Agricultural and Food Chemistry* 53(18), 7274–7278.

Chao, S.C., Young, D.G. and Oberg, C.J. 2000. Screening for inhibitory activity of essential oils on selected bacteria, fungi and viruses. *Journal of Essential Oil Research* 12(5), 639–649.

Chen, Y.F., Wang, Y.W., Huang, W.S., Lee, M.M., Wood, W.G., Leung, Y.M. and Tsai, H.Y. 2016. Trans-cinnamaldehyde, an essential oil in cinnamon powder, ameliorates cerebral ischemia-induced brain injury via inhibition of neuroinflammation through attenuation of iNOS, COX-2 expression and NFκ-B signaling pathway. *Neuromolecular Medicine* 18, 322–333.

Das, G., Gonçalves, S., Heredia, J.B., Romano, A., Jiménez-Ortega, L.A., Gutiérrez-Grijalva, E.P., Shin, H.S. and Patra, J.K. 2022. Cardiovascular protective effect of cinnamon and its major bioactive constituents: An update. *Journal of Functional Foods* 105045.

Diviyagahage, C.M., Thuvaragan, S., Gnanakarunyan, T.J. and Srikaran, R. 2021. Formulation and characterization of essential oils based antibacterial hand sanitizer gels. *Pharmaceutical Journal of Sri Lanka* 11(1).

Dolgacheva, L.P., Berezhnov, A.V., Fedotova, E.I., Zinchenko, V.P. and Abramov, A.Y. 2019. Role of DJ-1 in the mechanism of pathogenesis of Parkinson's disease. *Journal of Bioenergetics and Biomembranes* 51, 175–188.

Dos Santos, D.S., Boito, J.P., Santos, R.C., Quatrin, P.M., Ourique, A.F., Dos Reis, J.H., Gebert, R.R., Glombowsky, P., Klauck, V., Boligon, A.A. and Baldissera, M.D. 2017. Nanostructured cinnamon oil has the potential to control Rhipicephalus microplus ticks on cattle. *Experimental and Applied Acarology* 73, 129–138.

Doughari, J.H. 2012. Phytochemicals: Extraction methods, basic structures and mode of action as potential chemotherapeutic agents. Rijeka, Croatia: INTECH Open Access Publisher 1–33.

Friedman, M., Henika, P.R., Levin, C.E. and Mandrell, R.E. 2004. Antibacterial activities of plant essential oils and their components against Escherichia coli O157: H7 and salmonella enterica in apple juice. *Journal of Agricultural and Food Chemistry* 52(19), 6042–6048.

Ghodki, B.M. and Goswami, T.K. 2016. Optimization of cryogenic grinding process for cassia (*Cinnamomum loureirii* Nees L.). *Journal of Food Process Engineering* 39(6), 659–675.

Goel, B. and Mishra, S. 2020. Medicinal and nutritional perspective of cinnamon: A mini-review. Eur. *Journal of Medicinal Plants* 31, 10–16.

Hamid, A.A., Aiyelaagbe, O.O. and Usman, L.A. 2011. Essential oils: Its medicinal and pharmacological uses. *International Journal of Current research* 33(2), 86–98.

Han, X. and Parker, T.L. 2017. Antiinflammatory activity of cinnamon (Cinnamomum zeylanicum) bark essential oil in a human skin disease model. *Phytotherapy Research* 31(7),1034–1038.

Hosny, K.M., Khallaf, R.A., Asfour, H.Z., Rizg, W.Y., Alhakamy, N.A., Sindi, A.M., Alkhalidi, H.M., Abualsunun, W.A., Bakhaidar, R.B., Almehmady, A.M. and Abdulaal, W.H. 2021. Development and optimization of cinnamon oil nanoemulgel for enhancement of solubility and evaluation of antibacterial, antifungal and analgesic effects against oral microbiota. *Pharmaceutics* 13(7), 1008.

Inouye, S., Takizawa, T. and Yamaguchi, H. 2001. Antibacterial activity of essential oils and their major constituents against respiratory tract pathogens by gaseous contact. *Journal of Antimicrobial Chemotherapy* 47(5), 565–573.

Jawale, A., Datusalia, A.K., Bishnoi, M. and Sharma, S.S. 2016. Reversal of diabetes-induced behavioral and neurochemical deficits by cinnamaldehyde. *Phytomedicine* 23(9), 923–930.

Jayaprakasha, G.K. and Rao, L.J.M. 2011. Chemistry, biogenesis, and biological activities of *Cinnamomum zeylanicum*. *Critical Reviews in Food Science and Nutrition* 51(6), 547–562.

Khan, M.S.A. and Ahmad, I. 2012. Antibiofilm activity of certain phytocompounds and their synergy with fluconazole against Candida albicans biofilms. *Journal of Antimicrobial Chemotherapy* 67(3), 618–621.

Kim, S.I., Yi, J.H., Tak, J.H. and Ahn, Y.J. 2004. Acaricidal activity of plant essential oils against Dermanyssus gallinae (Acari: Dermanyssidae). *Veterinary Parasitology* 120(4), 297–304.

Kim, Y.G., Lee, J.H., Kim, S.I., Baek, K.H. and Lee, J. 2015. Cinnamon bark oil and its components inhibit biofilm formation and toxin production. *International Journal of Food Microbiology* 195, 30–39.

Lee, H.S., Kim, B.S. and Kim, M.K. 2002. Suppression effect of cinnamomum cassia bark-derived component on nitric oxide synthase. *Journal of Agricultural and Food Chemistry* 50(26), 7700–7703.

Li, J.E., Futawaka, K., Yamamoto, H., Kasahara, M., Tagami, T., Liu, T.H. and Moriyama, K. 2015. Cinnamaldehyde contributes to insulin sensitivity by activating PPARδ, PPARγ, and RXR. *The American Journal of Chinese Medicine* 43(05), 879–892.

Li, X., Lu, H.Y., Jiang, X.W., Yang, Y., Xing, B., Yao, D., Wu, Q., Xu, Z.H. and Zhao, Q.C. 2021. Cinnamomum cassia extract promotes thermogenesis during exposure to cold via activation of brown adipose tissue. *Journal of Ethnopharmacology* 266, 113413.

Makimori, R.Y., Endo, E.H., Makimori, J.W., Zanqueta, E.B., Ueda-Nakamura, T., Leimann, F.V., Gonçalves, O.H. and Dias Filho, B.P. 2020. Preparation, characterization and anti-dermatophytic activity of free-and microencapsulated cinnamon essential oil. *Journal de Mycologie Médicale* 30(2), 100933.

Matan, N., Rimkeeree, H., Mawson, A.J., Chompreeda, P., Haruthaithanasan, V. and Parker, M. 2006. Antimicrobial activity of cinnamon and clove oils under modified atmosphere conditions. *International Journal of Food Microbiology* 107(2), 180–185.

Mohammed, K.A., Ahmed, H.M., Sharaf, H.A., El-Nekeety, A.A., Abdel-Aziem, S.H., Mehaya, F.M. and Abdel-Wahhab, M.A. 2020. Encapsulation of cinnamon oil in whey protein counteracts the disturbances in biochemical parameters, gene expression, and histological picture of the liver and pancreas of diabetic rats. *Environmental Science and Pollution Research* 27, 2829–2843.

Muhammad, D.R.A. and Dewettinck, K. 2017. Cinnamon and its derivatives as potential ingredient in functional food: A review. *International Journal of Food Properties* 20(sup2), 2237–2263.

Mukerjee, A., Pandey, H., Tripathi, A.K. and Singh, S.K. 2019. Development, characterization and evaluation of cinnamon oil and usnic acid blended nanoemulsion to attenuate skin carcinogenicity in Swiss albino mice. *Biocatalysis and Agricultural Biotechnology* 20, 101227.

Niu, C. and Gilbert, E.S. 2004. Colorimetric method for identifying plant essential oil components that affect biofilm formation and structure. *Applied and Environmental Microbiology* 70(12), 6951–6956.

Opdyke, D.L.J. 1979. Monographs on fragrance raw materials. *Food and Cosmetics Toxicology* 17(4), 357–390. https://doi.org/10.1016/0015-6264(79)90330-4

Park, I.K., Park, J.Y., Kim, K.H., Choi, K.S., Choi, I.H., Kim, C.S. and Shin, S.C. 2005. Nematicidal activity of plant essential oils and components from garlic (*Allium sativum*) and cinnamon (*Cinnamomum verum*) oils against the pine wood nematode (*Bursaphelenchus xylophilus*). *Nematology* 7(5), 767–774.

Pathirana, L.S.S. 2007. Factors affecting bark yield components of cinnamon. *Bulletin of the Rubber Research Institute of Sri Lanka* 48, 43–48.

Ping, H., Zhang, G. and Ren, G. 2010. Antidiabetic effects of cinnamon oil in diabetic KK-Ay mice. *Food and Chemical Toxicology* 48(8–9), 2344–2349.

Prajapati, V., Tripathi, A.K., Aggarwal, K.K. and Khanuja, S.P.S. 2005. Insecticidal, repellent and oviposition-deterrent activity of selected essential oils against Anopheles stephensi, Aedes aegypti and Culex quinquefasciatus. *Bioresource Technology* 96(16), 1749–1757.

Przygodzka, M., Zielińska, D., Ciesarová, Z., Kukurová, K. and Zieliński, H. 2014. Comparison of methods for evaluation of the antioxidant capacity and phenolic compounds in common spices. *LWT-Food Science and Technology* 58(2), 321–326.

Rao, P.V. and Gan, S.H. 2014. Cinnamon: A multifaceted medicinal plant. *Evidence-Based Complementary and Alternative Medicine* 2014, 642942.

Ravindran, P.N., Nirmal-Babu, K. and Shylaja, M. eds. 2003. Cinnamon and cassia: The genus cinnamomum. CRC press.

Salman, A.S., Al-Shaikh, T.M., Hamza, Z.K., El-Nekeety, A.A., Bawazir, S.S., Hassan, N.S. and Abdel-Wahhab, M.A. 2021. Matlodextrin-cinnamon essential oil nanoformulation as a potent protective against titanium nanoparticles-induced oxidative stress, genotoxicity, and reproductive disturbances in male mice. *Environmental Science and Pollution Research* 28, 39035–39051.

Sangwan, N.S., Farooqi, A.H.A., Shabih, F. and Sangwan, R.S. 2001. Regulation of essential oil production in plants. *Plant Growth Regulation* 34, 3–21.

Shi, W., Yan, R. and Huang, L. 2022. Preparation and insecticidal performance of sustained-release cinnamon essential oil microemulsion. *Journal of the Science of Food and Agriculture* 102(4), 1397–1404.

Singh, G., Maurya, S., DeLampasona, M.P. and Catalan, C.A. 2007. A comparison of chemical, antioxidant and antimicrobial studies of cinnamon leaf and bark volatile oils, oleoresins and their constituents. *Food and Chemical Toxicology* 45(9), 1650–1661.

Stevens, N. 2020. Cinnamon Bark Essential Oil and a Novel Essential Oil Blend as Potential Modulators of Glucose Metabolism (Doctoral dissertation, University of Miami).

Surburg, H. and Panten, J. 2016. Common fragrance and flavor materials: Preparation, properties and uses. John Wiley & Sons.

Tanaka, T., Matsuo, Y., Yamada, Y. and Kouno, I. 2008. Structure of polymeric polyphenols of cinnamon bark deduced from condensation products of cinnamaldehyde with catechin and procyanidins. *Journal of Agricultural and Food Chemistry* 56(14), 5864–5870.

Tanu, B. and Harpreet, K. 2016. Benefits of essential oil. *Journal of Chemical and Pharmaceutical Research* 8(6), 143–149.

Tisserand, R. and Young, R. 2013. Essential oil safety: A guide for health care professionals. Elsevier Health Sciences.

Tung, Y.T., Yen, P.L., Lin, C.Y. and Chang, S.T. 2010. Anti-inflammatory activities of essential oils and their constituents from different provenances of indigenous cinnamon (Cinnamomum osmophloeum) leaves. *Pharmaceutical Biology* 48(10), 1130–1136.

Vangalapati, M., Satya, N.S., Prakash, D.S. and Avanigadda, S. 2012. A review on pharmacological activities and clinical effects of cinnamon species. *Research Journal of Pharmaceutical, Biological and Chemical Sciences* 3(1), 653–663.

Vasconcelos, N.G., Croda, J. and Simionatto, S. 2018. Antibacterial mechanisms of cinnamon and its constituents: A review. *Microbial Pathogenesis* 120, 198–203.

Veerasophon, J., Sripalakit, P. and Saraphanchotiwitthaya, A. 2020. Formulation of anti-acne concealer containing cinnamon oil with antimicrobial activity against propionibacterium acnes. *Journal of Advanced Pharmaceutical Technology & Research* 11(2), 53.

Wijesekera, R.O.B. and Chichester, C.O. 1978. The chemistry and technology of cinnamon. *Critical Reviews in Food Science & Nutrition* 10(1), 1–30.

Yang, X.Q., Zheng, H., Ye, Q., Li, R.Y. and Chen, Y. 2015. Essential oil of cinnamon exerts anti-cancer activity against head and neck squamous cell carcinoma via attenuating epidermal growth factor receptor-tyrosine kinase. *Journal of BUON* 20(6), 1518–1525.

Yostawonkul, J., Nittayasut, N., Phasuk, A., Junchay, R., Boonrungsiman, S., Temisak, S., Kongsema, M., Phoolcharoen, W. and Yata, T. 2021. Nano/microstructured hybrid composite particles containing cinnamon oil as an antibiotic alternative against foodborne pathogens. *Journal of Food Engineering*, 290, 110209.

Zainol, N.A., Ming, T.S. and Darwis, Y. 2015. Development and characterization of cinnamon leaf oil nanocream for topical application. *Indian Journal of Pharmaceutical Sciences* 77(4), 422.

Zhang, H., Zhou, W., Zhang, W., Yang, A., Liu, Y., Jiang, Y.A.N., Huang, S. and Su, J. 2014. Inhibitory effects of citral, cinnamaldehyde, and tea polyphenols on mixed biofilm formation by foodborne Staphylococcus aureus and Salmonella enteritidis. *Journal of Food Protection* 77(6), 927–933.

Zhao, H., Wu, H., Duan, M., Liu, R., Zhu, Q., Zhang, K. and Wang, L. 2021. Cinnamaldehyde improves metabolic functions in streptozotocin-induced diabetic mice by regulating gut microbiota. *Drug Design, Development and Therapy* 2339–2355.

# 13 Pharmacological Aspects of *Ocimum Basilicum* Essential Oil
## Current and Future Trends

*Yogita Ale, Shivani Rawat,*
*Nidhi Nainwal, and*
*Vikash Jakhmola*

## 13.1 INTRODUCTION

Drug-resistance and adverse effects of synthetic medicines have developed the interest in medicinal plants and herbs extracts, metabolites, and their essential oils among the scientists and the public over the world. With their non-toxic nature, these plants are suitable for use in clinical and medical practice to treat a wide range of health problems (Salehi et al., 2019). Their metabolites and phytoconstituents are being proven scientifically and promoted across the world in the form of various pharmaceutical and cosmeceutical formulations (Tiwari et al., 2013). Also, they have shown potent activity through their many and varied health benefits. For example, some of these include antimicrobial, antiviral, antioxidant, and immunomodulatory activities, and they also protect against blood pressure, diabetes, digestive problems, obesity, kidney problems, and other health problems (Tiwari et al., 2018).

Among the holistic herbal plants is *Ocimum basilicum*, which has many different possible phytoconstituents that give it medicinal properties.

In the genus *Ocimum*, which is in the family *Lamiaceae*, there are many fragrant shrubs and herbs, such as *O. tenuiflorum* (Tulsi or holy basil), *O. gratissimum* (African basil), *O. basilicum* (sweet basil), *O. campechianum* (Amazonian basil), etc. Studies have shown that *Ocimum basilicum* has many biomedical, therapeutic, pharmacological, and other health-related uses (Purushothaman et al., 2018). This plant grows all over the world in areas with tropical, subtropical, and temperate climates, such as India, Africa, West Asia, Pakistan, Nepal, etc., and is used for many different things in everyday life (Dhama et al., 2015). In mythology, this species is also called the "God of Spices," and it is an important part of the Ayurvedic and Unani medical systems (Sharifi et al., 2020).

Basil is a very nutritious herb. It has fats, vitamins like C, A, E, K, B1 (thiamine), B2 (riboflavin), B3 (niacin), and B5 (pantothenic acid); proteins; carotene; and choline; along with minerals like calcium, phosphorus, iron, magnesium, zinc, potassium, and sodium. It also has various secondary metabolites like essential oils (Yatoo et al., 2018). It shows various therapeutic activity including analgesic, antioxidant, antimicrobial, anti-inflammatory, hypoglycaemic, antihyperlipidemic, hepatoprotective, anti-ulcerative, antihypertensive, hepatoprotective, cytoprotective, cardioprotective, immunomodulatory, cardio stimulant, hypnotic, sedative, anti-nociceptive, chemo-preventative, anti-cancer, chemo modulatory, and mosquito larvicidal (Bilal et al., 2012; Kumar et al., 2013). Moreover, antimicrobial effects on both Gram-positive and Gram-negative bacteria, such as *S. epidermidis*, *Listeria monocytogenes*, *S. aureus*, *P. aeruginosa*, *Shigella sp.*, *P. putida*, *E. coli*, and fungi such as aflatoxin-producing *Aspergillus* (Miraj and Kiani, 2016).

## 13.2 CHEMICAL PROFILE OF *OCIMUM BASILICUM*

*Ocimum basilicum* has been known for being high in essential oils content. These oils are extracted from the herb's leaves and stems using a technique called hydrodistillation. With the help of gas chromatography along with mass spectrometry, 36 chemical compounds are found in the essential oils (Rubab et al., 2017). The main ingredient was found to be linalool, 1,8-cineole, p-allylanisole, geraniol, transbergamotene, and neryl acetate. The major chemical constituents identified in the essential oil are methyl eugenol, linalool, methyl chavicol, geraniol, and 1,8-cineol. Figure 13.1 represents the various phytoconstituents present in *Ocimum basilicum* (Sestili et al., 2018; Tantiwatcharothai et al., 2019).

## 13.3 PHARMACOLOGICAL ACTIVITIES OF *OCIMUM BASILICUM*

### 13.3.1 ANTI-INFLAMMATORY ACTIVITY

Anti-inflammatory effects have been associated with the presence of methyl eugenol, estragole, α-cadinol, methyl eugenol, α-bergamotene, and linoleic acid. Anti-inflammatory activity happens when pro-inflammatory mediators are turned off and anti-inflammatory cytokines are turned on (Eftekhar et al., 2019). The plant extract inhibit Raw 264.7 cells stimulated by LPS from producing cytokines such as IL-6, TNF-α, and IL-β by stopping the genes that make these cytokines from being expressed (Shiwakoti et al., 2017). An *in vitro* study found that extracts even stopped the nitric oxide production and inducible nitric oxide synthase. Aye et al. (2019) found that the *O. basilicum* ethanolic extract of leaf and callus showed anti-inflammatory effect in an *in vitro* test on LPS-stimulated RAW 264.7 macrophage cells by lowering nitric oxide production. At an 8 mg/mL concentration, research by Bayala et al. (2014) showed that the anti-inflammatory effect of essential oil of *O. basilicum* is caused by the inhibition of the lipoxygenase enzyme by 98.2%. The elevated concentration of eugenol, limonene, and linalool in the essential oil are responsible for better fighting of any inflammation. Since most tests of *O. basilicum*'s anti-inflammatory activity are done in an *in vitro* setting, the outcomes cannot be fully extrapolated to its clinical use. To confirm the *in vivo* activity, more research needs to be done (Guez et al., 2017).

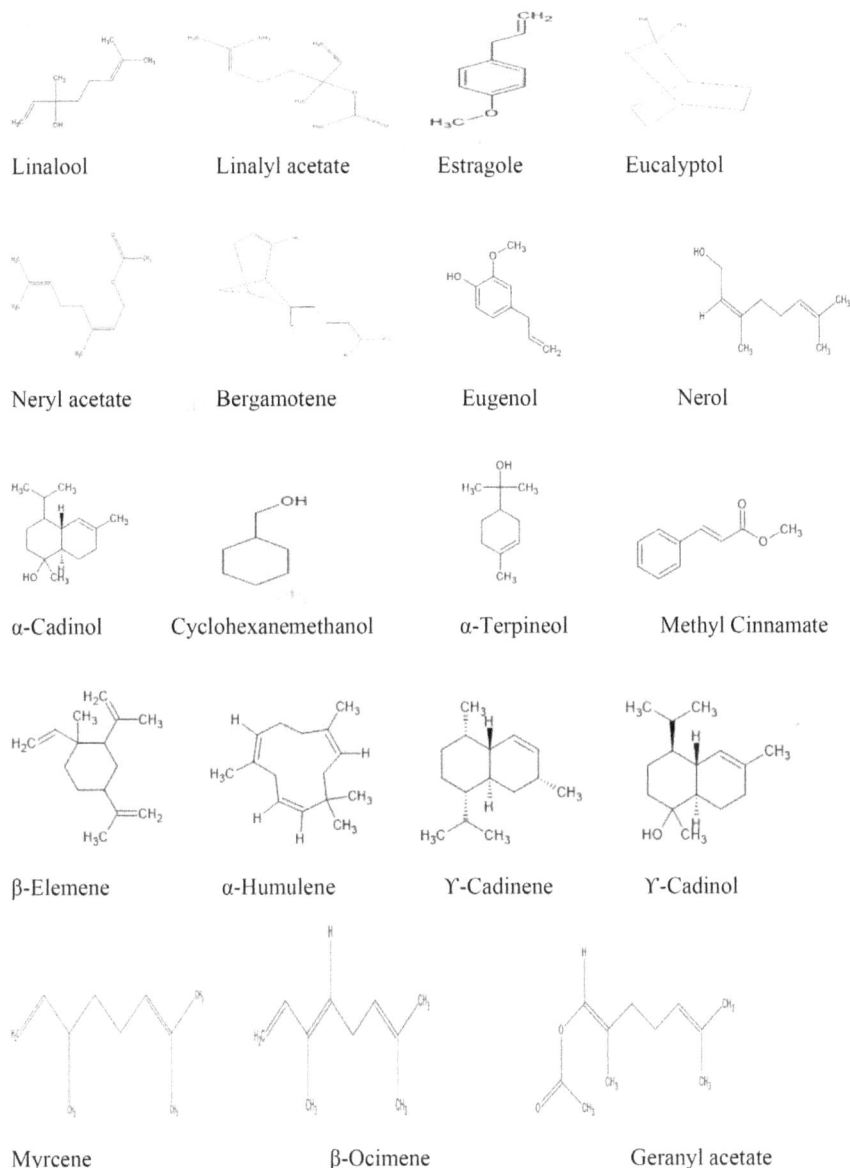

FIGURE 13.1    Structures of phytoconstituents present in basil (*Ocimum basilicum*).

## 13.3.2    ANTI-BACTERIAL ACTIVITY

Gram-positive as well as Gram-negative bacteria were killed with the extract of *O. basilicum*, which is a positive indication. Gram-negative bacteria like *P. mirabilis*, *Proteus vulgaris*, and *Pseudomonas aeruginosa* were killed by *O. basilicum* essential oil and Gram-positive bacteria including *M. luteus, Bacillus subtilis, Micrococcus flavus, Streptococcus faecalis, Staphylococcus aureus,* and *S. epidermidis* were also killed (Adam et al., 2015). Adiguzel et al. (2005) studied the *in vitro* antimicrobial effect of *O. basilicum* extracts from methanol, ethanol, and hexane. The hexane extract was the most effective at killing bacteria. The methanol and ethanol extracts, which were also used, killed 10%, 9%, and 6% of the 146 bacterial strains that were examined, respectively. MICs for hexane were between 125 and 250 μg/mL, methanol was between 62.5and 500 μg/mL, and the ethanol extracts were between 125 and 250 μg/mL. Based on the results of this study, *O. basilicum* extract may contain chemicals that kill bacteria and fungi that cause diseases. Al Abbasy et al. (2015) used the agar well diffusion method to test the anti-bacterial effect of *O. basilicum* essential oil, which was extracted from aerial parts of plant. Studies revealed that the essential oil stopped the growth of *S. aureus, B. cereus, S. typhimurium,* and *E. coli,* but showed no effect on *S. epidermidis* and *K. pneumoniae* (Joshi, 2014; Nabrdalik and Grata, 2016).

### 13.3.3 ANTI-VIRAL ACTIVITY

Antiviral medicines from herbal sources are becoming more widely used for a variety of reasons, such as the absence of suitable drug candidates, the rise in antiviral drug resistance, and the fact that new and old viral pathogens keep reappearing (Chattopadhyay et al., 2007). The antiviral activity of *O. basilicum* extracts was examined against various viral pathogens, such as hepatitis B virus (HBV), adenoviruses (ADV), coxsackievirus B1 (CVB1), herpes simplex viruses (HSV), and enterovirus 71 (EV71). Romeilah et al. (2010) demonstrate that *in vitro* analysis results show that these compounds were effective against herpes simplex virus. Studies found (Chiang et al., 2005) that the bovine viral diarrhoea virus (BVDV) was interrupted by testing the anti-viral power of *O. basilicum* essential oil in a test tube. Even though the essential oil reduced plaque by 90%, the virucidal dose which would be required to achieve this result is too high to be practical. Several phytoconstituents found in *O. basilicum* were very effective at killing viruses. Major important constituents are linalool, apigenin, and ursolic acid. Among these, ursolic acid has been shown to fight viruses like ADV-8, EV71, CVB1, and HSV-1 (Romeilah et al., 2010).

### 13.3.4 ANTIOXIDANT ACTIVITY

*O. basilicum* extract has a potent antioxidant effect that protects against oxidative effects by boosting the levels of defensive antioxidative enzymes and lowering lactate dehydrogenase activity as well as lipid peroxidation. There are different types of antioxidants in basil leaves, such as glutathione, vitamin C, and fat-loving components (vitamin E and carotenoids). Also, the increased levels of linalool and eugenol present in *O. basilicum* essential oil help to boost its ability to fight free radicals. Studies have shown that the *O. basilicum* methanolic extract shows significant antioxidant effect (Kaurinovic et al., 2011). This was observed in the DPPH free radical-scavenging test by the change in absorbance. Flavonoids may have a property that makes them able to get rid of 1,1-diphenyl-2-picrylhydrazyl radicals. The antioxidant properties of five different extracts (Et2O, CHCl3, EtOAc, *n*-BuOH, and H2O) of *Ocimum basilicum* L. and *Origanum vulgare* L. were studied. Results showed that

EtOAc, *n*-BuOH, and H2O extracts of *O. basilicum* and *O. vulgare* expressed very strong scavenger activity, as well as the mentioned extracts showed notable inhibition of LPx. However, Et2O and CHCl3 extracts showed much weaker effect in the neutralization of DPPH, NO, and O2•– radicals and the neutralization of H2O2. When examining the production of OH radicals and inhibition of LPx, the Et2O and CHCl3 extracts showed weak prooxidative properties. The observed differences in antioxidant activity could be partially explained by the levels of phenolics and flavonoids in the investigated *O. basilicum* and *O. vulgare* extracts (Kaurinovic et al., 2011; Al-Ali et al., 2013).

### 13.3.5 ANTI-NEOPLASTIC AND ANTICANCER PROPERTIES

Plants from the *Ocimum* family have been used to treat cancer for a long time. The active chemical in *Ocimum basilicum* for anticancer activity is eugenol. On reviewing various research studies, when eugenol is introduced to breast cancer cells, the expression of p53 mRNA goes up and the expression of the bcl-2 gene goes down. Several studies have come to the conclusion that eugenol kills breast cancer cells. In an interesting way, eugenol stops cancer cells from growing by causing apoptosis and stopping cell division in the G2 or M phase. Aside from eugenol, the most important phytochemicals in basil that might help fight cancer are caffeic acid, rosmarinic acid, and isoeugenol (Jaganathan and Supriyanto, 2012). All of these, as well as linalool, have strong anticancer effects on SKOV3 cells (human ovary-based cancer cell line). Eugenol and isoeugenol are the potent inhibitors for DNA synthesis and show powerful cytotoxic effects against the tumour cell line of salivary gland. Isoeugenol destroys cells because it contains radicals that interact with the cell membrane. The presence of active phenolic content (p-hydroxy benzoic acid, benzoic acid, chlorogenic acid, caffeic acid, cinnamic acid, gallic acid, ferulic acid, kaempferol, p-coumaric acid, quercetin, and ellagic acid) had a strong cytotoxic effect on colon carcinoma (HCT116) as well as liver cell lines (HEPG2) (Zarlaha et al., 2014). The growth of a human breast cancer cell line (MCF-7) was slowed down. The anticancer activity of the essential oil was evaluated on three different cancer cell lines. The IC50 values were 431.215.3 g/ml for U-87 MG (glioblastoma cell line), 432.332.2 g/ml for MDA-MB-231 (triple negative human breast cancer cells), and 320.423.2 g/ml for MCF7 (breast cancer) (Torres et al., 2018).

### 13.3.6 CARDIOPROTECTIVE AND HEPATOPROTECTIVE PROPERTIES

The aqueous as well as organic extracts of the *Ocimum* reduce the cholesterol level in blood thus resulting in effective at treatment of both atherosclerosis and hyperlipidaemia. Researchers have found that isoproterenol made the ST-segment rise on an electrocardiogram, but ethanolic leaf extract lowered this rise. Also, the extract helped to improve myocardial necrosis and fibrosis, as well as the pressure and contractility of the left ventricle at the end of diastole. Moreover, malondialdehyde levels were reduced in the serum and myocardium (Tabassum and Ahmad, 2011). It normalizes systolic, diastolic, as well as blood pressure in dose-dependent way with 30 mg/Kg being the median effective dose. Eugenol, which is thought to be a natural calcium channel blocker, is thought to be the reason why *O. basilicum* protects the heart (Muralidharan and Dhananjayan, 2004, Fathiazad et al., 2012).

Hepatoprotective and antioxidant effects of *O. basilicum* were examined in the acetaminophen liver damage model in rats. There was a significant drop in amounts of liver enzymes present in serum-like aspartate aminotransferase, alanine aminotransferase, and alkaline phosphatase. Additionally, bilirubin and blood urea nitrogen levels in the serum also decreased. It was found that the reduction was much greater when *O. basilicum* whole plant extracts were used than when chloroform, diethyl ether, or ethyl acetate extracts were used. It was found that methanolic extracts of the whole plant of *O. basilicum* were better at protecting the liver than silymarin, which is a mixture of flavonoid lignans taken from milk thistle (*Silybum marianum* Gaertneri) (Abatan and Asala, 2016).

### 13.3.7  ANTI-FUNGAL ACTIVITY

*Ocimum basilicum* is found to be very effective against various pathogenic fungus including *A. flavus, C. albicans, Aspergillus, Cryptococcus, Trichophyton, Aureobasidium pullulans, Microsporum gypseum, Trichoderma viride, Aspergillus niger, Aspergillus fumigatus, Penicillium chrysogenum*, etc.

The research finding of Ahmad et al. (2016) states that methanolic extract of *O. basilicum* proved potent effects against plant-killing chemicals and fungi such as *A. flavus, Penicillium, A. niger, A. alternata, A. fumigates*, and *Rhizopus solani*. These fungi were significantly slowed down by the methanolic extract of this plant. *Candida albicans* and *Curvularia lunata* were the least affected. At a concentration of 1,000 mg/L of oil, the growth of fungi was completely stopped, and the amount of aflatoxin B1 produced dropped at concentration of oil at 500 mg/L and1,000 mg/L. *Candida albicans* and *C. glabrata* isolates were killed and stopped from growing by the *O. basilicum* essential oil. The way it works is by stopping the transition from yeast to mycelial form (Oxenham et al., 2005).

### 13.3.8  INSECTICIDAL AND ANTI-PARASITIC ACTIVITY

The essential oil obtained from *O. basilicum* leaf extract was strong in killing the larvae of *Aedes albopictus, Culex tritaeniorhynchus, Anopheles subpictus*, etc. Essential oil can be utilized to kill mosquito larvae in a way that is safe, effective, and easy to find in nature. *O. basilicum* essential oil can be utilized instead of conventional insecticides because it kills insects very well (Govindarajan et al., 2013).

### 13.3.9  ANTICONVULSANT ACTIVITY

Research studies have revealed that the *O. basilicum* essential oil treated convulsions caused by pentylenetetrazole and picrotoxin. Research studies (Modaresi et al., 2014) reported the hydroalcoholic extract had the same effect on anxiety as diazepam, with 150 mg/kg being the least effective dose. It's interesting to observe that the sedative effect of the essential oil as compared to that of the whole plant was much stronger; this was mostly due to phenol and terpenoid contents. Geraniol is also a major constituent of the essential oil. It slows down the activity of the CNS, causing ataxia and ptosis in addition to the sedative effect. When *O. basilicum* extract of leaves was used to treat people, it was found that their memories and motor skills got better. It also reduced the brain damage and oxidative stress in mice, resulting in better function after an ischemic stroke, which makes it a possible neuroprotective agent (Hirai and Ito, 2019).

The various pharmacological activities of *Ocimum basilicum* are summarized in Table 13.1.

---

**TABLE 13.1**

## Phytochemical Constituents of *Ocimum basilicum* with Their Pharmacological Activities

| S. No. | Phytochemical Constituents | Pharmacological Activity | Mechanisms |
|--------|---------------------------|--------------------------|------------|
| 1. | Eugenol<br>Ursolic acid<br>Linalool<br>Isoeugenol | Anticancer and antineoplastic | Induce apoptosis.<br>Inhibit DNA synthesis.<br>Exhibits potent cytotoxicity against tumour cell. |
| 2. | Eugenol<br>Linalool<br>Rosmarinic acid<br>Linoleic acid<br>Methyl cinnamate | Antioxidant activity | Scavenge free radicals.<br>Increase antioxidative defence enzyme level. |
| 3. | Eugenol<br>Linalool<br>Rosmarinic acid | Cardio- and hepatoprotective activity | Prevent hyperlipidaemia.<br>Prevent hepatic fibrosis. |
| 4. | Estragole<br>Methyl eugenol<br>Linalool<br>Eugenol<br>Methyl cinnamate<br>Linoleic acid | Anti-inflammatory activity | Inhibit pro-inflammatory mediators cyclooxygenase and lipoxygenase enzymes.<br>Stimulate cytokines. |
| 5. | Linalool<br>Eugenol<br>Estragole<br>α-terpineol<br>1,8-cineole | Anti-bacterial activity | Damage bacterial cell wall and cytoplasmic protein membrane. |
| 6. | Apigenin<br>Eugenol<br>Linalool<br>Ursolic acid | Anti-viral activity | Prevent virus attachment.<br>Interfere with hepatitis B replication. |
| 7. | Estragole<br>Linalool<br>Eugenol<br>Methyl cinnamate | Anti-fungal activity | React with ROS.<br>Inhibit mycelium and spore germination. |

*(Continued)*

**TABLE 13.1** (*Continued*)
**Phytochemical Constituents of *Ocimum basilicum* with Their Pharmacological Activities**

| S. No. | Phytochemical Constituents | Pharmacological Activity | Mechanisms |
|--------|---------------------------|--------------------------|------------|
| 8. | Linalool<br>2-decanone<br>Pulegone | Anti-parasitic activity | Defence mechanisms against insects and other arthropods. |
| 9. | Eucalyptol<br>Linalool<br>Methyl eugenol<br>Estragole | Immunomodulatory activity | Proliferate immune cells.<br>Stimulate cytokines. |
| 10. | Apigenin<br>Linalool<br>Eugenol | Anti-osteoporotic effect | Induce apoptosis in mature osteoclasts.<br>Inhibit bone resorption. |
| 11. | Methyl eugenol<br>Anthocyanins<br>1,8-cineole | Anti-ulcer activity | Reduce pepsin production.<br>Inhibit lipoxygenase. |
| 12. | Apigenin<br>Diosmetin<br>Genistein<br>Kaempferol<br>Luteolin | Hypoglycaemic activity | Utilize increased glucose.<br>Promote glycogen in liver.<br>Stimulate insulin secretion. |
| 13. | Linalool<br>Eugenol | Analgesic activity | Inhibit cyclooxygenase.<br>Inhibit pain mediators. |

## 13.4 ADVANCED FORMULATIONS OF *OCIMUM BASILICUM*

Advanced formulations of *Ocimum basilicum* have been formulated for various therapeutic activities and pharmaceutical application, mentioned in Table 13.2.

## 13.5 CONCLUSION AND FUTURE PERSPECTIVES

*Ocimum basilicum*, which is more commonly known as basil, has many proven therapeutic properties including analgesic, antioxidant, antimicrobial, anti-inflammatory, hypoglycaemic, antihyperlipidaemic, hepatoprotective, anti-ulcerative, antihypertensive, cytoprotective, etc., due to the presence of its various active chemical components 1,8-cineole, linalool, eugenol, and chavicol. Most of *O. basilicum*'s activities are confirmed by researchers by *in vitro* and *in vivo* evaluations. Clinical studies have also proven *Ocimum basilicum* shows a wide range of activities but more of these kinds of evaluations are needed to figure out and confirm *O. basilicum*'s ethnopharmacological profile. It's important to remember that herbal medicines or their extracts have no side effects, unlike some other medicines used in the treatment of same disease. Future research should focus on finding the active parts of

**TABLE 13.2**

**Advanced Formulations of *Ocimum basilicum***

| S. No. | Formulation | Part Used | Activity | Key Finding | Reference |
|---|---|---|---|---|---|
| 1. | Silver nanoparticles | aqueous leaf extract | Antibacterial Antimicrobial | Control the diabetic-induced bacterial infections, occurring due to peripheral neuropathy. *In vitro* result states potent inhibition action against both Gram-negative and Gram-positive bacteria. | Malapermal et al., 2017 |
| 2. | Nano emulsion | essential oil | Antibacterial Antioxidant Larvicidal | Potential applications in drug delivery, biomedical field, cosmetics, pharmaceuticals, and food industry. | Sundararajan et al., 2018 |
| 3. | Basil seed gum nanoparticles | basil seed gum mucilage | In drug delivery systems As commercial hydrocolloids in food industry | Used as polymer in antibacterial wound dressing; shows non-cytotoxic and non-adherent nature. | Pirtarighat et al., 2019 |

*O. basilicum*, making them on a large scale, figuring out their chemical properties, therapeutic potential, and toxicity profile, allowing molecular changes to be made to the active compounds so that suitable therapeutic formulations can be prepared for commercial scale. Another alternative is to include *O. basilicum* as an additive to chemotherapeutic drugs thereby reducing the doses of the synthetic drugs and making them less harmful. Also, some explanatory mechanism-of-action studies should be done to find out how this revered medicinal herb works on the inside. Strengthening the current methods of extracting for the herb, the protocols for standardizing drugs, and future clinical studies on the health-promoting properties of this plant would help to increase its usefulness.

## REFERENCES

Abatan, M. O.; Asala, M. T. The Hepatoprotective Effects of Whole Plant Extracts of *Ocimum basilicum* in Experimentally Induced Liver Damage in Rats. Fed Am Soc. Exp Biol J. 2016, 30, 932–939.

Adam, Z. A.; Omer, A. A. Antibacterial Activity of *Ocimum basilicum* (Rehan) Leaf Extract against Bacterial Pathogens in Sudan. Am. J. Res. Commun. 2015, 3(8), 94–99.

Adiguzel, A.; Gulluce, M.; Sengul, M.; Ogutcu, H.; Sahin, F.; Karaman, I. Antimicrobial Effects of *Ocimum basilicum* (Labiatae) Extract. Turk J Biol. 2005, 29, 155–160.

Ahmad, K.; Khalil, A. T.; Somayya, R. Antifungal, Phytotoxic and Hemagglutination Activity of Methanolic Extracts of *Ocimum basilicum*. J Tradit Chin Med. 2016, 36(6), 794–798.

Al Abbasy, D. W.; Pathare, N.; Al-Sabahi, J. N.; Khan, S. A. Chemical Composition and Antibacterial Activity of Essential Oil Isolated from Omani Basil (*Ocimum basilicum* Linn.). Asian Pacific J Trop Dis. 2015, 5(8), 645–649.

Al-Ali, K. H.; El-Beshbishy, H. A.; El-Badry, A. A.; Alkhalaf, M. Cytotoxic Activity of Methanolic Extract of Menthalongi Folia and *Ocimum basilicum* against Human Breastcancer. Pak. J. Biol. Sci. 2013, 16(23), 1744–1750.

Aye, A.; Jeon, Y. D.; Lee, J. H.; Bang, K. S. Anti-Inflammatory Activity of Ethanol Extract of Leaf and Leaf Callus of Basil (*Ocimum basilicum* L.) On RAW 264.7 Macrophage Cells. Orient. Pharm. Exp. Med. 2019, 19(2), 217–226.

Bayala, B.; Bassole, I. H.; Gnoula, C.; Nebie, R.; Yonli, A.; Morel, L.; Figueredo, G.; Nikiema, J. B.; Lobaccaro, J. M.; Simpore, J. Chemical Composition, Antioxidant, Anti-Inflammatory and Anti-Proliferative Activities of Essential Oils of Plants from Burkina Faso. PLoS One. 2014, 9(3), e92122.

Bilal, A.; Jahan, N.; Ahmed, A.; Bilal, S. N.; Habib, S.; Hajra, S. Phytochemical and Pharmacological Studies on *Ocimum basilicum* Linn-A Review. Int J Curr Res Rev. 2012, 4(23), 73–83.

Chattopadhyay, D.; Naik, T. N. Antivirals of Ethnomedicinal Origin: Structure-activity Relationship and Scope. Mini. Rev. Med. Chem. 2007, 7(3), 275–301.

Chiang, L. C.; Ng, L. T.; Cheng, P. W.; Chiang, W.; Lin, C. C. Antiviral Activities of Extracts and Selected Pure Constituents of *Ocimum basilicum*. Clin. Exp. Pharmacol. Physiol. 2005, 32(10), 811–816.

Dhama, K.; Latheef, S. K.; Mani, S.; Samad, H. A.; Karthik, K.; Tiwari, R.; Khan, R. U.; Alagawany, M.; Farag, M. R.; Alam, G. M.; et al. Multiple Beneficial Applications and Modes of Action of Herbs in Poultry Health and Production: A Review. International Journal of Pharmacology. 2015, 11(3), 152–176.

Eftekhar, N.; Moghimi, A.; MohammadianRoshan, N.; Saadat, S.; Boskabady, M. H. Immunomodulatory and Anti-Inflammatory Effects of Hydro-Ethanolic Extract of *Ocimum basilicum* Leaves and Its Effect on Lung Pathological Changes in an Ovalbumin-Induced Rat Model of Asthma. BMC Complement. Altern. Med. 2019, 19(1), 349. DOI: 10.1186/s12906-019-2765-4.

Fathiazad, F.; Matlobi, A.; Khorrami, A.; Hamedeyazdan, S.; Soraya, H.; Hammami, M.; Maleki-Dizaji, N.; Garjani, A. Phytochemical Screening and Evaluation of Cardioprotective Activity of Ethanolic Extract of *Ocimum basilicum* L. (Basil) against Isoproterenol Induced Myocardial Infarction in Rats. Daru. 2012, 20, 87.

Govindarajan, M.; Sivakumar, R.; Rajeswary, M.; Yogalakshmi, K. Chemical Composition and Larvicidal Activity of Essential Oil from *Ocimum basilicum* (L.) against Culex Tritaeniorhynchus, Aedes Albopictus and Anopheles Subpictus (Diptera: Culicidae). Exp Parasitol. 2013, 134(1), 7–11.

Guez, C. M.; Souza, R. O.; Fischer, P.; Leão, M. F.; Duarte, J. A.; Boligon, A. A.; Athayde, M. L.; Zuravski, L.; Oliveira, L. F.; Machado, M. M. Evaluation of Basil Extract (*Ocimum basilicum* L.) On Oxidative, Anti-genotoxic and Anti-Inflammatory Effects in Human Leukocytes Cell Cultures Exposed to Challenging Agents. Braz. J. Pharm. Sci. 2017, 53(1), 1–12.

Hirai, M.; Ito, M. Sedative Effects of the Essential Oil and Headspace Air of *Ocimum basilicum* by Inhalation in Mice. J Nat Med. 2019, 73(1), 283–288. DOI: 10.1007/s11418-018-1253-3.

Jaganathan, S. K.; Supriyanto, E. Antiproliferative and Molecular Mechanism of Eugenol-Induced Apoptosis in Cancer Cells. Molecules. 2012, 17(6), 6290–6304. DOI: 10.3390/molecules17066290.

Joshi, R. K. Chemical Composition and Antimicrobial Activity of the Essential Oil of *Ocimum basilicum* L. (Sweet Basil) from Western Ghats of North West Karnataka, India. Ancient Sci. Life. 2014, 33(3), 151–156.

Kaurinovic, B.; Popovic, M.; Vlaisavljevic, S.; Trivic, S. Antioxidant Capacity of *Ocimum basilicum* L. And Origanum Vulgare L. Extracts. Molecules. 2011, 16(9), 7401–7414.

Kumar, A.; Rahal, A.; Chakraborty, S.; Tiwari, R.; Latheef, S. K.; Dhama, K. Ocimum Sanctum (Tulsi): A Miracle Herb and Boon to Medical Science: A Review. Int. J Agron Plant Prod. 2013, 4(7), 1580–1589.

Malapermal, V.; Botha, I.; Krishna, S. B.; Mbatha, J. N. Enhancing Antidiabetic and Antimicrobial Performance of *Ocimum basilicum*, and Ocimum Sanctum (L.) Using Silver Nanoparticles. Saudi J. Biol. Sci. 2017, 24(6), 1294–1305.

Miraj, S.; Kiani, S. Study of Pharmacological Effect of *Ocimum basilicum*: A Review. Der Pharmacia Lettre. 2016, 8, 276–280.

Modaresi, M.; Pouriyanzadeh, A.; Asadi-Samani, M. Antiepileptic Activity of Hydroalcoholic Extract of Basil in Mice. J Herb Med Pharmacol. 2014, 3, 57–60.

Muralidharan, A.; Dhananjayan, R. Cardiac Stimulant Activity of *Ocimum basilicum* Linn. Extracts. Indian J Pharmacol. 2004, 36, 163–166.

Nabrdalik, M.; Grata, K. Antibacterial Activity of *Ocimum basilicum* L. Essential Oil against Gram-Negative Bacteria. Post Fitoter. 2016, 17(2), 80–86.

Oxenham, S. K.; Svoboda, K. P.; Walter, D. R. Antifungal Activity of the Essential Oil of Basil (*Ocimum basilicum*). J. Phytopathol. 2005, 153(3), 174–180.

Pirtarighat, S.; Ghannadnia, M.; Baghshahi, S. Biosynthesis of Silver Nanoparticles Using *Ocimum basilicum* Cultured under Controlled Conditions for Bactericidal Application. Mater Sci Eng C Mater Biol Appl. 2019, 98, 250–255. DOI: 10.1016/j.msec.2018.12.090.

Purushothaman, B.; Srinivasan, P.; Suganthi, R.; Ranganathan, P.; Gimbun, B.; Shanmugam, K. A Comprehensive Review on *Ocimum Basilicum*. J Nat Remedies. 2018, 18, 71–85.

Romeilah, R. M.; Fayed, S. A.; Mahmoud, G. I. Chemical Compositions, Antiviral and Antioxidant Activities of Seven Essential Oils. J. Appl. Sci. Res. 2010, 6(1), 50–62.

Rubab, S.; Hussain, I.; Khan, B. A.; Unar, A. A.; Abbas, K. A.; Khich, Z. H.; Khan, M.; Khanum, S.; Khan, K. U.H. Biomedical Description of *Ocimum basilicum* L. J Islamic Int Med Colleg. 2017, 12, 59–67.

Salehi, B.; Ata, A.; Anil Kumar, V. N.; Sharopov, F.; Ramírez-Alarcón, K.; Ruiz-Ortega, A.; Abdulmajid Ayatollahi, S.; Tsouh Fokou, P. V.; Kobarfard, F.; Amiruddin Zakaria, Z.; Rahman, A.-U.; Choudhary, M. I.; Cho, W. C; Sharifi-Rad, J.; et al. Antidiabetic Potential of Medicinal Plants and Their Active Components. Biomolecules. 2019, 9(10), 551.

Sestili, P; Ismail, T; Calcabrini, C; Guescini, M; Catanzaro, E; Turrini, E; Layla, A; Akhtar, S; Fimognari, C. The Potential Effects of *Ocimum basilicum* on Health: A Review of Pharmacological and Toxicological Studies. Expert. Opin. Drug Metab Toxicol. 2018, 14(7), 679–692.

Shiwakoti, S.; Saleh, O.; Poudyal, S.; Barka, A.; Qian, Y.; Zheljazkov, V. D. Yield, Composition and Antioxidant Capacity of the Essential Oil of Sweet Basil and Holy Basil as Influenced by Distillation Methods. Chem. Biodivers. 2017, 14(4). DOI: 10.1002/cbdv.201600417.

Sundararajan, B.; Moola, A. K.; Vivek, K.; Kumari, B. R. Formulation of Nanoemulsion from Leaves Essential Oil of *Ocimum basilicum* L. And Its Antibacterial, Antioxidant and Larvicidal Activities (Culexquinquefasciatus). Microb. Pathogenesis. 2018, 125, 475–485.

Tabassum, N.; Ahmad, F. Role of Natural Herbs in the Treatment of Hypertension. Phcog. Rev. 2011, 5, 30–40.

Tantiwatcharothai, S.; Prachayawarakorn, J. Characterization of an Antibacterial Wound Dressing from Basil Seed (*Ocimum basilicum* L.) Mucilage-ZnOnanocomposite. Int J Biol Macromolecules. 2019, 135, 133–140.

Tiwari, R.; Chakraborty, S.; Dhama, K.; Rajagunalan, S.; Singh, S. V. Antibiotic Resistance: An Emerging Health Problem: Causes, Worries, Challenges and Solutions: A Review. Int J Curr Res. 2013, 5(7), 1880–1892.

Tiwari, R.; Latheef, S. K.; Ahmed, I.; Iqbal, H. M. N.; Bule, M. H.; Dhama, K.; Samad, H. A.; Karthik, K.; Alagawany, M.; El-Hack, M. E. A.; Yatoo, M. I.; et al. Herbal Immunomodulators: A Remedial Panacea for Designing and Developing Effective Drugs and Medicines: Current Scenario and Future Prospects. Curr. Drug Metab. 2018, 19(3), 264–301.

Torres, R. G.; Casanova, L.; Carvalho, J.; Marcondes, M. C.; Costa, S. S.; Sola-Penna, M.; Zancan, P. *Ocimum basilicum* but Not Ocimum Gratissimum Present Cytotoxic Effects on Human Breast Cancer Cell Line MCF-7, Inducing Apoptosis and Triggering mTOR/ Akt/p70S6K Pathway. Journal of Bioenergetics and Biomembranes. 2018, 50(2), 93–105. DOI: 10.1007/s10863-018-9750-3.

Yatoo, M. I.; Gopalakrishnan, A.; Saxena, A.; Parray, O. R.; Tufani, N. A.; Chakraborty, S.; Tiwari, R.; Dhama, K.; Iqbal, H. M. N. Anti-Inflammatory Drugs and Herbs with Special Emphasis on Herbal Medicines for Countering Inflammatory Diseases and Disorders: A Review. Recent Pat Inflamm Allergy Drug Discov. 2018, 12(1), 39–58.

Zarlaha, A.; Kourkoumelis, N.; Stanojkovic, T. P.; Kovala-Demertzi, D. Cytotoxic Activity of Essential Oil and Extracts of *Ocimum basilicum* against Human Carcinoma Cells. Molecular Docking Study of Isoeugenol as a Potent COX and LOX Inhibitor. Digest J Nanomat Biostr. 2014, 9, 907–917.

# 14 Exploration of the Pharmacological Aspects of *Thymus Vulgaris* Essential Oil (TEO)

*Kiran Dobhal, Shalu Verma, Alka Singh, Ruchika Garg, and Vikash Jakhmola*

## 14.1 INTRODUCTION

A bioactive compound of plants viz. *Jasminum grandiflorum, Olea europaea, Fraxinus americana, Syringa vulgare, Ligustrum vulgare, Forsythia viridissima, Cinnamomum zeylanicum, Mentha piperita, Curcuma longa, Withania somnifera, Ocimum basilicum, Origanum vulgare, Piper nigrum, Rosmarinus officinalis*, and *Thymus vulgaris* has been explored for various chronic ailments. The plant extract has been used as a spice to enhance the taste of food, medicine, preservatives, like clove and anise essential oil, etc. (Abeer M et al. 2019). Naturally occurring products draw the attention of consumers and manufacturing hubs because they come under the GRAS (generally recognized as safe) alternative of synthesized products. Thyme is the utmost exhausted species explored for its ethnopharmacological aspects and bioactive components (Singletary 2016; Mohamed 2022; Hammoudi et al. 2022). *Th. vulgaris* (thyme) comes under the shadow of the *Lamiaceae* (Labiate) family and *Thymus* L. genus; extensively noticed as a spice in the western Mediterranean region (Stahl-Biskup and Sáez 2002). It is native to southern Europe, Spain, Italy, and Lebanon. The popular name thyme means strength derived from the Greek word "thymos". It is a perennial, evergreen herb with a straight attitude along with a woody stem (Stahl-Biskup and Venskutonis 2012). The leaves are the most consuming part of the plant, having an oval shape with a pleasing aroma (Salehi et al. 2018; Kowalczyk et al. 2020).

## 14.2 CHEMICAL COMPONENTS OF THYME

Numerous secondary metabolites and essential oils compose thyme, which relies on the climate, soil, harvesting period, and geographical circumstances. GC and GC-MS techniques were developed to identify the chemical fingerprint in the leaf extracts of *Ocimum basilicum* L. (basil) and *Th. Vulgaris* L. (thyme). Dominant volatile components of basil oil found were linalool, estragole, methyl cinnamate, eugenol, and 1,8-cineole, whereas thymol, carvacrol, linalool, α-terpineol, and 1,8-cineole were

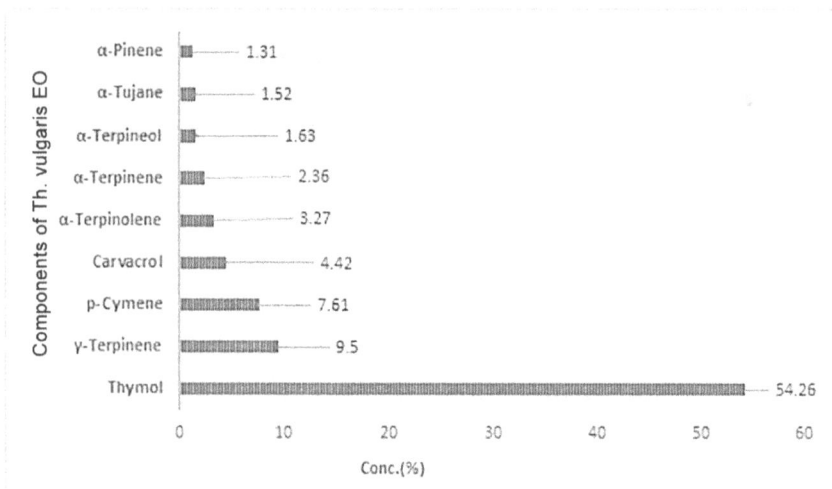

**FIGURE 14.1** Concentrations of components of *Th. vulgaris* essential oil.

the chief components in thyme oil. These volatile components further subjected to evaluate antioxidant potential via aldehyde and carboxylic acid assay. Eugenol, thymol, carvacrol, and 4-allylphenol exposed more intense antioxidant activities than others (Prasanth et al. 2014; Lee et al. 2005).

Thyme is blessed with phytonutrients, minerals, and vitamins, responsible for good quality health and the inhibition of disease. *Th. vulgaris* essential oil (TEO) is a naturally occurring assortment at different concentrations (Hoodia et al. 2002; Fecka and Turek 2008). TEOs are completely natural mixtures of thymol, carvacrol (cymophenol), p-cymene, γ-terpinene, linalool, β-myrcene, and terpinen-4-ol (Dauqan and Abdullah 2017; Agili 2014).

Other miscellaneous components are camphene, δ-3-carene, 1,8-cineol, geranic acid, 3-hexanol, myrcene, octadecenoic acid, cis-ocimene, β-ocimene, 3-octanol, α-phellandrene, α-pinene, cis-sabinene, sylvestrene, α-terpinene, and γ-terpinene. Thymol is the most abundant compound at approximately 54.26%, followed by 9.5%, 7.61%, and 4.42% of γ-terpinene, p-cymene, and carvacrol content respectively. Thymol and carvacrol are isomers of each other (Raudone et al. 2017; Aprotosoaie et al. 2019; Aljabeili et al. 2018).

The fresh herb of thyme possesses the highest level of minerals and vitamins which are excellent for good health. Thyme is a plentiful resource of vitamins A, C, and B-complex; it is particularly rich in $B_6$ (pyridoxine), K, E, β-carotene, and $B_{12}$. The leaves contain potassium, calcium, manganese, iron, magnesium, and selenium (Lorenzo et al. 2019; Vlaicu et al. 2022). Most of the bioactive components are extracted through a methanolic medium, although extraction carried out by another organic solvent like butanol, ethyl acetate, and hexane confirms the presence of saponins, steroids, flavonoids, alkaloids, and tannins. Luteolin, hesperidin, rutin, quercetin 7-o-glucoside, kaempferol, kaempferol-3-o-rutinoside, naringenin, and apigenin are the flavonoids present in thyme. Rosmarinic acid, p-Coumaric acid, caffeic acid, syringic acid, quercetin, ferulic acid,

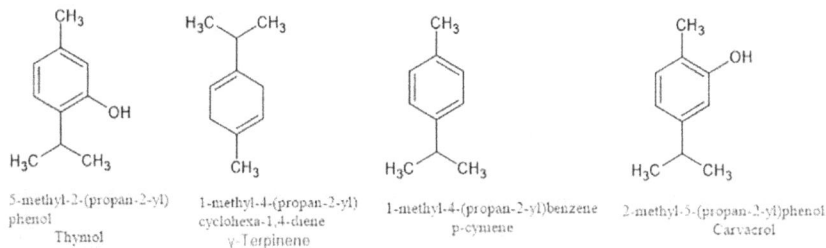

**FIGURE 14.2**    Chemical structures of four components of *Th. Vulgaris* essential oil.

carnosic acid, quinic acid, and caffeoylquinic are the numerous phenolic acids present explored for astringent, anti-allergic, anti-mutagen, antioxidative, etc. effects (Youdim and Deans 2000; Abeer et al. 2019; Mohammadzadeh and Pirzad 2021).

Maceration, Soxhlet, ultrasound-assisted extraction, and rapid solid–liquid dynamic extraction were employed to find out the bioactive compounds from *Th. vulgaris* L. (thyme), *Cannabis sativa* L. (industrial hemp), and *Coriandrum sativum* L. (coriander). GC-MS and HPLC-UV were employed to characterize the aromatic component and total polyphenolic component. Soxhlet techniques revealed the polyphenolic constituent viz. rosmarinic acid, apigenin, and luteolin in dry extract of thyme (Palmieri et al. 2020).

## 14.3    PHARMACOLOGICAL ASPECTS OF *TH. VULGARIS*

Antioxidants have been crucial for the defense and promotion of human health against free radicals, which cause numerous diseases. Essential oils high in oxygenated monoterpenes and/or sesquiterpenes have been presumed to have significant antioxidative properties. Oxidation or loss of electrons in our body produces free radicals, causing unwanted uninterrupted biochemical reactions in our body. TEO is rich in oxygenated monoterpenes, behaving as an antioxidant by removing free radicals. Thyme leaf has been used as a spice, a taste enhancer, and a preservative in our diet. Traditionally it is used to cure respiratory disorders, and as antifungal, analgesic, antipyretic, carminative, fumigants, memory enhancer, stress reliever, antispasmodic, antiseptic, anthelmintic, and anticancer. It is a treasure of iron, calcium, manganese, magnesium, and selenium; it boosts the entire body system. *Th. vulgaris* is quite an expensive spice compared to other thyme species; therefore other thyme species can be alternatives of TEO for the preparation of pharmaceutical dosage forms viz. ointment, syrup, tincture, etc. The leafy parts of thyme and TEO have been consumed in foods for scents, and preservation in traditional scripts (Singletary 2016).

### 14.3.1    ANTIOXIDANT ASPECTS OF TEO

A study on TEO evaluated its antioxidative effect against aflatoxin-induced oxidative stress in mature male Sprague-Dawley rats. The dosing of TEO was 5 mg/kg and 7.5 mg/kg. Aflatoxin interrupts the lipid content in serum, raises creatinine, uric acid, and nitric oxide in serum, and lipid peroxidase enzyme in the hepatic and renal systems, leading to serious metabolic disorders. Aflatoxin induces serious antioxidant action in our bodies. TEO is composed of carvacrol, thymol, β-phellandrene, linalool, humulene, α-phellandrene, and myrcene, a phenolic compound. Although a single dose of TEO was not effective against the aflatoxin-induced oxidative stress, a combined dose produced a remarkable antioxidant effect in all biochemical and histological reports. It means the antioxidant effect was dose-dependent (El-Nekeety et al. 2011). TEO was used to prepare a nano-emulsion by whey protein isolate and evaluated its antioxidant activity against the malfunctioning of hepatic and renal systems, lipid abnormality, mutagenicity, biochemical changes, oxidative stress, and DNA damage due to titanium dioxide nanoparticles (TNPs). TNPs have been extensively employed as medicinal and industrial agents, still mysterious about the safety criteria in living organisms. GC-MS characterization of TEO confirmed the presence of thymol and carvacrol. The average particle size was measured at $230 \pm 3.7$ accompanying $-24.17$ mV zeta potential (Sallam et al. 2022).

The brain is responsible for regulating polyunsaturated fatty acid (PUFA) which protects biological cells against free radicals; it can be maintained by TEO consumption in the diet. Docosahexaenoic acid (DHA) is the important PUFA content that regulates brain activity. Alteration of aging leads to the disturbance of antioxidative enzymes viz. superoxide dismutase (SOD) and glutathione peroxidase, entire antioxidant, and membrane phospholipid. The elevated antioxidant level of superoxide dismutase and glutathione peroxidase enzymes in the brains of aged male Wistar rats was monitored with treatment of TEO. A declining level of these antioxidative enzymes causes aging. In the clinical report, TEO in the diet raises the DHA in the relevance of another dietary supplement: thymol, a major constituent of thyme oil was claimed for it (Youdim and Deans 2000).

Chitosan nanoparticles of TEO were evaluated for beef burger's stability. Burgers that have TEO encapsulated exhibited the reduction of *Enterobacteriaceae* and *Staphylococcus aureus* (Ghaderi-Ghahfarokhi et al. 2016). TEO was obtained from leaves of *Th. vulgaris* by hydro-distillation techniques in Muscat, Sultanate of Oman. GS-MS were confirmed the presence of thymol, geraniol, carvacrol, α-terpineol, thujanol-4, linalool, etc., while carvacrol and α-terpinene were the main fingerprint region present in TEO as the aromatic volatile content in TEO. *In vitro* antioxidant activity of Omani TEO investigated by colorimetric method with 1,1 diphenyl picrylhydrazyl radical as a reference reducing agent and the effect was moderate. TEO disclosed the improved antimicrobial action than the β-lactam antibiotic ampicillin to counteract *S. aureus* and *E. coli* by disc diffusion method. The carvacrol was account for the reducing potential and antibacterial action of Omani thyme oil. It could be the promising *in situ* antibacterial candidate in future eras; however, exhausted research should be proposed in *in vivo* studies and animal models (Alsaraf et al. 2020). TEO was investigated for antioxidant activity of peroxidase, catalase, and SOD enzyme. Thymol, the chief component of TEO, claimed the raising of SOD and catalase, as well as reducing the THP-1 cells human monocyte/macrophage cell line which was stimulated by *Pseudomonas aeruginosa* invasion. TEO behaves as a potent scavenging radical reagent and alters the antioxidant enzyme potential. TEO obtained from the initial flowering of thyme revealed the maximum total antioxidant action and enzyme triggering function while TEO obtained from the ending of flowering elevated the antioxidant effect exerted due to enzyme and non-enzyme chemicals like glutathione (Pandur et al. 2022).

Thyme (*Th. vulgaris*), oregano (*Origanum vulgare* L.), and marjoram (*Origanum majorana* L.) were subjected to the 95% ethanolic solvent extraction, to prepare the phenolic extract of the respective plant. These extracts were further subjected to the various antioxidant and radical-scavenging potential experiments on the prepared extracts employing colorimetric assays and linoleic acid-ferric thiocyanate model system; precisely focused on the total phenolics content, reduction potential in a model system, scavenging outcome on 2,2'-diphenyl-1-picrylhydrazyl radical, and hydroxyl radical-scavenging action via electron paramagnetic resonance spectroscopy. Furthermore, the antioxidant potential of these extracts was evaluated in a realistic consuming food product, i.e., the preservation of butter against oxidation (Amarowicz et al. 2009).

Essential oil obtained from Moldavian *Thymus* species viz. *Th. vulgaris*, *Th. citriodorus*, *Th. calcareus*, and cultivars species, i.e., *Th. vulgaris* "Faustini", *Th. citriodorus* "Aureus", subjected to identify chemical component and *in vitro* antifungal action. Thymol was found in the *Th. vulgaris* and *Th. citriodorus* EOs, whereas lavandulol was found in *Th. citriodorus* EO, and geraniol in *Th. citriodorus* "Aureus" and *Th. vulgaris* "Faustini" EOs correspondingly. *Th. vulgaris* and *Th. calcareus* EOs accompanied the highest scavenging action and revealed substantial suppression action to counteract aflatoxin-producing *Aspergillus flavus* fungus at 0.25 µL/mL MIC. They concluded that these Moldavian *Thymus* species could be worthy resources of EOs for pharmaceutical and food industries viz. *Th. vulgaris* and *Th. calcareus* as well as for aroma industries viz. *Th. citriodorus*, *Th. citriodorus* "Aureus", and *Th. vulgaris* "Faustini" (Aprotosoaie et al. 2017).

## 14.3.2 Anticancer Activity

Most anticancer drugs are of natural origin. It has been postulated that naturally occurring phytochemical mixtures discovered in plant foods possess cancer-suppressive attributes. Approximately 2–3% of people die due to head and neck squamous cell carcinoma (HNSCC) globally. TEO was investigated against the HNSCC cell line and $IC_{50}$ was reported at 369 µg/mL. The interferon triggering, N-glycan biosynthesis, and stimulation of extracellular signal-regulated kinase 5 pathway were the active mechanism for the accounting of its anticancer action. However, further investigation is required against the molecular mode of anticancer activity of TEO (Sertel et al. 2011).

*In vivo* and *in vitro* chemically induced breast mammary cancer in the syngeneic 4T1 mouse models was investigated in form of haulm of dried thyme in the diet. Through autopsy, histopathological and molecular analyses after the consumption of thyme indicate the reduction of 4T1 cancer by 85% and 84% for 0.1% and 1% in the diet respectively (Kubatka et al. 2019). *In vitro* clinical testing was investigated on breast adenocarcinoma MCF-7, lung carcinoma H460, and acute lymphoblastic leukemia MOLT-4 by MTT assay. GS-MS analysis revealed the presence of thymol

(36.7%), p-cymene (30.0%), γ-terpinene (9.0%), and carvacrol (3.6%). A brine shrimp lethality test was carried out. Anticancer action is produced on a dose-dependent basis whereas $IC_{50}$ ranges from 52.65–228.78 µg/mL in vitro (Niksic et al. 2021).

TEO studied DLD-1 colorectal cancer cell line employing the real-time cell analyzing system (xCELLigence System). The anticancer effect was dependent on dose criteria; $IC_{50}$ was reported at 0.347 mg/mL. When the antineoplastic and free radical scavenging effects of TEO are considered, it is feasible to conclude that TEO may be a viable option for a colorectal cancer cure (Çetinus et al. 2013). *Rosmarinus officinalis, Th. vulgaris* L., and *Lavandula x intermedia* evaluated the anticancer effects on MCF-7 cells via MTT (3-[4,5-dimethylthiazol-2-yl]-2,5-diphenyl tetrazolium bromide) bioassay. TEO revealed more effectiveness at 400 µg/mL whereas *R. officinalis* and *L. x intermedia* was effective at 800 µg/mL and 400 µg/mL respectively against MCF-7 cells. Furthermore, TEO could be safer and more potent as an anticancer agent (Tabatabaei et al. 2018). TEO investigated HeLa (human epithelial cervical cancer) and MCF-7 (human breast carcinoma) cell lines at 6.25, 12.5, 25, 50, 100, and 200 ppm conc. At 200 ppm conc., 78.67% and 83.60% reductions were reported for HeLa and MCF-7 respectively. $IC_{50}$ against HeLa and MCF-7 cell lines was 34.63 and 27.66 ppm, respectively. Although the MCF-7 cell line showed higher sensitivity against TEO than the HeLa cell line (Khalaf and Abed 2021).

TEO was incorporated by blending whey protein isolate, maltodextrin, and gum Arabic. Zinc oxide nanoparticles caused oxidative stress, DNA impairment, biochemical and histopathological changes, and cytotoxicity; treatment with encapsulated TEO was given to male Sprague-Dawley rats. It revealed that treatment of encapsulated TEO exhibited a synergistic effect on cytotoxicity due to zinc oxide nanoparticles (Hassan et al. 2021).

### 14.3.3 ANTIVIRAL ACTION

Inhalation of essential oils from thyme, orange, clove bud, and frankincense improve energy levels in post-COVID-19 female patients through a double-blind random clinical trial in the United States at the end of 2021 (Hawkins et al. 2022). TEO investigated several RNA viruses including the coronavirus against feline infectious peritonitis in cats *in vitro*; 27 µg/mL–270 µg/mL of TEO was able to inhibit the transcription of coronavirus (Catella et al. 2021). Viricidal action of TEO was demonstrated against airborne coronavirus. Carvacrol is responsible for virucidal action in solution and in the air; 99.99% of the airborne virus are deactivated by TEO, and such a finding could be a potent outcome for future implications (Şakalar and Ertürk 2023).

TEO was consumed by 83 patients in form of syrup. Results revealed the reduction of fever, dizziness, cough, dyspnea, muscular pain, headache, anorexia, weakness and lethargy, fatigue, and chest wall pain, whereas blood urea nitrogen, neutrophil, and calcium declined. Lymphocyte numbering was raised remarkably (Sardari et al. 2021). An influenza virus is capable of causing threatening infection globally. Anti-influenza action of EOs obtained from *Citrus bergamia, Eucalyptus globulus, Pelargonium graveolens, Cinnamomum zeylanicum, Cymbopogon flexuosus,* and *Th. vulgaris* was evaluated in both liquid and vapor phase. *Cinnamomum zeylanicum*, *Citrus bergamia*, *Cymbopogon flexuosus*, and *Th. vulgaris* were used in liquid form and exhibited complete inhibition of virus infection at 3.1 μL/mL (Vimalanathan and Hudson 2014).

Essential oils from anise, hyssop, thyme, ginger, chamomile, and sandalwood were investigated against herpes simplex virus type 2 (HSV-2) *in vitro* on RC-37 cells through a plaque reduction assay. $IC_{50}$ was secured at 0.016%, 0.0075%, 0.007%, 0.004%, 0.003%, and 0.0015% for anise oil, hyssop oil, thyme oil, ginger oil, chamomile oil, and sandalwood oil, respectively. Dose-dependent action was extorted more than 90% with viral envelope (Koch et al. 2008).

## 14.3.4 ANTIFUNGAL ACTION

TEO and peppermint oil were investigated against *Aspergillus*, *Penicillium*, *Fusarium*, and *Saccharomyces* genera fungi in boiler houses. TEO reduces the *Aspergillus* by 75%, whereas 46% reduction is done by peppermint oil relevant to the standard (Witkowska et al. 2016). TEO, summer savory, and clove essential oils were investigated against *Aspergillus flavus* fungi in a liquid medium and tomato paste. TEO and summer savory oil exhibited excellent inhibition at 350 ppm and 500 ppm, correspondingly (Omidbeygi et al. 2007).

Antifungal oleogel of TEO exhibited an antifungal effect against *Candida albicans*, *Staphylococcus aureus*, *Salmonella typhimurium*, *Pseudomonas aeruginosa*, *Escherichia coli*, *Klebsiella pneumoniae*, and *Enterococcus faecalis*. Antifungal action was secured at 5 to 20 μL/mL. GS-MS confirms the presence of thymol and carvacrol in TEO. Oleogel containing TEO demonstrated antifungal activity against *Candida albicans*. Oleogel with TEO is a skin-care product that can be used for overall skin protection as well as a natural antiseptic with pharmaceutical applications (Kasparaviciene et al. 2018). TEO was evaluated against *Trichophyton interdigitale* on sheepskins for footwear lining and was revealed as a safe method to sanitize infected footwear (Chirilă et al. 2017).

## 14.3.5 NEURODEGENERATIVE ACTION

Several central nervous system diseases can be triggered by neuroinflammation. Geraniol, thujanol, and linalool, a chemical constituent of TEO, were evaluated for lipopolysaccharide-induced BV-2 microglia. It declines the concentration of tumor necrosis factor and interleukin-6 proinflammatory cytokines which were computed by the western blot method. Furthermore, by conducting exhaustive research, TEO can be an alternative candidate against neuroinflammation (Horváth et al. 2021). Alzheimer's disease is a neurodegenerative condition that develops over time. It has a broad spectrum of clinical markers and biomarkers, as well as many genetic and environmental components are believed to be responsible for its etiology and advancement. TEO was evaluated to raise cognitive cholinergic neurotransmitter function induced by using the scopolamine-induced zebrafish (*Danio rerio*) model of memory impairments. Scopolamine is an antimuscarinic antagonist. TEO improved anticholinesterase enzyme function and reduced oxidative stress in the brain.

Different concentrations of TEO, i.e., 25, 150, and 300 µL/L, was employed for more than two weeks to zebrafish. Space-based memory and novel object recognition test evaluated by the Y-maze test while anxiety and depression were measured in the novel tank diving test. GC-MS employed to study the phytochemical component of TEO. TEO augmented the acetylcholine degradation and oxidative stress response in the zebrafish's CNS. It was concluded that TEO could be the better option in cognitive management and amnesia in the treatment of Alzheimer's disease (Capatina et al. 2020).

### 14.3.6 MICROBIOLOGICAL BIOFILM ACTION AND ANTIBIOTIC RESISTANCE

Biofilm is a sort of polysaccharide protective layer in microorganisms which causes resistance against antimicrobial agents. Antibiofilm protection activity was evaluated against methicillin-resistant *S. aureus* and other bacterial strains. It was revealed that 0.01% and 0.05% of TEO concentration reduced 53% and 76% of the biofilm formation against *Streptococcus pyogenes* and *Escherichia coli*. Thymol was the key content for this action (Kryvtsova et al. 2019). Thymol, the chief constituent of thyme, exhibited antimicrobial inhibition against *E. coli*, *Listeria monocytogenes*, *Pseudomonas putida*, and *S. aureus* by reduction of biofilm formation (Kerekes et al. 2019). Hospital-acquired infection caused by *Klebsiella pneumonia* has the tendency to form biofilm against antimicrobial agents. Treatment of TEO revealed 80.1% to 98% of biofilm formation inhibition. Accompanied by ciprofloxacin, thymol showed a synergistic effect (Mohamed et al. 2018).

## 14.4 TEO AND ITS NEW THERAPEUTIC APPROACHES

It is critical to find a consistent approach for delivering both synthetic and natural agents to the disease's target cells to take benefit from their therapeutic activity. When in interaction with body enzymes, TEOs and their components may lose due to irritative effects. Consumption of TEO can be possible through blending with a natural and synthetic polymer, microfibers, etc. For example, excellent biocompatibility was reported of thymol with lignosulfonate. Lignosulfonate is also an antioxidant agent like thymol, which leads to a synergistic effect. This combination is used in microvesicles for targeted drug delivery systems and sustained release systems for high lipophilic drugs. Thymol can be fused in a porous membrane of cellulose acetate, revealing good inhibition against *S. aureus* and *E. coli*. Such an approach can be employed in wound healing material in the future. Glycerol liposomes and propylene glycol vesicles with TEO were found to be effective against *S. mutans*. Methylcellulose microspheres could enhance poor absorption and hide the irritating taste. Thymol is known as an excellent chronic wound healer in earlier studies. Blending target-release antimicrobial drugs into the dressing will be more effective in chronic wound therapy. A sophisticated dressing approach was integrated: mesoporous silicon dioxide loaded with thymol into electro-spun polycaprolactone microfibers. Therefore, more studies and innovations in techniques for creating therapeutically active microvesicles are anticipated (Kowalczyk et al. 2020; Kosakowska et al. 2020).

## 14.5  CONCLUSION

Currently, European Pharmacopoeia X have standardized the thyme herb and essential oil preparations for the manufacturing of pharmaceutical agents. Thyme herb is recognized as entire leaves and dried stems of *Th. vulgaris* or *Th. zygis*, composed of thymol and its isomer carvacrol. TEO is obtained by steam distillation of fresh flowering aerial sections of both species, varying concentrations of thymol (37–55%) and carvacrol (0.5–5.5%). The broad range of biological and therapeutic properties of thymol and TEO are confirmed by previous studies. *E. coli*, *L. monocytogenes*, *P. putida*, *S. aureus*, and methicillin-resistant *S. aureus* (MRSA) are some of the bacteria that certainly can break down biofilms. Furthermore, fungi strains viz. *Fusarium spp.*, *Aspergillus spp.*, *Candida spp.*, as well as yeast strains viz. *C. neoformans* and *C. laurentii* were characterized by their resistance to conventional treatment due to their capacity to form biofilms; therefore there is a need to develop effective natural treatment to counteract the biofilm formation. TEO is the better alternative to counteract the biofilm inhibition. TEO revealed the antiviral properties against viruses viz. influenza virus, coronavirus, herpes simplex virus 1 and 2, and HIV-1. Studies conducted *in silico* on thymol's anti-Sars-CoV-2 efficacy are likewise highly encouraging. Unfortunately, their preponderance of them lacks a well-established molecular mechanism of action. Furthermore, their new therapeutic formulations, including nanocapsules, microspheres, advanced dressing, and liposomes that include these ingredients, can be beneficial in medical training and open doors for their widespread use. Even though it needs more investigation, the widespread use of thymol and thyme essential oil in the healthcare sector is quite promising.

## ACKNOWLEDGMENT

Authors convey special thanks to Mr. Jitender Joshi, Chancellor, and Dr. Dharam Buddhi, Vice Chancellor of Uttaranchal University for encouragement in writing this communication.

## CONFLICT OF INTEREST

The authors declare that there is no conflict of interest.

## REFERENCES

Abeer M, Ahlam R, Marwa H. Impact of anise, clove, and thyme essential oils as feed supplements on the productive performance and digestion of Barki ewes. Australian Journal of Basic and Applied Science. 2019 Jun;13:1–3.

Agili FA. Chemical composition, antioxidant and antitumor activity of Thymus vulgaris L. essential oil. Middle-East Journal of Scientific Research. 2014;21(10):1670–1676.

Aljabeili HS, Barakat H, Abdel-Rahman HA. Chemical composition, antibacterial and antioxidant activities of thyme essential oil (Thymus vulgaris). Food and Nutrition Sciences. 2018 May 10;9(05):433.

Alsaraf S, Hadi Z, Al-Lawati WM, Al Lawati AA, Khan SA. Chemical composition, in vitro antibacterial and antioxidant potential of Omani thyme essential oil along with in silico studies of its major constituent. Journal of King Saud University-Science. 2020 Jan 1;32(1):1021–1028.

Amarowicz R, Żegarska Z, Rafałowski R, Pegg RB, Karamać M, Kosińska A. Antioxidant activity and free radical-scavenging capacity of ethanolic extracts of thyme, oregano, and marjoram. European Journal of Lipid Science and Technology. 2009 Nov;111(11):1111–1117.

Aprotosoaie AC, Miron A, Ciocârlan N, Brebu M, Roşu CM, Trifan A, Vochiţa G, Gherghel D, Luca SV, Niţă A, Costache II. Essential oils of Moldavian Thymus species: Chemical composition, antioxidant, anti-Aspergillus and antigenotoxic activities. Flavour and Fragrance Journal. 2019 May;34(3):175–186.

Capatina L, Todirascu-Ciornea E, Napoli EM, Ruberto G, Hritcu L, Dumitru G. *Thymus vulgaris* essential oil protects zebrafish against cognitive dysfunction by regulating cholinergic and antioxidants systems. Antioxidants (Basel). 2020 Nov 4;9(11):1083.

Catella C, Camero M, Lucente MS, Fracchiolla G, Sblano S, Tempesta M, Martella V, Buonavoglia C, Lanave G. Virucidal and antiviral effects of Thymus vulgaris essential oil on feline coronavirus. Res Vet Sci. 2021 Jul;137:44–47.

Çetinus E, Temiz T, Ergül M, Altun A, Çetinus Ş, Kaya T. Thyme essential oil inhibits proliferation of DLD-1 colorectal cancer cells through antioxidant effect. Cumhuriyet Medical Journal. 2013 Mar 22;35(1):14–24.

Chirilă C, Deselnicu V, Berechet MD. Footwear protection against fungi using thyme essential oil. Revista de Pielarie Incaltaminte. 2017;17(3):173.

Dauqan EM, Abdullah A. Medicinal and functional values of thyme (Thymus vulgaris L.) herb. Journal of Applied Biology and Biotechnology. 2017 Mar 20;5(2):0–2.

El-Nekeety AA, Mohamed SR, Hathout AS, Hassan NS, Aly SE, Abdel-Wahhab MA. Antioxidant properties of Thymus vulgaris oil against aflatoxin-induce oxidative stress in male rats. Toxicon. 2011 Jun 1;57(7–8):984–991.

Fecka I, Turek S. Determination of polyphenolic compounds in commercial herbal drugs and spices from Lamiaceae: Thyme, wild thyme and sweet marjoram by chromatographic techniques. Food Chemistry. 2008 Jun 1;108(3):1039–1053.

Ghaderi-Ghahfarokhi M, Barzegar M, Sahari MA, Azizi MH. Nanoencapsulation approach to improve antimicrobial and antioxidant activity of thyme essential oil in beef burgers during refrigerated storage. Food and Bioprocess Technology. 2016 Jul;9:1187–1201.

Hammoudi Halat D, Krayem M, Khaled S, Younes S. A focused insight into thyme: Biological, chemical, and therapeutic properties of an indigenous Mediterranean herb. Nutrients. 2022 Jan;14(10):2104.

Hassan ME, Hassan RR, Diab KA, El-Nekeety AA, Hassan NS, Abdel-Wahhab MA. Nanoencapsulation of thyme essential oil: a new avenue to enhance its protective role against oxidative stress and cytotoxicity of zinc oxide nanoparticles in rats. Environmental Science and Pollution Research. 2021 Oct;28(37):52046–52063.

Hawkins J, Hires C, Keenan L, Dunne E. Aromatherapy blend of thyme, orange, clove bud, and frankincense boosts energy levels in post-COVID-19 female patients: A randomized, double-blinded, placebo-controlled clinical trial. Complementary Therapies in Medicine. 2022 Aug;67:102823.

Hoodia M, Speroni E, Di Pietra AM, Cavrini V. GC/MS evaluation of thyme (Thymus vulgaris L.) oil composition and variations during the vegetative cycle. Journal of Pharmaceutical and Biomedical Analysis. 2002 Jul 20;29(4):691–700.

Horváth G, Horváth A, Reichert G, Böszörményi A, Sipos K, Pandur E. Three chemotypes of thyme (Thymus vulgaris L.) essential oil and their main compounds affect differently the IL-6 and TNFα cytokine secretions of BV-2 microglia by modulating the NF-κB and C/EBPβ signalling pathways. BMC Complementary Therapies in Medicine. 2021 May 22;21(1):148.

Kasparaviciene G, Kalveniene Z, Pavilonis A, Marksiene R, Dauksiene J, Bernatoniene J. Formulation and characterization of potential antifungal oleogel with essential oil of thyme. Evidence-Based Complementary and Alternative Medicine. 2018 Jan 1;2018.

Kerekes EB, Vidács A, Takó M, Petkovits T, Vágvölgyi C, Horváth G, Balázs VL, Krisch J. Anti-biofilm effect of selected essential oils and main components on mono-and poly-microbic bacterial cultures. Microorganisms. 2019 Sep 12;7(9):345.

Khalaf AN, Abed IJ. Evaluating the in vitro cytotoxicity of Thymus vulgaris essential oil on MCF-7 and HeLa cancer cell lines. Iraqi Journal of Science. 2021 Sep 30:2862–2871.

Koch C, Reichling J, Schneele J, Schnitzler P. Inhibitory effect of essential oils against herpes simplex virus type 2. Phytomedicine. 2008 Jan 25;15(1–2):71–78.

Kosakowska O, Bączek K, Przybył JL, Pawełczak A, Rolewska K, Węglarz Z. Morphological and chemical traits as quality determinants of common thyme (Thymus vulgaris L.), on the example of 'Standard Winter'cultivar. Agronomy. 2020 Jun 25;10(6):909.

Kowalczyk A, Przychodna M, Sopata S, Bodalska A, Fecka I. Thymol and thyme essential oil – new insights into selected therapeutic applications. Molecules. 2020 Sep 9;25(18):4125.

Kryvtsova MV, Salamon I, Koscova J, Bucko D, Spivak M. Antimicrobial, antibiofilm and biochemichal properties of Thymus vulgaris essential oil against clinical isolates of opportunistic infections. Biosystems Diversity. 2019;27(3):270–275.

Kubatka P, Uramova S, Kello M, Kajo K, Samec M, Jasek K, Vybohova D, Liskova A, Mojzis J, Adamkov M, Zubor P. Anticancer activities of Thymus vulgaris L. in experimental breast carcinoma in vivo and in vitro. International Journal of Molecular Sciences. 2019 Apr 9;20(7):1749.

Lee SJ, Umano K, Shibamoto T, Lee KG. Identification of volatile components in basil (Ocimum basilicum L.) and thyme leaves (Thymus vulgaris L.) and their antioxidant properties. Food Chemistry. 2005 Jun 1;91(1):131–137.

Lorenzo JM, Mousavi Khaneghah A, Gavahian M, Marszałek K, Eş I, Munekata PE, Ferreira IC, Barba FJ. Understanding the potential benefits of thyme and its derived products for food industry and consumer health: From extraction of value-added compounds to the evaluation of bioaccessibility, bioavailability, anti-inflammatory, and antimicrobial activities. Critical Reviews in Food Science and Nutrition. 2019 Oct 11;59(18):2879–2895.

Mohamed SH, Mohamed MS, Khalil MS, Azmy M, Mabrouk MI. Combination of essential oil and ciprofloxacin to inhibit/eradicate biofilms in multidrug-resistant Klebsiella pneumoniae. Journal of Applied Microbiology. 2018 Jul 1;125(1):84–95.

Mohamed SH. Role of moringa, thyme and licorice leave extracts on productive performance of growing rabbits. Annals of Agricultural Science, Moshtohor. 2022 Dec 1;60(4):1077–1090.

Mohammadzadeh S, Pirzad A. Biochemical responses of mycorrhizal-inoculated Lamiaceae (lavender, rosemary, and thyme) plants to drought: A field study. Soil Science and Plant Nutrition. 2021 Jan 2;67(1):41–49.

Niksic H, Becic F, Koric E, Gusic I, Omeragic E, Muratovic S, Miladinovic B, Duric K. Cytotoxicity screening of Thymus vulgaris L. essential oil in brine shrimp nauplii and cancer cell lines. Scientific Reports. 2021 Jun 23;11(1):13178.

Omidbeygi M, Barzegar M, Hamidi Z, Naghdibadi H. Antifungal activity of thyme, summer savory and clove essential oils against Aspergillus flavus in liquid medium and tomato paste. Food control. 2007 Dec 1;18(12):1518–1523.

Palmieri S, Pellegrini M, Ricci A, Compagnone D, Lo Sterzo C. Chemical composition and antioxidant activity of thyme, hemp and coriander extracts: A comparison study of maceration, Soxhlet, UAE and RSLDE techniques. Foods. 2020 Sep 2;9(9):1221.

Pandur E, Micalizzi G, Mondello L, Horváth A, Sipos K, Horváth G. Antioxidant and anti-inflammatory effects of thyme (Thymus vulgaris L.) essential oils prepared at different plant phenophases on Pseudomonas aeruginosa LPS-activated THP-1 macrophages. Antioxidants. 2022 Jul 6;11(7):1330.

Prasanth Reddy V, Ravi Vital K, Varsha PV, Satyam S. Review on Thymus vulgaris traditional uses and pharmacological properties. Med Aromat Plants. 2014;3(164):2167–0412.

Raudone L, Zymone K, Raudonis R, Vainoriene R, Motiekaityte V, Janulis V. Phenological changes in triterpenic and phenolic composition of Thymus L. species. Industrial Crops and Products. 2017 Dec 15;109:445–451.

Şakalar Ç, Ertürk M. Inactivation of airborne SARS-CoV-2 by thyme volatile oil vapor phase. Journal of Virological Methods. 2023 Feb 1;312:114660.

Salehi B, Mishra AP, Shukla I, Sharifi-Rad M, Contreras MD, Segura-Carretero A, Fathi H, Nasrabadi NN, Kobarfard F, Sharifi-Rad J. Thymol, thyme, and other plant sources: Health and potential uses. Phytotherapy Research. 2018 Sep;32(9):1688–1706.

Sallam MF, Ahmed HMS, Diab KA, El-Nekeety AA, Abdel-Aziem SH, Sharaf HA, Abdel-Wahhab MA. Improvement of the antioxidant activity of thyme essential oil against biosynthesized titanium dioxide nanoparticles-induced oxidative stress, DNA damage, and disturbances in gene expression in vivo. Journal of Trace Elements in Medicine and Biology. 2022 Sep;73:127024.

Sardari S, Mobaiend A, Ghassemifard L, Kamali K, Khavasi N. Therapeutic effect of thyme (Thymus vulgaris) essential oil on patients with COVID19: A randomized clinical trial. Journal of Advances in Medical and Biomedical Research. 2021 Feb 10;29(133):83–91.

Sertel S, Eichhorn T, Plinkert PK, Efferth T. Cytotoxicity of Thymus vulgaris essential oil towards human oral cavity squamous cell carcinoma. Anticancer Research. 2011 Jan;31(1):81–87.

Singletary K. Thyme: History, applications, and overview of potential health benefits. Nutrition Today. 2016 Jan 1;51(1):40–49.

Stahl-Biskup E, Sáez F, editors. Thyme: The genus Thymus. CRC Press;2002 Sep 5.

Stahl-Biskup E, Venskutonis RP. Edited by Peter KV. Thyme. In Handbook of herbs and spices (pp. 499–525). Woodhead Publishing; 2012 Jan 1.

Tabatabaei SM, Kianinodeh F, Nasiri M, Tightiz N, Asadipour M, Gohari M. In vitro inhibition of MCF-7 human breast cancer cells by essential oils of Rosmarinus officinalis, Thymus vulgaris L., and Lavender x intermedia. Archives of Breast Cancer. 2018 May 1:81–89.

Vimalanathan S, Hudson J. Anti-influenza virus activity of essential oils and vapors. American Journal of Essential Oils and Natural Products. 2014;2(1):47–53.

Vlaicu PA, Untea AE, Turcu RP, Saracila M, Panaite TD, Cornescu GM. Nutritional composition and bioactive compounds of basil, thyme and sage plant additives and their functionality on broiler thigh meat quality. Foods. 2022 Apr 12;11(8):1105.

Witkowska D, Sowińska J, Żebrowska JP, Mituniewicz E. The antifungal properties of peppermint and thyme essential oils misted in broiler houses. Brazilian Journal of Poultry Science. 2016 Oct;18:629–638.

Youdim KA, Deans SG. Effect of thyme oil and thymol dietary supplementation on the antioxidant status and fatty acid composition of the ageing rat brain. British Journal of Nutrition. 2000 Jan;83(1):87–93.

# 15 Copaifera Oil-Resin as a Potential Therapeutic Source

*M.R. Furlan, D. Garcia,*
*A.D. de Souza, and R.F. de Assis*

## 15.1 INTRODUCTION

In addition to being the gateway to supporting the conservation of natural resources in developing countries, using natural compounds derived from biodiversity and ethnobotanical knowledge is vital to developing new medicines (Nogueria, Cerqueira, and Soares 2010). The possibility of finding new medicines from natural sources is one of the most cited reasons for preserving biodiversity (Barreiro 2019).

Brazil is one of the countries with the greatest biodiversity on Earth, with an advantageous location (between 5°N and 33°S and between 35°E and 74°W) and a large continental dimension, with the title of largest country in the southern hemisphere and the fifth largest place in the world in total area (Alves and Azevedo 2018). Within the Americas, Brazil has the most diverse flora, with 33,161 species, followed by Colombia (23,104) and Mexico (22,969) (Ulloa et al. 2017). For Dutra et al. (2016), Brazil has the highest total biodiversity in the world, comprising more than 45,000 species of higher plants (20% to 22% of the total existing on the planet).

Secondary metabolites play a crucial role in plants regulating, balancing, adapting to habitats, physical and climatic factors, and protecting against pathogens and predators (Valli, Russo and Bolzani 2018). According to these authors, Brazilian plants developed extraordinary chemical diversity because of their geographical extent and the Brazilian habitats to which they had to adapt during their evolution, which has not been explored sufficiently and may be used to develop bio-commodities such as pharmaceuticals, cosmetics, food supplements and agricultural pesticides.

Among other reasons, the disclosure of Brazilian biodiversity is justified by the intense destruction of all its ecosystems, including the Amazon Rainforest, which was the result of monocultures of sugar cane, soy, eucalyptus and livestock, resulting in the process of genetic and cultural erosion (Palhares et al. 2021). The Amazon Basin is the habitat of the largest tropical forest in the world, covering eight countries in South America, as well as an overseas territory of France (Codeço et al. 2021).

Protecting the Amazonian ecosystems is essential for preserving biodiversity, climate regulation, energy production and food and water security. It is crucial to pollination, natural or biological control of pests, the region's economy and human health, without forgetting its aesthetic and cultural value. For urbanized communities, among other benefits, the Amazon rainforest is a source of food, chemical compounds for developing medicines and raw materials for the most diverse industries (Codeço et al. 2021).

In recent centuries, indigenous communities have used, in medical practices, medicines derived from native Brazilian plants included in the European Pharmacopoeia. Among these plants was *Carapichea ipecacuanha* (Brot.) L. Andersson ("ipecacuanha") (*Rubiaceae*), which produces the emetic and amoebicidal alkaloid emetine (Ricardo et al. 2018). Through a review, the authors evaluated the use of preparations containing barbatimão bark and copaiba oil. *Copaifera spp.* (copaiba oleoresin) can be considered effective in the treatment of wounds. They also warn of the need to improve the quality of formulations as defined by the WHO.

Traditional communities in Brazil widely use species of the genus *Copaifera*. For example, the oleoresins originating from species of the genus *Copaifera* are widely used in folk medicine to treat various diseases. The most used species is *C. langsdorffii*. Its leaves are rich in phenolic compounds with potential biological activities, such as antioxidants and chelating agents.

## 15.2   BOTANICAL ASPECTS

*Copaifera* is a genus of species belonging to the *Fabaceae* family, including 72 tree species. Also present in Africa (Congo, Cameroon, Guinea and Angola), it is in Latin America where most species can be found, 17 of which are endemic to the Amazon (Venezuela, Colombia, Guianas), North (Amazonia, Para), Midwest (Mato Grosso, Mato Grosso do Sul and Goiás), Southeast (Sao Paulo and Minas Gerais) and South (Parana) regions of Brazil, according to the Index Kewensis (Oxford University 1996).

From 106 specific names (www.theplantlist.com), 49 are considered valid, 2 are misapplied, 49 are synonyms, and 6 are unresolved (The Plant List *Copaifera* 2023). Regarding the folk names, "Copaíba" is the common name in Brazil, and some of the most frequently species found in these regions are *Copaifera officinalis* L., *C. reticulata* Ducke and *C. langsdorffii* Desf. The popular name comes from the Tupi Guarani language "kupa'iwa", that means "reservoir/deposit tree", in reference to the oil-resin highly presented in its trunk.

*Copaifera officinalis*, also known as copaiba balsam or copaiba, is native to northern South America in tropical countries, especially Venezuela, Guyana and Brazil (Campos et al. 2022).

The bark of *C. langsdorffii* is thin, dark reddish-brown, exfoliated in irregular flakes. It is very dense, with highly lignified cells and abundant sclereids, and cellular fillings of a phenolic nature. It includes a poorly developed rhytidome and a periderm with thick and thin-walled phellem cells (Portella et al. 2015).

The oil-resin is a liquid with variable viscosity and color, ranging from yellow to light brown, composed by a solid phase or resin with a non-volatile portion comprising mainly acid diterpenes, and a volatile oil part consisting of a mixture of sesquiterpenes. The tree can reach up to 40 m in height, its trunk is rough and dark in color, it can reach 4 m in diameter and can reach an age of 400 years. The bark, reddish when it is young and brown when it reaches the adult age, is 17 mm thick, and the inner bark exudes a bitter-tasting oil-resin. It occurs naturally both in well-drained fertile soils, such as humid land in riparian forests, and in poor soils in the Brazilian *cerrado* biome (Arruda et al. 2019).

The wood of the genus *Copaifera* generally has characteristics of high resistance to moisture and attack by phytopathogens, which makes it of great interest to the timber market, because in addition to high durability, it presents desirable organoleptic characteristics and high commercial value. But its oil-resin is the main product, and most often used as raw material for various forms of pharmaceutical preparations, from ointments to capsules (Pieri et al. 2009), commonly called "the universal remedy of the Amazon" due to its versatility of use and the large number of pharmacological activities.

Copaiba oil is an example of a medicinal product widely used by the Brazilian population, being sold in street markets and by herbalists, pharmacies, health food stores and others. Its medicinal use was approved by the FDA (Food and Drug Administration), the US government's drug and food regulation agency, in 1972 (Cascon 2004).

Currently, the oil-resin is widely used for various therapeutic purposes by people living in forest interiors, such as "Quilombolas", indigenous people, riverside dwellers, as well as by the populations of the big Brazilian cities in the treatment of numerous health disorders. Copaiba oil-resin is widely employed in the pharmaceutical and cosmetic industries in the development of soaps, ointments, pills, perfumes and others. Its market value is low, due to the abundance of trees found in Brazil. Each 1 ml of oil-resin can cost up to US$3 in the normal market. Research with copaiba is still rare and insufficient, which hinders the production of new phytopharmaceuticals and large-scale agricultural production.

## 15.3   USES OF SPECIES OF THE GENUS *COPAIFERA*

The oil resin of *C. officinalis*, called copaiba oil, ranges from golden yellow to brown. Historically, indigenous peoples have used it against insect bites and skin disorders due to its high healing power (Campos et al. 2022). In folk medicine, it is an anti-inflammatory in rheumatism, skin ulcers, wounds and dermatoses. The oil has also been used internally as a diuretic and expectorant, aiding respiratory, urinary and genital problems. Creams and soaps that treat acne contain this ingredient.

The sesquiterpenes and diterpenes present in the oil are different for each *Copaifera* species and have been associated with several reported biological activities, ranging from antitumor to embryotoxic effects (Leandro et al. 2012). According to the authors, perfumery and cosmetics industries have shown great interest in the sesquiterpenic fraction, responsible for the aroma of copaiba oleoresin.

## 15.4   CLINICAL TRIALS

Regarding randomized and controlled clinical studies, research with species of *Copaifera* is still rare. In the search for clinical research in the last five years, only works with the species *C. langsdorffii* and *C. officinalis* are found. Musale and Soni

(2016) conclude that *C. langsdorffii* resin oil is efficacious as a pulpotomy agent for deciduous teeth for up to one year. Further clinical studies with long-term follow-up could confirm its efficacy as a pulpotomy agent.

Valadas et al. (2021) found that three annual applications of copaiba (*C. langsdorffii*) varnish provide significant antimicrobial activity against *Streptococcus mutans* for up to 12 months in children at high risk of caries. Fluoride and copaiba varnishes had good results in preventing dental caries, but the authors recommend further studies to establish the use of varnish in preventing caries.

In one study, peptic ulcer healing was 65% to 75% with copaiba oil versus 100% in the omeprazole group, with no significant adverse effects; two had nausea, and three had epigastric pain (Arroyo-Acevedo et al. 2011). Patients were randomly distributed into three groups of 20 cases each, according to the order of arrival. The first two groups received copaiba oil capsules at 80 mg and 120 mg, respectively, and a third group received omeprazole at 20 mg. The treatments were administered on an empty stomach, once in the morning, 30 minutes before ingesting the first meal.

Da Silva et al. (2012) verified a significant decrease in the surface affected with acne in the areas treated with an application of essential oil of *C. langsdorffii* at 1.0%, compared to placebo. The essential oil comprised 48 substances, of which 14 were the major components, representing 95.80% of the total composition, with cis-tujopsene being the main component, with 46.96% of the entire composition of the essential oil.

When evaluating the efficacy and safety of *C. officinalis* L. "copaíba" oil suppositories in 60 patients with a final diagnosis of acute hemorrhoidal crisis, Arroyo Acevedo et al. (2013) concluded that the suppository with *C. officinalis* oil is an effective and safe alternative in the treatment of critical hemorrhoidal problems.

### 15.4.1 TESTS WITH ANIMAL MODELS

In most animal studies with *Copaifera* oil species, the purpose was to verify their efficacy as cures. However, numerous variables can influence the content of active ingredients in *Copaifera*, generating contradictory results and strengthening the need to conduct further tests.

Caryophyllene is common in copaiba oil-resin (*Copaifera officinalis*); perhaps the biggest revelation about caryophyllene as a selective full agonist at CB2 (100 nM), which makes it the first proven phytocannabinoid beyond the *Cannabis* genus. Subsequent work demonstrated that this dietary component produced anti-inflammatory analgesic activity at the lowest dose of 5 mg·kg$^{-1}$ in wild-type mice, but not in CB2 knockout mice (Gertsch 2008). Given the lack of psychoactivity attributed to CB2 agonists, caryophyllene offers great promise as a therapeutic compound, either systemically or in dermatological applications such as contact dermatitis. With its rapid and direct binding to CB2, β-caryophyllene is a powerful constituent with the potential to promote wellness in many ways.

Teixeira et al. (2017) verified in research with Wistar rats that *C. reticulata* oleoresin reduces chronic inflammation and inhibits macrophage activity. However, in the study by Wagner et al. (2017), topical administration of *C. reticulata* oleoresin, although secure, did not accelerate the healing process in Wistar rats.

Senedese et al. (2019) verified the chemopreventive activity of *C. reticulata* oleoresin in colon carcinogenesis. They suggested diterpene acid between the anti-inflammatory acts through nitric oxide and concluded that this oil could potentially suppress colon carcinogenesis. When testing in rats, Teixeira et al. (2019) found that *Copaifera officinalis* oil does not reduce intestinal mucosa injury after hypovolemic shock.

In a test with 45 Wistar, Alvarenga et al. (2020) demonstrated that the systemic application of *C. reticulata* oleoresin is safe, promotes oral wound healing, provides early anti-inflammatory activity and accelerates wound resolution. Compared to corticosteroids and control, copaiba-treated injuries revealed a smaller wound area, decreased acute inflammatory reaction and greater precipitating. The levels of renal and liver function evidence did not disclose the presence of post-tract damage.

Becker et al. (2020), in a study with copaiba oleoresin (did not specify the species), verified topical antinociceptive activity in the firing mode of UVB radiation-induced skin. In a study performed on mice, it was concluded that copaiba oleoresin might be of value in treating inflammation-related pain. In horses, Kauer et al. (2020) observed that hydroalcoholic extract of *C. langsdorffii* and oleoresin creams are promising for healing these lesions.

According to Waibel et al. (2021), in a randomized, double-blind, placebo-controlled study, copaiba oil (species not mentioned) in silicone-based gel reduced abnormal scar formation during the healing process. It significantly improved color, contour, distortion and texture for different scar types.

*C. reticulata* oleoresin with high β-bisabolene concentration showed anti-inflammatory activity, reducing vascular permeability and consequently the formation of edema in Wistar rats (140–220 g) at 8 to 12 weeks, reducing cell migration and the production of inflammatory cytokines, confirming their traditional use by local Amazonian communities (Almeida Júnior et al. 2021).

The chitosan membrane containing copaiba oil contents (*Copaifera* spp.) In 0.1%, 0.5%, 1.0% and 5.0% doses, it revealed fluid absorption capacity, hydrophilic surface and moisture and other characteristics that favor wound treatment (Paranhos et al. 2021).

After evaluating the toxic effects of copaiba oil-resin and copaiba oil-resin vaginal cream (*Copaifera duckei*) in the subacute phase of treatment, in Wistar rats treated orally and intravaginally (ivag), Lima et al. (2017) concluded that treatment with copaiba resin (orally and intravaginally) and the cream was effective and did not cause clinical signs of toxicity.

Systemic administration of copaiba oleoresin (*C. reticulata*) in ligature-induced periodontitis in rats considerably reduced the inflammatory profile, limited alveolar bone loss and increased trabecular thickness and bone tissue bone-volume ratio, decreasing trabeculae compared to the untreated experimental periodontitis group (Santos et al. 2022).

Copaiba oil extracted from the trunk of *C. langsdorffii* and linseed oil extracted from the seeds of *Linum usitatissimum* L. tested in rats (Heck et al. 2022) were not mutagenic and provided an antimutagenic effect against the damage-inducing agent cyclophosphamide.

Reis et al. (2023), after a systematic review of the use of essential oils in women's health for the herbal treatment of candidiasis, with emphasis on the potential of copaiba oil (*Copaifera sp.*), concluded that although *Copaifera officinalis* does not entirely inhibit *Candida albicans*, it can reduce biofilm adhesion, suggesting its prophylactic use against candidiasis.

According to Gomes et al. (2023), the dentin modifier based on *Copaifera multijuga* oil has demonstrated antibacterial, anti-inflammatory and metalloproteinase inhibitory activity, which may help the adhesion of restorative materials to the tooth structure. They suggest that the biological properties of the 10% copaiba emulsion have an advantage over the 2% chlorhexidine digluconate, because it is a natural product with less cytotoxicity. In the research carried out by the authors, the treatment of the collagen of the demineralized dentin matrix with emulsion based on copaiba was the group that presented more excellent stability of the modulus of elasticity (SM) values over the evaluated storage time, being effective in maintaining the ME of the dentin in values like those described in the literature.

Martínez et al. (2023) demonstrated that the hydroalcoholic extract and the oleoresin of *C. multijuga* could be a target for establishing a new therapeutic strategy for congenital toxoplasmosis.

In veterinary medicine, Campanholi et al. (2022) tested a gel filled with a bioadhesive emulsion containing a high amount of *C. reticulata* oil-resin for the treatment of wounds and prevention of myiasis. *In vivo* evaluations carried out through a case report for treating ulcerative cutaneous injuries aggravated by myiasis in calves and heifers showed healing, anti-inflammatory and repellent performance for the gel filled with emulsion. They concluded that the low-cost emulgel preparation shows promise as a medicine for treating wounds.

Campanholi et al. (2023) evaluated copaiba oil resin extracted from *C. reticulata* to treat bovine mastitis. The formulation consisted of an emulgel with a high concentration of oil resin. Monitoring the treated inflammatory response showed that the extract prevents mastitis. They observed that the formulation could form a thin gel film on the application site, avoiding the proliferation of flies and significantly reducing the pathogen load.

A preclinical study with galloylquinic acid compounds from *Copaifera lucens* demonstrated potent antifungal activity against induced vaginal candidiasis in a murine model through multi-target modes of action (Al-Madboly et al. 2022).

## 15.5   CHEMICAL COMPOSITION OF *COPAIFERA* SPECIES

The phytochemical composition of essential oils and most bioactive compounds in plants may vary, for example, as a function of genetics; environmental factors such as temperature, humidity, and photoperiod; the form of cultivation; the harvest time and how the processing is carried out.

According to Santiago, Santos and Martins (2021), oleoresin, a liquid found in the trunks of copaiba trees, acts as a defense against animals and microorganisms. The authors report that the oleoresin can be extracted from the interior of the tree trunk by three forms of extraction: total, traditional and rational, the first two of which are not recommended because they cause significant damage to the tree and do not allow future extractions. In rational extraction, the most sustainable way to obtain oleoresin, a small hole is made in the trunk of the tree, and a small pipe is inserted that leads the oleoresin to the outside of the tree. After extraction, the hole is sealed, which will allow reopening for future extractions.

The diterpenes in the oil resins of *Copaifera* species have kaurane, labdane and clerodane skeletons (Santos et al. 2020). Oleoresin is a solution of diterpenoids, mainly mono and diacids, solubilized by sesquiterpene hydrocarbons (Leandro et al. 2012). The main sesquiterpenes in *Copaifera* species are β-caryophyllene, caryophyllene oxide, α-humulene, δ-cadinene, α-cadinol, α-cubebene, α and β-selinene, β-elemene, trans-α-bergamotene and β-bisabolene (Pinto et al. 2000).

Veiga-Junior and Pinto (2002) warn that despite hundreds of studies published in several languages, results regarding the chemical composition and pharmacological activity of copaiba oil are contradictory, because there are errors in the botanical identification and chemical composition of copaiba oils, which are also often mixed with other oils and adulterated.

In the essential oil of *C. officinalis* purchased commercially with a purity certificate above 99.9%, according to research by Campos et al. (2022), 14 compounds were identified, with β-caryophyllene (61.7%), α-humulene (8.4%), α-bergamotene (6.3%), α-copaene (6.3%) compounds (3.9%), germacrene D (2.8%), β-bisabolene (2.8%) and δ-cadinene (2.1%), representing 88% of the total.

In research by Pasquel-Reátegui et al. (2022), β-caryophyllene (39.61%) was also the primary compound of oleoresin from *C. officinalis*, followed by α-bergamotene (14.07%) among sesquiterpenes, while the significant diterpenic acid was copalic acid (7.82%).

For *C. reticulata*, Costa and Lameira (2021) verified through the oleoresin chemical analysis that the components' percentages varied between individuals. The main compounds of this species in this research were β-bisabolene (21.83%), α-bergamotene (18.43%), α-bisabolene (6.27%) and caryophyllene (6.23%).

Fractionation of the oil-resin of *C. reticulata*, carried out by chromatography on a column of silica gel impregnated with KOH, made it possible to obtain the three metabolites that make up the oil-resin (sesquiterpene hydrocarbons, oxygenated sesquiterpenes and diterpene acids) (Santos et al. 2020). Preparative high-performance liquid chromatography (HPLC) allowed isolating of four diterpenic acids: copalic acid, ent-agatic acid, polyaltic acid and 3-hydroxypalic acid.

After analysis of the chemical composition of the oil-resin of *C. reticulata* by GC-MS, significant constituents containing sesquiterpene hydrocarbons are β-bisabolene (48.9%), trans-α-bergamotene (23.4%) and β-caryophyllene (12.0%). The oxygenated sesquiterpene fraction contains β-bisabolol (16.7%), caryophyllene oxide (11.8%) and allo-himachalol (9.8%) (Santos et al. 2020).

In the volatile fraction of the oil-resin of *C. reticulata* from the state of Pará, Brazil, obtained through hydro-distillation with a Clevenger apparatus, the primary constituents for sesquiterpene hydrocarbons were identified as β-bisabolene (24.91%), trans-α-bergamotene (21.99%) and β-selinene (12.17%). Regarding oxygenated sesquiterpenes, only α-bisabolol (0.17%) and caryophyllene oxide (0.21%) were reported (Bardají et al. 2016).

The *C. multijuga* oil-resin was fractionated by chromatography on a silica gel column impregnated with a methanolic KOH solution, using hexane, chloroform and methanol as eluents. In the hexane fraction, trans-β-caryophyllene was the primary compound, followed by α-humulene, β-bergamotene, δ-cadinene, γ-muurolene, germacrene D, bicyclogermacrene, α-elemene and α-copaene. In the minor chloroform fraction, the oxygenated sesquiterpenes identified were caryophyllene oxide, τ-muurolol, δ-cadinol, α-cadinol and (Z)-α-santalol. In the methanol fraction, copalic acid was the most abundant acidic diterpene and was identified by co-injection with the previously isolated methylated standard. Methyl esters of collagenic acid, ent-agatic acid, hydroxycopalic acid and acetoxycopalic acid were also identified (Gomes et al. 2010). Chemical analysis of the HF and CF fractions showed 83% and 4% of the total composition of oleoresins (hydrocarbons and oxygenated sesquiterpenes, respectively), while MF, representing 9% of the entire composition, showed free diterpene acids.

Veiga Junior et al. (2007) show that among the diterpenes observed in *Copaifera* species, copalic acid was the main component from *C. multijuga* (6.2%) and was found in all the oleoresins studied in *C. cearensis*, clorechinic (11.3%) and hardwickiic acids (6.2%) were the significant diterpenes while kaurenoic (3.9%) and kolavenic acids (3.4%) predominated in *C. reticulata*.

A literature review did not reveal any findings concerning the composition of oils produced by *C. confertiflora* and *C. coriacea*.

GC/MS analysis of hydro-distilled essential oils from leaves, root bark, fruit bark, trunk bark, trunk wood, root wood and fruits of *C. langsdorffii* obtained yields of 0.04%, 0.01%, 0.7%, 0.003%, 0.008%, 0.07% and 0.3%, respectively, and from copaiba balsam (7.3%), allowed the identification of 40 different constituents. The main compounds were as follows: leaf and fruit oils: β-caryophyllene (16.6% and 14.8%) and γ-muurolene (25.2% and 29.8%); fruit peel oil: caryophyllene oxide (47.3%); wood root oil: caryophyllene oxide (40.5%) and 4-α-copaenenol (17.6%); root bark oil: caryophyllene oxide (30.7%) and kaurene (8.2%); trunk wood oil: γ-muurolene (8.3%), caryophyllene oxide (31.0%) and kaurene (30.2%); trunk bark oil: β-bisabolol (30.5%), kaurene (16.7%) and kaurenal (31.9%); copaiba balsam oil: β-caryophyllene (53.3%) (Nilce; Gramosa and Silveira 2005).

Research revealed that the average chemical composition of *C. langsdorffii* bark was ash 3.7%, total extractives 21.3%, corresponding mainly to polar compounds soluble in ethanol and water, suberin 0.8% and lignin 36.6%. The polysaccharides showed a predominance of glucose and xylose (66.4% and 23.5% of the total monosaccharides, respectively). The ethanol-water extract of the bark showed a high phenolic content: total phenolics 589.2 mg gallic acid/g extract, flavonoids 441.9 mg catechin/g extract and tannins 54.8 mg catechin/g extract (Portella et al. 2015).

The dry and rainy seasons present in different formations in the Cerrado domain can promote changes in the composition of volatile compounds (terpenes) in the essential oil of copaiba (*C. langsdorffii* Desf.) (Santos et al. 2022).

Antonio et al. (2022), using a non-targeted metabolomics approach to evaluate the chemical variability of *C. langsdorffii* from Brazilian biomes with contrasting climates, the Atlantic Forest and the semi-arid Cerrado, identified 11 compounds in the species, including glycosylated flavonoids and derivatives of galloylquinic acid. In this research, the authors demonstrated the influence of the ecosystem on the production of bioactive compounds in *C. langsdorffii*. The Cerrado population had significantly higher galloylquinic acid derivative concentrations than the rainforest biome.

The Atlantic Forest populations had a higher flavonol content, while the semi-arid biome reduced the concentration of flavonoids, mainly concerning quercetin and kaempferol derivatives. However, in this biome, the flavonoids were more diverse. They concluded that both chemical classes were relevant to be used as chemical markers of geographic origin due to qualitative and quantitative characteristics.

Santos et al. (2022) also demonstrated that the biome affects the chemical composition of the essential oil of the *C. langsdorffii* resin. Comparing areas of Cerradão (one of the Cerrado ecosystems), Carrasco (belonging to the Caatinga) and Mata Úmida, they verified that there was variation in the chemical composition both among the phytophysiognomies and among the individuals of the same locality. However, β-caryophyllene was the majority for all areas studied.

## 15.6   CONCLUSION

South American biodiversity is considered a rich source of native and exotic plant species with great potential for therapeutic properties. However, there is still a need for clinical trials with these species, which are essential to determine the efficacy and safety of a plant to be made available in the pharmaceutical market as a phyto-therapy or plant medicine.

Species of the *Copaifera* genus, known as copaiba, despite their wide use in tra-ditional medicine and with significant research in pre-clinical trials, still need to be researched in clinical trials, as observed in the literature surveyed. The various ethnopharmacological records on copaiba justify conducting clinical trials.

Therefore, research indicates that the species of the *Copaifera* genus have the potential for various applications in the pharmaceutical industries and should receive more attention regarding applied research.

## REFERENCES

Al-Madboly, L. A., M. A. Abd El-Salam, J. K. Bastos, S. H. El-Shorbagy, and R. M. El-Morsi. 2022. Novel preclinical study of galloylquinic acid compounds from *Copaifera lucens* with potent antifungal activity against vaginal candidiasis induced in a murine model via multitarget modes of action. *Microbiology Spectrum*, 10(5). https://doi.org/10.1128/spectrum.02724-21

Almeida Júnior, J. S., E. B. S. da Silva, T. M. P. Moraes, A. A. M. Kasper, A., Baratto, L. C. Sartoratto, E. C. P. de Oliveira, E. Oliveira, L. E. S. Barata, A. H. H. Minervino, and W. P. Moraes. 2021. Anti-inflammatory potential of the oleoresin from the Amazonian tree *Copaifera reticulata* with an unusual chemical composition in rats. *Veterinary Sciences*, 8(12): 320. https://doi.org/10.3390/vetsci8120320

Alvarenga M. O. P., L. O. Bittencourt, P. F. S. Mendes, J. T. Ribeiro, O. A. Lameira, M. C. Monteiro C. A. G. Barboza, M. D. Martins, and R. R. Lima. 2020. Safety and effective-ness of copaiba oleoresin (*C. reticulata* Ducke) on inflammation and tissue repair of oral wounds in rats. *International Journal of Molecular Sciences*, 21(10): 3568. https://doi.org/10.3390/ijms21103568

Alves, A. A. C., and V. C. R. Azevedo. 2018. Embrapa network for Brazilian plant genetic resources conservation. *Biopreservation and Biobanking*, 16(5): 350–360. https://doi.org/10.1089/bio.2018.0044

Antonio, A. S., L. O. Franco, S. R. S. Cardoso, G. R. C. Dos Santos, H. M. G. Pereira, L. S. M. Wiedemann, P. C. G. Ferreira, and V. F. Veiga-Junior. 2022. Chemical variability of *Copaifera langsdorffii* Desf. from environmentally contrasting populations. *Natural Product Research*, 1–5. Advance online publication. https://doi.org/10.1080/14786419. 2022.2043856

Arroyo Acevedo, J. L., M. Q. Florentini, P. O. Miranda, J. M. Heredia, Y. A. Pinedo, C. B. Cisneros Hilario, and B. J. Teixeira. 2013. Efecto protector del supositorio de aceite de *Copaifera officinalis* L. "copaiba" en pacientes con hemorroides. *Conocimiento para el Desarrollo*, 4(1). https://revista.usanpedro.edu.pe/index.php/CPD/article/view/181

Arroyo-Acevedo, J., M. Quino-Florentini, J. Martínez-Heredia, Y. Almora-Pinedo, Yuan, A. Alba-González, and M. Condorhuamán-Figueroa. 2011. Efecto cicatrizante del aceite de *Copaifera officinalis* (copaiba), en pacientes con úlcera péptica. *Anales de la Facultad de Medicina*, 72(2): 113–117. www.scielo.org.pe/scielo. php?script=sci_arttext&pid=S1025-55832011000200004&lng=en&tlng=es

Arruda, C., J. A. A., Mejía, V. P. Ribeiro, C. H. G. Borges, C. H. G. Martins, R. C. S. Veneziani, S. R. Ambrósio, and J. K. Bastos. 2019. Occurrence, chemical composition, biological activities and analytical methods on *Copaifera* genus-A review. *Biomedicine & Pharmacotherapy*, 109: 1–20. https://doi.org/10.1016/j.biopha.2018.10.030

Bardají, D. K. R., J. J. M. Silva, T. C. Bianchi, D. S. Eugênio, P. F. Oliveira, L. F. Leandro, H. L. G. Rogez, R. C. S. Venezianni, S. R. Ambrosio, D. C. Tavares, J. K. G. Bastos, and C. H. Martins. 2016. *Copaifera reticulata* oleoresin: Chemical characterization and antibacterial properties against oral pathogens. *Anaerobe*, 40: 18–27. www.sciencedirect. com/science/article/abs/pii/S1075996416300440

Barreiro, E. J. 2019. What is hidden in the biodiversity? The role of natural products and medicinal chemistry in the drug discovery process. *Anais da Academia Brasileira de Ciencias*, 91(supp 3): e20190306. https://doi.org/10.1590/0001-3765201920190306

Becker, G., I. Brusco, R. Casoti, M. C. L. Marchiori, L. Cruz, G. Trevisan, and S. H. Oliveira. 2020. Copaiba oleoresin has topical antinociceptive activity in a UVB radiation-induced skin-burn model in mice. *Journal of Ethnopharmacology*, 250: 112476. https:// doi.org/10.1016/j.jep.2019.112476

Campanholi, K. D. S. S., R. C. D. S. Junior, R. S. Gonçalves, J. B. da Silva, F. A. P. de Morais, R. S. dos Santos, B. H. Vilsinski, G. L. M. Oliveira, M. S. D. S. Pozza, M. L. Bruschi, B. B. Saraiva, C. V. Nakamura, and W. Caetano. 2022. Design and optimization of a natural medicine from *Copaifera reticulata* Ducke for skin wound care. *Polymers*, 14(21): 4483. https://doi.org/10.3390/polym14214483

Campanholi, K. D. S. S., R. C. D. Silva Junior, F. A. P. Morais, R. S. Gonçalves, B. M. Rodrigues, M. S. D. S. Pozza, L. V. Castro-Hoshino, S. M., Leite, O. A. Capeloto, M. L. Baesso, P. C. Pozza, and W. Caetano. 2023. Copaiba oil-based emulsion as a natural chemotherapeutic agent for the treatment of bovine mastitis: *In vivo* studies. *Pharmaceutics*, 15(2): 346. https://doi.org/10.3390/pharmaceutics15020346

Campos, D. N., P. E. E. Chaves, J. R. D. Messa, J. A. V. Costa, M. M. Machado, and L. Zuravski. 2022. Identificação e quantificação do óleo essencial do bálsamo de copaíba (*Copaifera officinalis*). *SIEPE* [Internet], 23° de novembro de, 2(14). https://periodicos. unipampa.edu.br/index.php/SIEPE/article/view/113613

Cascon, V. 2004. Copaíba – *Copaifera* spp. In: Fitoterápicos antiinflamatórios: aspectos químicos, farmacológicos e aplicações terapêuticas. ed. J. C. T. Carvalho. Ribeirão Preto: Tecmedd.

Codeço, C. T., A. P. Dal'Asta, A. C. Rorato, R. M. Lana, T. C. Neves, C. S. Andreazzi, M. Barbosa, M. I. S. Escada, D. A. Fernandes, D. L. Rodrigues, I. C. Reis, M. Silva-Nunes, A. B. Gontijo, F. C. Coelho, and A. M. V. Monteiro. 2021. Epidemiology, biodiversity, and technological trajectories in the Brazilian Amazon: From malaria to COVID-19. *Frontiers in Public Health*, 9: 647754. https://doi.org/10.3389/fpubh.2021.647754

Costa, A. S., and O. A. Lameira. 2021. Estudo fitoquímico da oleorresina extraída de *Copaifera reticulata* Ducke (Leguminosae-Caesalpiniosidade) em área de manejo sustentável. *Investigação, Sociedade e Desenvolvimento*, 10(16): e154101622305, 2021. http://dx.doi.org/10.33448/rsd-v10i16.22305

da Silva, A. G., P. F. Puziol, R. N. Leitao, T. R. Gomes, R. Scherer, M. L. Martins, A. S. Cavalcanti, and L. C. Cavalcanti. 2012. Application of the essential oil from copaiba (*Copaifera langsdori* Desf.) for acne vulgaris: A double-blind, placebo-controlled clinical trial. *Alternative Medicine Review: A Journal of Clinical Therapeutic*, 17(1): 69–75. https://pubmed.ncbi.nlm.nih.gov/22502624/

Dutra, R. C., M. M. Campos, A. R. Santos, and J. B. Calixto. 2016. Medicinal plants in Brazil: Pharmacological studies, drug discovery, challenges and perspectives. *Pharmacological Research*, 112: 4–29. https://doi.org/10.1016/j.phrs.2016.01.021

Gertsch, J., M. Leonti, S. Raduner I. Racz, J. Z. Chen, X. Q. Xie, K. Altmann, M. Karsak, and A. Simmer. 2008. Beta-caryophyllene is a dietary cannabinoid. *Proceedings of the National Academy of Sciences of USA*, 105(26): 9099–9104. https://doi.org/10.1073/pnas.0803601105

Gomes, L., G. Lima, A. L. Mota, V. Passos, M. F. Bandeira, N. Conde, and C. Toda. 2023. Influence of *Copaifera multijuga* hayne oil-based emulsion on the stability of the dentin matrix. *Concilium*, 23(3): 560–577. https://doi.org/10.53660/CLM-929-23B68

Gomes, N. M., C. M. de Rezende, S. P. Fontes, M. E. Matheus, A. C. Pinto, and P. D. Fernandes. 2010. Characterization of the antinociceptive and anti-inflammatory activities of fractions obtained from *Copaifera multijuga* hayne. *Journal of Ethnopharmacology*, 128(1): 177–183. https://doi.org/10.1016/j.jep.2010.01.005

Gramosa, N. V., and E. R. Silveira. 2005. Volatile constituents of *Copaifera langsdorffii* from the Brazilian Northeast. *Journal of Essential Oil Research*, 17(2): 130–132. https://doi.org/10.1080/10412905.2005.9698853

Heck, M. C., M. Yoshimoto-Higaki, M. A. F. Godoy, D. E. A. Mendonça, and V. E. P. Vicentini. 2022. Efeitos antimutagênicos dos óleos de copaíba (*Copaifera langsdorffii* Desf.) e linhaça (*Linum usitatissimum* L.) contra o clastogênio – ciclofosfamida, em ratos Wistar. *Pesquisa, Sociedade e Desenvolvimento*, 11(11): e567111133539. https://doi.org/10.33448/rsd-v11i11.33539

Kauer, D. P., J. M. Alonso, L. F. S. Gushiken, M. Lemos, C. R. Padovani, C. A. Rodrigues, A. L. G. Alves, M. J. Watanabe, J. K. Bastos, C. H. Pellizzon, and C. A. Hussni. 2020. Experimental skin wound treatment with *Copaifera langsdorffii* Desf Kuntze (Leguminosae) extract and oil-resin in horses. *Brazilian Journal of Veterinary Research and Animal Science*, 57(3): e166095. https://doi.org/10.11606/issn.1678-4456.bjvras.2020.166095

Leandro, L. M., F. S. Vargas, P. C. Barbosa, J. K. Neves, J. A. da Silva, and V. F. da Veiga-Junior. 2012. Chemistry and biological activities of terpenoids from copaiba (*Copaifera* spp.) oleoresins. *Molecules (Basel, Switzerland)*, 17(4): 3866–3889. https://doi.org/10.3390/molecules17043866

Lima, C. S., U. D. A. Silva, L. D. M. Góes, B. M. S. Hyacienth, H. O. Carvalho, C. P. Fernandes, A. N. Castro, and J. C. T. Carvalho. 2017. Non-clinical toxicity study of the oil-resin and vaginal cream of copaiba (*Copaifera duckei*, Dwyer). *Cogent Biology*, 3: 1394510. https://doi.org/10.1080/23312025.2017.1394510

Martínez, A. F. F., S. C. Teixeira, G. de Souza, A. M. Rosini, J. P. L. Júnior, G. N. Melo, K. O. E. Blandón, A. O. Gomes, S. R. Ambrósio, R. C. S. Veneziani, J. K. Bastos, C. H. G. Martins, E. A. V. Ferro, and B. F. Barbosa. 2023. Leaf hydroalcoholic extract and oleoresin from *Copaifera multijuga* control *Toxoplasma gondii* infection in human trophoblast cells and placental explants from third-trimester pregnancy. *Frontiers in Cellular and Infection Microbiology*, 13: 1113896. https://doi.org/10.3389/fcimb.2023.1113896

Musale, P. K., and A. S. Soni. 2016. Clinical pulpotomy trial of *Copaifera langsdorffii* oil resin versus formocresol and white mineral trioxide aggregate in primary teeth. *Pediatric Dentistry*, 38(2): 5–12. www.ingentaconnect.com/openurl?genre=article& issn=1942-5473&volume=38&issue=2&spage=5&aulast=Musale

Nogueira, R. C., H. F. Cerqueira, and M. B. Soares. 2010. Patenting bioactive molecules from biodiversity: The Brazilian experience. *Expert Opinion on Therapeutic Patents*, 20(2): 145–157. https://doi.org/10.1517/13543770903555221

Oxford University. 1996. *Index Kewensis*. Supplement XX Oxford: Clarendon Press.

Palhares, R. M., L. C. Baratto, M. Scopel, F. L. B. Mügge, and Brandão M. G. L. 2021. Medicinal plants and herbal products from Brazil: How can we improve quality? *Frontiers in Pharmacology*, 27(11): 606623. https://doi.org/10.3389/fphar.2020.606623

Paranhos, S. B., E. S. Ferreira, C. A. Canelas, S. P. A. Paz, M. F. Passos, C. E. F. Costa, A. C. R. Silva, S. N. M., and V. S. Cândido. 2021. Chitosan membrane containing copaiba oil (*Copaifera* spp.) for skin wound treatment. *Polymers* (Basel), 14(1): 35. https://doi.org/10.3390/polym1401003526

Pasquel-Reátegui, J. L., L. C. Santos, F. M. Barrales, V. L. Grober, M. B. S. Forte, A. Sartoratto, C. L. Queiroga, and J. Martínez. 2022. Fractionation of sesquiterpenes and diterpenic acids from copaiba (*Copaifera officinalis*) oleoresin using supercritical adsorption. *The Journal of Supercritical Fluids*, 184: 105565–105565. http://dx.doi.org/10.1016/j.supflu.2022.105565

Pieri, F. A., M. C. Mussi, and M. A. S. Moreira. 2009. Óleo de copaíba (*Copaifera* sp.): histórico, extração, aplicações industriais e propriedades medicinais. *Revista brasileira de plantas medicinais*, 11(4): 2009. https://doi.org/10.1590/S1516-05722009000400016

Pinto, A. C., W. F. Braga, C. M. Rezende, F. M. S. Garrido, V. F. Veiga Jr., L. Bergter, M. L. Patitucci, and O. A. C. Antunes. 2000. Separation of acid diterpenes of *Copaifera cearensis* Huber ex Ducke by flash chromatography using potassium hydroxide impregnated silica gel. *Journal of the Brazilian Chemical Society*, 11(4): 355–360. https://doi.org/10.1590/S0103-50532000000400005

Portella, R. O., R. Facanali, M. O. M. Marques, and L. F. R. Almeida. 2015. Composição química dos óleos essenciais das estruturas vegetativas e reprodutivas de *Copaifera langsdorffii* Desf. *Natural Product Research*, 29(9): 874–878. https://doi.org/10.1080/14786419.2014.987145

Reis, H. D., T. R. Bezerra, R. F. Gonçalves, C. C. Lievore, B. T. Vidal, M. B. S. Filha, F. C. Q. S. Anjos, P. F. Bessa, and N. G. F. Bessa. 2023. Clinical utility of essential oils in women's health for phytotherapeutic treatment of candidiasis: A systematic review with emphasis on the potential of copaiba oil (*Copaifera* sp) from Brazilian biodiversity and technological perspectives applied to biomedicine. *Collection of International Topics in Health Science*, 1: 639–665. http://sevenpublicacoes.com.br/index.php/editora/article/view/244

Ricardo, L. M., B. M. Dias, F. L. B. Mügge, V. V. Leite, and M. G. L. Brandão. 2018. Evidence of traditionality of Brazilian medicinal plants: The case studies of *Stryphnodendron adstringens* (Mart.) Coville (barbatimão) barks and *Copaifera* spp. (copaíba) oleoresin in wound healing. *Journal of Ethnopharmacology*, 219: 319–336. https://doi.org/10.1016/j.jep.2018.02.042

Santiago, M. B., R. A. Santos, and C. H. G. Martins. 2021. *Guia das copaíbas*: pra quê serve? Recife: Observa PICS, ISBN 978-65-996091-0-7. http://observapics.fiocruz.br/wp-content/uploads/2022/01/Guia-das-Copaibas-ObservaPICS.pdf

Santos, D. G., V. S. Castro, C. Conte Junior, C. A. Pinto, T. M. Uekane, and C. N. Rezende. 2020. *Copaifera reticulata*: Chemical characterization and bactericidal activity against pathogens in foods. *Revista Virtual de Química*, 12(2): 474–491. http://dx.doi.org/10.21577/1984-6835.20200038

Santos, M. O., C. J. Camilo, D. A. Ribeiro, J. G. F. Macedo, C. F. A. Nonato, F. F. G. Rodrigues, J. G. Martins da Costa, and M. M. A. Souza. 2022. Chemical composition variation of essential oils of *Copaifera langsdorffii* Desf. from different vegetational formations. *Natural Product Research*, 1–6. https://doi.org/10.1080/14786419.2022.2081849

Senedese, J. M., F. Rinaldi-Neto, R. A. Furtado, H. D. Nicollela, L. D. R. Souza, A. B. Ribeiro, L. S. Ferreira, G. M. Magalhães, I. Z. Carlos, J. J. M. da Silva, D. C. Tavares, and J. K. Bastos. 2019. Chemopreventive role of *Copaifera reticulata* Ducke oleoresin in colon carcinogenesis. *Biomedicine & Pharmacotherapy*, 111: 331–337. https://doi.org/10.1016/j.biopha.2018.12.091

Teixeira, F. B., R. B. Silva, O. A. Lameira, L. P. Webber, R. S. D'Almeida Couto, M. D. Martins, and R. R. Lima. 2017. Copaiba oil-resin (*Copaifera reticulata* Ducke) modulates the inflammation in a model of injury to rats' tongues. *BMC Complementary and Alternative Medicine*, 17(1): 313. https://doi.org/10.1186/s12906-017-1820-2

Teixeira, R. K. C., F. L. D. S. Costa, F. C. Calvo, D. R. D. Santos, E. Y. Yasojima, and M. V. H. Brito. 2019. Effect of copaiba oil in intestinal mucosa of rats submitted to hypovolemic shock. *Brazilian Archives of Digestive Surgery*, 32(3): e1451. https://doi.org/10.1590/0102-672020190001e1451

The Plant List *Copaifera*. 2023. www.theplantlist.org/tpl1.1/search?q=*Copaifera*. (Accessed 5 March 2023).

Ulloa, C. U., P. Acevedo-Rodríguez, S. Beck, M. J. Belgrano, R. Bernal, P. E. Berry, L. Brako, M. Celis, G. Davidse, R. C. Forzza, S. R. Gradstein, O. Hokche, B. León, S. León-Yánez, R. E. Magill, D. A. Neill, M. Nee, P. H. Raven, H. Stimmel, M. T. Strong, and P. M. Jørgensen. 2017. An integrated assessment of the vascular plant species of the Americas. *Science*, 358(6370): 1614–1617. https://doi.org/10.1126/science.aao0398

Valadas, L. A. R., P. L. D. Lobo, S. G. D. C. Fonseca, F. V. Fechine, E. M. Rodrigues Neto, M. M. F. Fonteles, L. R. A. Trévia, H. L. P. Vasconcelos, S. M. S. Lima, M. A. L., Lotif, A. M. B. Fernandes, and M. A. M. Bandeira. 2021. Clinical and antimicrobial evaluation of *Copaifera langsdorffii* Desf. dental varnish in children: a clinical study. *Evidence-Based Complementary and Alternative Medicine*, eCAM: 1–7. http://dx.doi.org/10.1155/2021/6647849

Valli, M., H. M. Russo, and V. S. Bolzani. 2018. The potential contribution of the natural products from Brazilian biodiversity to bioeconomy. *Anais da Academia Brasileira de Ciencias*, 90(1 Suppl 1): 763–778. https://doi.org/10.1590/0001-3765201820170653

Veiga J., V. F., E. C. Rosas, M. V. Carvalho, M. G. Henriques, and A. C. Pinto. 2007. Chemical composition and anti-inflammatory activity of copaiba oils from *Copaifera cearensis* Huber ex Ducke, *Copaifera reticulata* Ducke and *Copaifera multijuga* Hayne – a comparative study. *Journal of Ethnopharmacology*, 112(2): 248–254. https://doi.org/10.1016/j.jep.2007.03.005

Veiga Junior, V. F., and A. C. Pinto. 2002. O gênero *Copaifera* L. *Quím. Nova*, 25(2): 273–286. https://doi.org/10.1590/S0100-40422002000200016

Wagner, V. P., L. P. Webber, L. Ortiz, P. V. Rados, L. Meurer, O. A. Lameira, R. R. Lima, and M. D. Martins. 2017. Effects of copaiba oil topical administration on oral wound healing. *Phytotherapy Research*, 31(8): 1283–1288. https://doi.org/10.1002/ptr.5845

Waibel, J., H. Patel, E. Cull, R. Sidhu, and R. Lupatini. 2021. Prospective, randomized, double-blind, placebo-controlled study on efficacy of copaiba oil in silicone-based gel to reduce scar formation. *Dermatology and Therapy*, 11(6): 2195–2205. https://doi.org/10.1007/s13555-021-00634-5

# 16 Pharmacological Aspects of Turmeric Essential Oil

*Vipul Kumar, Reena Kaushik,*
*Pankaj Kumar Chaurasia, and*
*Sunita Singh*

## 16.1 INTRODUCTION

Turmeric or *Curcuma longa* L. is a rhizomatous perennial herbal plant belonging to the *Zingiberaceae* family which is widely cultured in the tropical and subtropical regions of Southeast Asia, mainly in India and China, as well as in some tropically warm and wet regions of Africa (Labban, 2014; Mehrotra et al., 2013). The *C. longa* tree grows to a height of about 91.44 cm, and its lance-shaped leaves include yellow flower prickles that ripen in either its underground stem or mushy rhizome. The orange pulp contained inside the rhizome is the source of turmeric medicinal powder (Kocaadam and Şanlier, 2017; Ulbricht et al., 2011). The plants of the *Curcuma* genus, which includes 70 identified species, are among those recognized for their therapeutic benefits. They have historically been employed as spices, food preservatives, and colouring agents, and also have highly significant therapeutic properties (Krup et al., 2013). There are different components of turmeric but curcumin is the major component that is responsible for the yellow colour. It is known by different names in different locations, like saffron or haridra (Sanskrit, Ayurvedic) in India and Arab nations, jianghuang (yellow ginger) in China, and kyoo or ukon in Japan (Goel et al., 2008). Curcumin is composed of various different compounds, including curcuminoids, which occur in three different categories as follows: 76.9% curcumin, 17.6% demethoxycurcumin, and 5.5% bis-demethoxycurcumin (Funk et al., 2006; Lawand and Gandhi, 2013). In addition, it includes resins, carbohydrates, proteins, and volatile oils (such as zingiberone, tumerone, and atlantone). Curcumin is a lipophilic polyphenol, and therefore it is weakly soluble in water and constant of the stomach's acidic pH (Jurenka, 2009). Curcuminoids have shown a wide range of bioactivities and potential outcomes in various studies. In particular, curcumin has proven to be a highly effective anticancer agent, exhibiting antioxidative, anti-inflammatory, and anti-Alzheimer's activity in both preclinical and clinical investigations. Additionally, curcumin has hepatoprotective, cardioprotective, hypoglycaemic, antirheumatic, neuroprotective, and anti-diabetic properties (Itokawa et al., 2008). Another important component of turmeric that contributes to its spicy and aromatic flavour is essential oil. Recent studies have shown that the biologically active components of the essential oil are ar-turmerone, α-turmerone, and β-turmerone, which have demonstrated their potential for antibacterial, antioxidant,

DOI: 10.1201/9781003389774-16

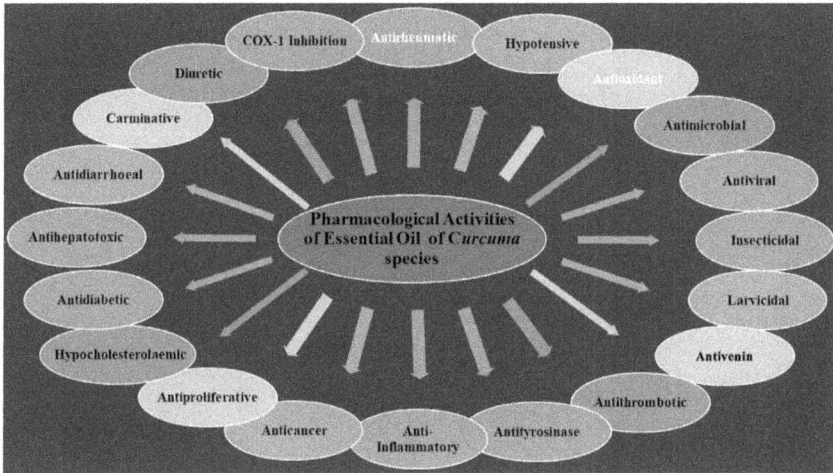

**FIGURE 16.1**  Pharmacological activities of essential oil of *Curcuma* species.

anti-inflammatory, and anticancer effects. Therefore, the core of turmeric's beneficial effects is composed of both curcuminoids and volatile compounds (Sikha and Harini, 2015; Afzal et al., 2013). A broad range of pharmacological activities are present in the essential oil (EO) of *Curcuma* species (Figure 16.1) (Mau et al., 2003; Herath et al., 2017; Chen et al., 2008; Reanmongkol et al., 2006; Wilson et al., 2005; Angel et al., 2014). Also, it is known that *Curcuma* oils can improve digestion and circulation of blood, speed up the removal of toxins, and boost immunity (Sacchetti et al., 2005; Raut and Karuppayil, 2014).

Typically, the fresh or dried rhizome is hydro- or steam-distilled to get the essential oils of *Curcuma* species. Moreover, the powdered rhizome of *Curcuma* has been used in solvent extraction or supercritical fluid extraction to recover the volatile components (Weiss, 2002; Gopalan et al., 2000). Gas chromatography-mass spectrometry is commonly used to distinguish the volatile components of various *Curcuma* species. Sesquiterpenes, monoterpenes, and other volatile aromatic chemicals are generally produced in large quantities by *Curcuma* species. Figure 16.2 presents the chemical constituents of the main volatile substances. *Curcuma* essential oils come in a wide variety of chemical make-ups. Different genotypes, varieties, geographic regions, climates, seasons, farming techniques, fertilizer uses, stresses encountered during growth or maturation, harvesting times, stages of maturation, storage, extraction, and analytical techniques could all affect the oil chemical profile differently. Nonetheless, some of the difference may be the result of incorrect identification of the plant species or a few of the parts (Singh et al., 2010; Dosoky, 2015; Sandeep et al., 2015; Srinivasan et al., 2016; Burt, 2004). This chapter summarizes various pharmacological aspects of turmeric essential oil and this work could serve as the theoretical framework for further research. We also anticipate that information will help to emphasize the significance of turmeric.

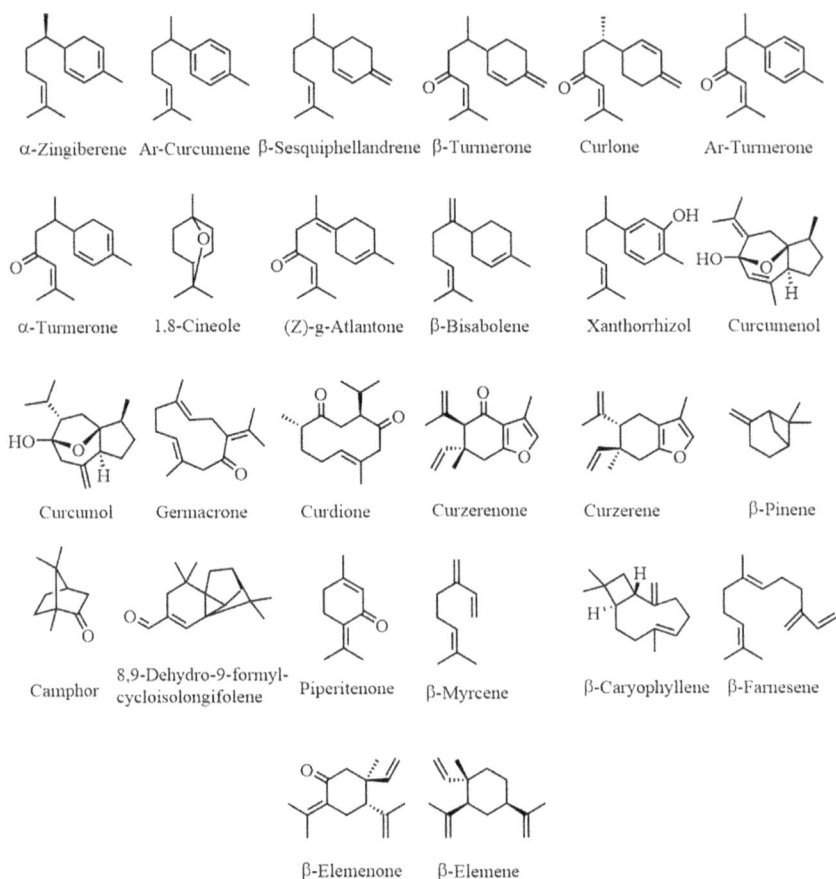

**FIGURE 16.2**  Major volatile chemical compounds in the essential oil obtained from the rhizomes of *Curcuma* species.

## 16.2  CHEMICAL EVALUATION OF THE *CURCUMA LONGA* (TURMERIC) ESSENTIAL OIL

Using the technique known as gas chromatography-mass spectrometry (GC-MS), the chemical constituents of the essential oil extracted from *C. longa* rhizomes have been extensively investigated. This is often used to investigate sesquiterpenoid compounds either on its own or in combination with a gas chromatography-flame ionization detector (GC-FID) to produce a quantitative analysis. Determining the chemical components is vital since the essential oil's constituents and concentrations may be compared to a fingerprint that confers unique qualities and features (Shang et al., 2019; Manzan et al., 2003; Stanojević et al., 2015; Pino et al., 2018; Afzal et al., 2013). The majority of sesquiterpenes and the main contributor of the pharmacological activities of turmeric essential oil have been shown to be oxygenated sesquiterpenes. Turmerones (α-, β-, and Ar-) are the three different and most significant

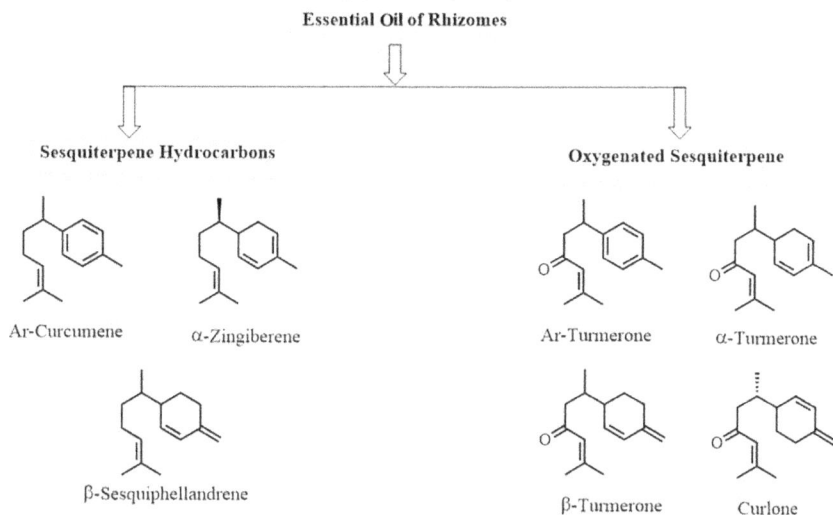

**FIGURE 16.3** Essential oils from turmeric's rhizomes contain the following primary substances.

chemical constituents (Figure 16.3). They provide *C. longa* essential oil with promising effects including anticancer, anti-inflammatory, antioxidant, and dementia prophylaxis. They even help other crucial turmeric constituents like curcumin be more active and bioavailable (Coy Barrera and Eunice Acosta, 2013; Jain et al., 2007; Bahl et al., 2014; Murakami et al., 2013; Yue et al., 2012; Yue et al., 2016). Ar-turmerone has a wide range of positive effects on human health, and many publications have commented on its medicinal potential. Moreover, Ar-turmerone has been found to be beneficial in the management and treatment of neurological and inflammatory illnesses, such as psoriasis (Ibáñez and Blazquez, 2021; Chen et al., 2018; Yang et al., 2020). The majority of the essential oils derived from the rhizome of other plants in the genus *Curcuma* are also mostly composed of oxygenated sesquiterpenes. As an example, *C. nankunshanensis*, *C. wenyujin*, and *C. kwangsiensis* all mostly contained curdione; both *C. leucorhiza* and *C. sichuanensis* contain germacrone; both *C. angustifolia* and *C. zedoaria* contain curzerenone; velleral in the *C. attenuata* and *C. xanthorhiza* contains xanthorrhizol (Zhang et al., 2017; Devi et al., 2012; Jantan et al., 2012; Singh et al., 2013a; Jena et al., 2017). Several samples of *C. longa* rhizome essential oil had lower concentrations of monoterpene hydrocarbons and oxygenated monoterpenes. On the other hand, they are the most prevalent group in the rhizome oils of other *Curcuma* species, including *C. amada*, as well as in the essential oils made from *C. longa*'s aerial parts. The chemical content of the essential oils from the leaf petiole, lamina, and rhizoid differed from the stem and rhizome oils, where turmerones predominated, while the quantity of *C. longa* essential oil differed throughout the leaves (23%), rhizomes (48%), and rhizoids (27%). While turmerones are only present in trace amounts, α-phellandrene, terpinolene, and 1,8-cineole

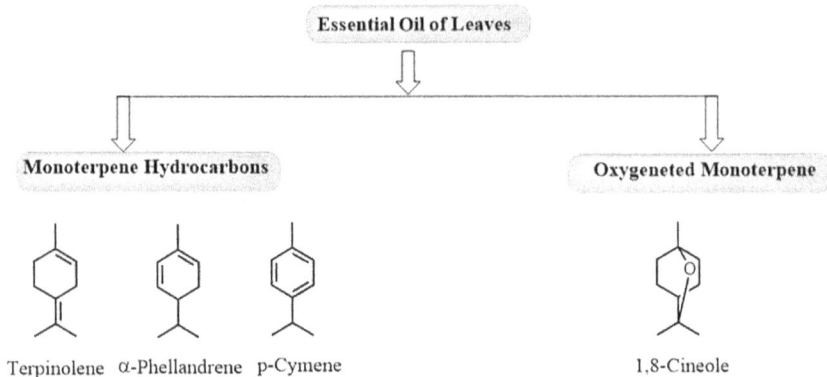

**FIGURE 16.4** Essential oils from turmeric's leaves contain the following primary substances.

are frequently the most prevalent chemicals discovered in the essential oil derived from the leaves of *C. longa* (Figure 16.4). The aerial part of *C. longa* also contains p-cymene, α-terpinene, myrcene, and pinenes (Tamta et al., 2016; Chane-Ming et al., 2002; Garg et al., 2002; Pande and Chanotiya, 2006; Sharma et al., 2019; Bansal et al., 2002; Sharma et al., 1997).

## 16.3 PHARMACOLOGICAL/BIOLOGICAL ACTIVITIES OF ESSENTIAL OIL (EO) OF *CURCUMA LONGA*

### 16.3.1 ANTIOXIDANT ACTIVITY

Food products that are kept in storage are susceptible to oxidation, which results in quality loss, changes to organoleptic characteristics and nutritive quality, as well as issues with food safety. There is great controversy regarding synthetic antioxidant preservatives, which are frequently used to prevent this process; thus, the agri-food industry increases its interest in plant-based preservatives.

Various essential oils and their constituents have already shown their potential to reduce storage losses and increase the shelf life of foods in the near future. Several are even currently being validated for use as flavour or food enhancers. The encapsulated essential oils are now being evaluated in an effort to maintain and possibly even increase their antioxidant action (B. Prakash et al., 2015; Santos-Sánchez et al., 2017). Turmeric essential oil (EO) exhibited great antioxidative activity as the scavenging activity of 1,1-diphenyl-2-picrylhydrazyl (DPPH) radical assay, the scavenging activity of superoxide anion radical assay, the activity of metal-chelating assay, the ferric reducing/antioxidant power (FRAP) assay, and phorbol-12-myristate-13-acetate-induced superoxide radical *in vivo* assay (Tsai et al., 2011; Zhao et al., 2010; Himaja et al., 2010; Zhang et al., 2017; Liju et al., 2011). The most serious effect of ischemic brain injury is cerebral edoema, which is thought to be inhibited by the antioxidative activity of turmeric EO (Dohare et al., 2008).

## 16.3.2 ANTIBACTERIAL ACTIVITY

Due to the reported harmful effects of synthetic preservatives as antimicrobial agents, nowadays consumers are demanding natural, eco-friendly, and safer alternatives. Essential oil constituents have shown powerful antimicrobial activity in individuals or combined with antibiotics (Santos-Sánchez et al., 2017; Sawicka and Egbuna, 2020; Schmidt et al., 2019). Turmeric EO also exhibited potential antimicrobial action against *Pseudomonas aeruginosa, Helicobacter pylori, Proteus mirabilis, Bacillus cereus, Vibrio parahaemolyticus, B. coagulans, Escherichia coli, B. subtilis*, and *Staphylococcus aureus* (Negi et al., 1999). *Aspergillus niger, Aspergillus flavus, Rhizoctonia solani, Trichoconis padwickii, Aspergillus parasiticum, Helminthosporium oryzae, Curvularia lunata, Fusarium oxysporum, Fusarium moniliforme*, and *Fusarium verticillioides* are also susceptible to turmeric EO's possible antifungal effects (Behura et al., 2000; Apisariyakul et al., 1995; Singh et al., 2010; Avanço et al., 2017).

## 16.3.3 ANTIHYPERLIPIDAEMIC ACTIVITY

Turmeric essential oil was reported as an antihyperlipidaemic effective on hyperlipidaemia in rats (Ling et al., 2012). Free fatty acids, triglycerides, serum total cholesterol, and low-density lipoprotein (LDL) cholesterol levels were all significantly reduced, while HDL cholesterol levels were significantly elevated. Moreover, turmeric EO reduced lipid-induced oxidative stress, vascular dysfunction, and platelet activation in hyperlipidaemic golden Syrian hamsters, which in turn had antihyperlipidaemic effects (Singh et al., 2013a). In diabetic rats, chronic food supplementation with turmeric EO (620 mg/kg/day) normalized blood glucose and produced antidiabetic and antihyperglycaemic effects (Nishiyama et al., 2005). Ingesting turmeric essential oil prevented obese diabetic mice from developing abdominal fat mass and prevented their blood glucose levels from rising (Honda et al., 2006).

## 16.3.4 ANTI-INSECTICIDAL/HERBICIDAL ACTIVITY

The primary issues resulting from the ongoing use of synthetic pesticides in worldwide agriculture for the development of weed tolerance and resistance to crop damage, or environmental degradation (Bhadoria, 2011; Busi et al., 2013). The study of natural sources, like essential oils, is necessary to develop eco-friendly, safer, and more sustainable insecticides without significantly reducing crop yields as compared to synthetic insecticides for weed management. A number of essential oils have shown significant insecticidal activities, reducing the germination of many weed seeds and/or the growth of their seedlings (Ramezani, 2008; Soltys et al., 2013). Turmeric EO showed significance in both insect repellent and insecticidal activity against white termites (*Odontotermes obesus*) (Fouad and da Camara, 2017). Both daytime and night-time biting mosquitoes were demonstrated to be repelled (Tawatsin et al., 2001). Isolated ar-turmerone and turmeric oil effective against mosquitos *Aedes aegypti* larvae (LD100 = 50 µg/mL) (Roth et al., 1998). Furthermore, the germination and growth of *Echinochloa crus-galli* (L.), *Avena fatua* L., and *Phalaris minor* Retz are inhibited by turmeric EO (Fagodia et al., 2017).

### 16.3.5 NEUROPROTECTIVE ACTIVITY

Turmeric EO demonstrated neuroprotective activity in the rat embolic-stroke model (Dohare et al., 2008). Turmeric EO inhibited free radical generation by exhibiting neuroprotective activity in the middle cerebral artery occlusion of the filament model (Rathore et al., 2008; Manhas et al., 2014). Its neuroprotective effects in rats during cardiac ischemia/reperfusion were achieved by decreasing endothelial cell-mediated inflammation (Manhas et al., 2014). It was also suggested that the ability of the oil to access the brain after stroke was via the transcellular lipophilic pathway (Dohare et al., 2008).

### 16.3.6 ANTICANCER ACTIVITY

The turmeric EO was reported to have anticancer activity. It was effective against mouse leukaemia (P388) cells and human mouth epidermal carcinoma (KB) cells, with corresponding $IC_{50}$ values of 1.088 and 0.084 mg/mL (Manosroi et al., 2006). Due to the presence of turmerone, ar-turmerone, $\alpha$-turmerone, ar-curcumene, curlone, $\beta$-sesquiphellandrene, and zingiberene, it was additionally cytotoxic to melanoma (B16), pancreatic cancer (PANC-1), human cervical adenocarcinoma, and prostate cancer (LNCaP) (Zhang et al., 2017; Jacob, 2016; Arora et al., 1971). Prostaglandin E2 (PGE2) and tumour necrosis factor (TNF) production in human leukaemia (HL-60) cells were inhibited by turmeric crude organic extracts ($IC_{50}$ = 15.2 g/mL and 0.92 g/mL, respectively) (Lantz et al., 2005). Turmeric EO's turmerones reduced inflammation-related mice colon carcinogenesis when combined with curcumin (Murakami et al., 2013) and protected patients against the precancerous situation for oral cancer and oral submucosal damage. Turmeric EO exhibited significant protective activity against benzo[a]pyrene-induced cytogenic damage (Joshi et al., 2003; Hastak et al., 1997).

### 16.3.7 ANTI-INFLAMMATORY ACTIVITY

Turmeric EO exhibits potential anti-inflammatory activity studied by a carrageenan-induced acute inflammatory model, dextran-induced inflammatory model, and formalin-induced chronic inflammatory model, by using the drug diclofenac sodium (10 mg/kg) with individual concentrations of turmeric EO (100,500, and 1000 mg/kg body weight) (Winter et al., 1962; Maity et al., 1998; Chau, 1989).

### 16.3.8 ANTIARTHRITIC ACTIVITY

Turmeric EO has significant antiarthritic activity with the presence of $\alpha$-turmerone, ar-turmerone, and $\beta$-turmerone major components. Thus, turmeric EO demonstrated protection against rheumatoid arthritis in the animal model and streptococcal cell wall (SCW)-induced arthritis in female rats (Funk et al., 2010).

## 16.3.9  HEPATOPROTECTIVE ACTIVITY

Turmeric EO reported significant hepatoprotective activity (Kiso et al., 1983). Turmeric EO (200 mg/kg) exhibits hepatoprotective and anti-fatty liver in rats by inhibiting the actions of serum enzymes, serum total cholesterol, serum triglyceride, and hepatic malondialdehyde level by increasing the level of reduced glutathione, effectively decreasing aspartate aminotransferase and alanine aminotransferase, and increasing albumin level (Nwozo et al., 2014). The studies showed that 100 mg/kg of turmeric EO may decrease *in vivo* CYP450 isoform CYP2C9 and CYP2D6 activities in rats, whereas 400 mg/kg of turmeric EO could stimulate CYP2C19 activity (Cheng et al., 2014).

## 16.3.10  ANTIPLATELET ACTIVITY

Turmeric EO consists of ar-turmerone as an active constituent having potential anti-platelet activity. Ar-turmerone prevents platelet aggregation induced by arachidonic acid ($IC_{50}$ 43.6 M), and collagen ($IC_{50}$ 14.4 M) with 50% inhibitory concentration ($IC_{50}$) values. Ar-turmerone, though, seemed to have no impact on thrombin-induced platelet aggregation or platelet-activating factor. Ar-turmerone is a significantly stronger platelet inhibitor than aspirin against platelet aggregation brought on by collagen. These results indicated that ar-turmerone might be useful for preventing platelet aggregation by collagen and arachidonic acid (Lee, 2006). Summary of pharmacological activities of essential oil of *Curcuma longa* is given in Table 16.1.

## TABLE 16.1
## Summary of Pharmacological Activities of Essential Oil of *Curcuma longa* (Turmeric)

| Pharmacological Activities | Description | References |
|---|---|---|
| Antioxidant activity | Antioxidant scavenging activity of 1,1-diphenyl-2-picrylhydrazyl (DPPH) assay, ferric reducing antioxidant power (FRAP), phorbol-12myristate-13-acetate-induced superoxide radical, meta chelating assay, and superoxide anion radical assay. | Tsai et al., 2011; Zhao et al., 2010; Himaja et al., 2010; Zhang et al., 2017; Liju et al., 2011 |
| Antibacterial activity | Antibacterial activity against *Pseudomonas aeruginosa, Helicobacter pylori, Proteus mirabilis, Bacillus cereus, Vibrio parahaemolyticus*, etc. | Negi et al., 1999 |
| Antihyperlipidaemic activity | Reduces triglycerides, serum total cholesterol, and low-density lipoprotein (LDL) cholesterol levels, thereby increasing high-density lipoprotein (HDL); antidiabetic and antihyperglycaemic effect. | Singh et al., 2013a; Nishiyama et al., 2005 |

*(Continued)*

**TABLE 16.1 (*Continued*)**
**Summary of Pharmacological Activities of Essential Oil of *Curcuma longa* (Turmeric)**

| Pharmacological Activities | Description | References |
|---|---|---|
| Anti-insecticidal/herbicidal activity | Ar-turmerone effective against mosquito repellent (*Aedes aegypti* larvae), reduces germination and growth of weed seed. | H.A. Fouad, C.A.G. da Camara, 2017; Roth et al., 1998; Fagodia et al., 2017 |
| Neuroprotective activity | Anti-neurotoxicity against rat embolic-stroke model, middle cerebral artery occlusion of the filament model. | Rathore et al., 2008; Manhas et al., 2014 |
| Anticancer activity | Cytotoxic to melanoma (B16), pancreatic cancer (PANC-1), human cervical adenocarcinoma, and prostate cancer (LNCaP). | Zhang et al., 2017; Jacob, 2016; Arora et al., 1971 |
| Anti-inflammatory activity | Carrageenan-induced acute inflammatory model, dextran-induced inflammatory model, and formalin-induced chronic inflammatory model. | Winter et al., 1962; Maity et al., 1998; Chau, 1989 |
| Antiarthritic activity | Streptococcal cell wall (SCW)-induced arthritis in the female rats model. | Funk et al., 2010 |
| Hepatoprotective activity | Turmeric EO (200 mg/kg) inhibits the actions of serum enzymes, serum total cholesterol, serum triglyceride, and hepatic malondialdehyde level. | Kiso et al., 1983 |
| Antiplatelet activity | Ar-turmerone preventing platelet aggregation by collagen and arachidonic acid. | Lee, 2006 |

## 16.4 CONCLUSION

From ancient times, traditional medicine has utilized turmeric to cure a wide range of medical conditions. It is also used as a flavouring ingredient. Because there are so many different potential pharmacological targets, essential oils have a medicinal potential that needs more and more scientific study. Bioactive compounds are abundant in essential oils. Key chemical components are widely mentioned as the substances that provide the oil its pharmacological characteristics. Furthermore, the combined activity of two or more chemicals in the oil might have an increased, synergistic, or inhibitory effect, which would have a negative impact on the oil's pharmacological function. To evaluate the potential therapeutic use of EOs' active ingredients, more research is necessary. To optimize their therapeutic effects for each target organ, it is still essential to ascertain the pharmacological profile of the identified EO active components as well as their bioavailability, potency, and safety.

# REFERENCES

Afzal, A., Oriqat, G., Akram Khan, M., Jose, J. and Afzal, M., 2013. Chemistry and biochemistry of terpenoids from Curcuma and related species. *Journal of Biologically Active Products from Nature*, 3(1), pp. 1–55.

Angel, G.R., Menon, N., Vimala, B. and Nambisan, B., 2014. Essential oil composition of eight starchy Curcuma species. *Industrial Crops and Products*, 60, pp. 233–238.

Apisariyakul, A., Vanittanakom, N. and Buddhasukh, D., 1995. Antifungal activity of turmeric oil extracted from Curcuma longa (Zingiberaceae). *Journal of Ethnopharmacology*, 49(3), pp. 163–169.

Arora RB, Kapoor V, Basu N, Jain AP, August 1971. Anti-inflammatory studies on Curcuma longa (turmeric). *The Indian Journal of Medical Research*, 59(8), pp. 1289–1295.

Avanço, G.B., Ferreira, F.D., Bomfim, N.S., Peralta, R.M., Brugnari, T., Mallmann, C.A., de Abreu Filho, B.A., Mikcha, J.M.G. and Machinski Jr, M., 2017. Curcuma longa L. essential oil composition, antioxidant effect, and effect on Fusarium verticillioides and fumonisin production. *Food Control*, 73, pp. 806–813.

Bahl, J.R., Bansal, R.P., Garg, S.N., Gupta, M.M., Singh, V., Goel, R. and Kumar, S., 2014. Variation in yield of curcumin and yield and quality of leaf and rhizome essential oils among Indian land races of turmeric Curcuma longa L. *Proceedings of the Indian National Science Academy*, 80, pp. 143–156.

Bansal, R.P., Bahl, J.R., Garg, S.N., Naqvi, A.A. and Kumar, S., 2002. Differential chemical compositions of the essential oils of the shoot organs, rhizomes and rhizoids in the tumeric Curcuma longa grown in Indo-Gangetic plains. *Pharmaceutical Biology*, 40(5), pp. 384–389.

Behura, C., Ray, P., Rath, C.C., Mishra, R.K., Ramachandraiah, O.S. and Charyulu, J.K., 2000. Antifungal activity of essential oils of Curcuma longa against five rice pathogens in vitro. *Journal of Essential Oil-Bearing Plants*, 3(2), pp. 79–84.

Bhadoria, P.B.S., 2011. Allelopathy: A natural way towards weed management. *American Journal of Experimental Agriculture*, 1(1), pp. 7–20.

Burt, S., 2004. Essential oils: Their antibacterial properties and potential applications in foods – a review. *International Journal of Food Microbiology*, 94(3), pp. 223–253.

Busi, R., Vila-Aiub, M.M., Beckie, H.J., Gaines, T.A., Goggin, D.E., Kaundun, S.S., Lacoste, M., Neve, P., Nissen, S.J., Norsworthy, J.K. and Renton, M., 2013. Herbicide-resistant weeds: From research and knowledge to future needs. *Evolutionary Applications*, 6(8), pp. 1218–1221.

Chane-Ming, J., Vera, R., Chalchat, J.C. and Cabassu, P., 2002. Chemical composition of essential oils from rhizomes, leaves and flowers of Curcuma longa L. from Reunion Island. *Journal of Essential Oil Research*, 14(4), pp. 249–251.

Chau TT., 1989. Analgesic testing in animal models. In: Chang JY, AJ Lewis, (Eds), *Pharmacological methods in the control of inflammation* (pp. 195–212). Alan R. Liss, Inc.

Chen, I.N., Chang, C.C., Ng, C.C., Wang, C.Y., Shyu, Y.T. and Chang, T.L., 2008. Antioxidant and antimicrobial activity of Zingiberaceae plants in Taiwan. *Plant Foods for Human Nutrition*, 63, pp. 15–20.

Chen, M., Chang, Y.Y., Huang, S., Xiao, L.H., Zhou, W., Zhang, L.Y., Li, C., Zhou, R.P., Tang, J., Lin, L. and Du, Z.Y., 2018. Aromatic-turmerone attenuates LPS-induced neuroinflammation and consequent memory impairment by targeting TLR4-dependent signaling pathway. *Molecular Nutrition & Food Research*, 62(2), p. 1700281.

Cheng, J.J., Yang, N.B., Wu, L., Lin, J.L., Dai, G.X. and Zhu, J.Y., 2014. Effects of zedoary turmeric oil on P450 activities in rats with liver cirrhosis induced by thioacetamide. *International Journal of Clinical and Experimental Pathology*, 7(11), p. 7854.

Coy Barrera, C.A. and Eunice Acosta, G., 2013. Actividad antibacteriana y determinación de la composición química de los aceites esenciales de romero (Rosmarinus officinalis), tomillo (Thymus vulgaris) y cúrcuma (Curcuma longa) de Colombia. *Revista Cubana de Plantas Medicinales*, 18(2), pp. 237–246.

Devi, L.R., Rana, V.S., Devi, S.I., Verdeguer, M. and Amparo Blázquez, M., 2012. Chemical composition and antimicrobial activity of the essential oil of Curcuma leucorhiza Roxb. *Journal of Essential Oil Research*, 24(6), pp. 533–538.

Dohare, P., Garg, P., Sharma, U., Jagannathan, N.R. and Ray, M., 2008. Neuroprotective efficacy and therapeutic window of curcuma oil: In rat embolic stroke model. *BMC Complementary and Alternative Medicine*, 8, pp. 1–20.

Dosoky, N.S. 2015. Isolation and Identification of Bioactive Compounds from Conradina canescens Gray. Ph.D. Dissertation, University of Alabama in Huntsville, Huntsville, AL.

Fagodia, S.K., Singh, H.P., Batish, D.R. and Kohli, R.K., 2017. Phytotoxicity and cytotoxicity of Citrus aurantiifolia essential oil and its major constituents: Limonene and citral. *Industrial Crops and Products*, 108, pp. 708–715.

Fouad, H.A. and da Camara, C.A., 2017. Chemical composition and bioactivity of peel oils from Citrus aurantiifolia and Citrus reticulata and enantiomers of their major constituent against Sitophilus zeamais (Coleoptera: Curculionidae). *Journal of Stored Products Research*, 73, pp. 30–36.

Funk, J.L., Frye, J.B., Oyarzo, J.N., Kuscuoglu, N., Wilson, J., McCaffrey, G., Stafford, G., Chen, G., Lantz, R.C., Jolad, S.D. and Sólyom, A.M., 2006. Efficacy and mechanism of action of turmeric supplements in the treatment of experimental arthritis. *Arthritis & Rheumatism: Official Journal of the American College of Rheumatology*, 54(11), pp. 3452–3464.

Funk, J.L., Frye, J.B., Oyarzo, J.N., Zhang, H. and Timmermann, B.N., 2010. Anti-arthritic effects and toxicity of the essential oils of turmeric (Curcuma longa L.). *Journal of Agricultural and Food Chemistry*, 58(2), pp. 842–849.

Garg, S.N., Mengi, N., Patra, N.K., Charles, R. and Kumar, S., 2002. Chemical examination of the leaf essential oil of Curcuma longa L. from the north Indian plains. *Flavour and Fragrance Journal*, 17(2), pp. 103–104.

Goel, A., Kunnumakkara, A.B. and Aggarwal, B.B., 2008. Curcumin as "Curecumin": From kitchen to clinic. *Biochemical Pharmacology*, 75(4), pp. 787–809.

Gopalan, B., Goto, M., Kodama, A. and Hirose, T., 2000. Supercritical carbon dioxide extraction of turmeric (Curcuma longa). *Journal of Agricultural and Food Chemistry*, 48(6), pp. 2189–2192.

Hastak, K., Lubri, N., Jakhi, S.D., More, C., John, A., Ghaisas, S.D. and Bhide, S.V., 1997. Effect of turmeric oil and turmeric oleoresin on cytogenetic damage in patients suffering from oral submucous fibrosis. *Cancer Letters*, 116(2), pp. 265–269.

Herath, I.C., Wijayasiriwardene, T.D.C.M.K. and Premakumara, G.A.S., 2017. Comparative GC-MS analysis of all Curcuma species grown in Sri Lanka by multivariate test. *Ruhuna Journal of Science*, 8(2).

Himaja, M., Anand, R., Ramana, M.V., Anand, M. and Karigar, A., 2010. Phytochemical screening and antioxidant activity of rhizome part of Curcuma zedoaria. *International Journal of Research in Ayurveda and Pharmacy (IJRAP)*, 1(2), pp. 414–417.

Honda, S., Aoki, F., Tanaka, H., Kishida, H., Nishiyama, T., Okada, S., Matsumoto, I., Abe, K. and Mae, T., 2006. Effects of ingested turmeric oleoresin on glucose and lipid metabolisms in obese diabetic mice: A DNA microarray study. *Journal of Agricultural and Food Chemistry*, *54*(24), pp. 9055–9062.

Ibáñez, M.D. and Blázquez, M.A., 2021. Curcuma longa L. rhizome essential oil from extraction to its agri-food applications. A review. *Plants*, *10*(1), p. 44.

Itokawa, H., Shi, Q., Akiyama, T., Morris-Natschke, S.L. and Lee, K.H., 2008. Recent advances in the investigation of curcuminoids. *Chinese Medicine*, *3*, pp. 1–13.

Jacob, J.N., 2016. Comparative studies in relation to the structure and biochemical properties of the active compounds in the volatile and nonvolatile fractions of turmeric (C. longa) and ginger (Z. officinale). *Studies in Natural Products Chemistry*, *48*, pp. 101–135.

Jain, V., Prasad, V., Singh, S. and Pal, R., 2007. HPTLC method for the quantitative determination of ar-turmerone and turmerone in lipid soluble fraction from Curcuma longa. *Natural Product Communications*, *2*(9), p. 1934578X0700200912.

Jantan, I., Saputri, F.C., Qaisar, M.N. and Buang, F., 2012. Correlation between chemical composition of Curcuma domestica and Curcuma xanthorrhiza and their antioxidant effect on human low-density lipoprotein oxidation. *Evidence-Based Complementary and Alternative Medicine*, *2012*.

Jena, S., Ray, A., Banerjee, A., Sahoo, A., Nasim, N., Sahoo, S., Kar, B., Patnaik, J., Panda, P.C. and Nayak, S., 2017. Chemical composition and antioxidant activity of essential oil from leaves and rhizomes of Curcuma angustifolia Roxb. *Natural Product Research*, *31*(18), pp. 2188–2191.

Joshi, J., Ghaisas, S., Vaidya, A., Vaidya, R., Kamat, D.V., Bhagwat, A.N. and Bhide, S., 2003. Early human safety study of turmeric oil (Curcuma longa oil) administered orally in healthy volunteers. *Journal-Association of Physicians of India*, *51*, pp. 1055–1060.

Jurenka, JS., 2009. Anti-inflammatory properties of curcumin, a major constituent of Curcuma longa: a review of preclinical and clinical research. *Alternative Medicine Review*, *14*(2), pp. 141–153.

Kiso, Y., Suzuki, Y., Watanabe, N., Oshima, Y. and Hikino, H., 1983. Antihepatotoxic principles of Curcuma longa rhizomes. *Planta Medica*, *49*(11), pp. 185–187.

Kocaadam, B. and Şanlier, N., 2017. Curcumin, an active component of turmeric (Curcuma longa), and its effects on health. *Critical Reviews in Food Science and Nutrition*, *57*(13), pp. 2889–2895.

Krup, V., Prakash, L.H. and Harini, A., 2013. Pharmacological activities of turmeric (Curcuma longa Linn): A review. *Journal of Homeopathy & Ayurvedic Medicine*, *2*(133), pp. 2167–1206.

Labban, L., 2014. Medicinal and pharmacological properties of turmeric (Curcuma longa): A review. *International Journal of Pharmaceutical and Biomedical Science*, *5*(1), pp. 17–23.

Lantz, R.C., Chen, G.J., Solyom, A.M., Jolad, S.D. and Timmermann, B.N., 2005. The effect of turmeric extracts on inflammatory mediator production. *Phytomedicine*, *12*(6–7), pp. 445–452.

Lawand, R.V. and Gandhi, S.V., 2013. Comparison of Curcuma caesia Roxb. with other commonly used Curcuma species by HPTLC. *Journal of Pharmacognosy and Phytochemistry*, *2*(4), pp. 126–131.

Lee, H.S., 2006. Antiplatelet property of Curcuma longa L. rhizome-derived ar-turmerone. *Bioresource Technology*, *97*(12), pp. 1372–1376.

Liju, V.B., Jeena, K. and Kuttan, R., 2011. An evaluation of antioxidant, anti-inflammatory, and antinociceptive activities of essential oil from Curcuma longa. L. *Indian Journal of Pharmacology*, *43*(5), p. 526.

Ling, J., Wei, B., Lv, G., Ji, H. and Li, S., 2012. Anti-hyperlipidaemic and antioxidant effects of turmeric oil in hyperlipidaemic rats. *Food Chemistry*, *130*(2), pp. 229–235.

Maity, T.K., Mandal, S.C., Mukherjee, P.K., Saha, K., Das, J., Pal, M. and Saha, B.P., 1998. Studies on antiinflammatory effect of Cassia tora leaf extract (fam. Leguminosae). *Phytotherapy Research: An International Journal Devoted to Pharmacological and Toxicological Evaluation of Natural Product Derivatives*, *12*(3), pp. 221–223.

Manhas, A., Khanna, V., Prakash, P., Goyal, D., Malasoni, R., Naqvi, A., Dwivedi, A.K., Dikshit, M. and Jagavelu, K., 2014. Curcuma oil reduces endothelial cell-mediated inflammation in postmyocardial ischemia/reperfusion in rats. *Journal of Cardiovascular Pharmacology*, *64*(3), pp. 228–236.

Manosroi, J., Dhumtanom, P. and Manosroi, A., 2006. Anti-proliferative activity of essential oil extracted from Thai medicinal plants on KB and P388 cell lines. *Cancer Letters*, *235*(1), pp. 114–120.

Manzan, A.C.C., Toniolo, F.S., Bredow, E. and Povh, N.P., 2003. Extraction of essential oil and pigments from Curcuma longa [L.] by steam distillation and extraction with volatile solvents. *Journal of Agricultural and Food Chemistry*, *51*(23), pp. 6802–6807.

Mau, J.L., Lai, E.Y., Wang, N.P., Chen, C.C., Chang, C.H. and Chyau, C.C., 2003. Composition and antioxidant activity of the essential oil from Curcuma zedoaria. *Food Chemistry*, *82*(4), pp. 583–591.

Mehrotra, S., Agnihotri, G., Singh, S. and Jamal, F., 2013. Immunomodulatory potential of Curcuma longa: A review. *South Asian Journal of Experimental Biology*, *3*(6), pp. 299–307.

Murakami, A., Furukawa, I., Miyamoto, S., Tanaka, T. and Ohigashi, H., 2013. Curcumin combined with turmerones, essential oil components of turmeric, abolishes inflammation-associated mouse colon carcinogenesis. *Biofactors*, *39*(2), pp. 221–232.

Negi, P.S., Jayaprakasha, G.K., Jagan Mohan Rao, L. and Sakariah, K.K., 1999. Antibacterial activity of turmeric oil: A byproduct from curcumin manufacture. *Journal of Agricultural and Food Chemistry*, *47*(10), pp. 4297–4300.

Nishiyama, T., Mae, T., Kishida, H., Tsukagawa, M., Mimaki, Y., Kuroda, M., Sashida, Y., Takahashi, K., Kawada, T., Nakagawa, K. and Kitahara, M., 2005. Curcuminoids and sesquiterpenoids in turmeric (Curcuma longa L.) suppress an increase in blood glucose level in type 2 diabetic KK-Ay mice. *Journal of Agricultural and food Chemistry*, *53*(4), pp. 959–963.

Nwozo, S.O., Osunmadewa, D.A. and Oyinloye, B.E., 2014. Anti-fatty liver effects of oils from Zingiber officinale and Curcuma longa on ethanol-induced fatty liver in rats. *Journal of Integrative Medicine*, *12*(1), pp. 59–65.

Pande, C. and Chanotiya, C.S., 2006. Constituents of the leaf oil of Curcuma longa L. from Uttaranchal. *Journal of Essential Oil Research*, *18*(2), pp. 166–167.

Pino, J.A., Fon-Fay, F.M., Pérez, J.C., Falco, A.S., Hernández, I., Rodeiro, I. and Fernández, M.D., 2018. Chemical composition and biological activities of essential oil from turmeric (Curcuma longa L.) rhizomes grown in Amazonian Ecuador. *Revista CENIC Ciencias Químicas*, *49*(1).

Prakash, B., Kedia, A., Mishra, P.K. and Dubey, N.K., 2015. Plant essential oils as food preservatives to control moulds, mycotoxin contamination and oxidative deterioration of agri-food commodities – potentials and challenges. *Food Control*, *47*, pp. 381–391.

Ramezani, S., Saharkhiz, M.J., Ramezani, F., Fotokian, M.H., 2008. Use of essential oils as bioherbicides. *Journal of Essential Oil-Bearing Plants* 11, 319–327.

Rathore, P., Dohare, P., Varma, S., Ray, A., Sharma, U., Jaganathanan, N.R. and Ray, M., 2008. Curcuma oil: Reduces early accumulation of oxidative product and is anti-apoptogenic in transient focal ischemia in rat brain. *Neurochemical Research, 33*, pp. 1672–1682.

Raut, J.S. and Karuppayil, S.M., 2014. A status review on the medicinal properties of essential oils. *Industrial Crops and Products, 62*, pp. 250–264.

Reanmongkol, W., Subhadhirasakul, S., Khaisombat, N., Fuengnawakit, P., Jantasila, S. and Khamjun, A., 2006. Investigation the antinociceptive, antipyretic and anti-inflammatory activities of Curcuma aeruginosa Roxb. extracts in experimental animals. *Songklanakarin Journal of Science and Technology, 28*(5), pp. 999–1008.

Roth, G.N., Chandra, A. and Nair, M.G., 1998. Novel bioactivities of Curcuma longa constituents. *Journal of Natural Products, 61*(4), pp. 542–545.

Sacchetti, G., Maietti, S., Muzzoli, M., Scaglianti, M., Manfredini, S., Radice, M. and Bruni, R., 2005. Comparative evaluation of 11 essential oils of different origin as functional antioxidants, antiradicals and antimicrobials in foods. *Food Chemistry, 91*(4), pp. 621–632.

Salas, M.L., Mounier, J., Valence, F., Coton, M., Thierry, A., & Coton, E. 2017. Antifungal microbial agents for food biopreservation—A review. *Microorganisms, 5*(3), 37.

Sandeep, I.S., Sanghamitra, N. and Sujata, M., 2015. Differential effect of soil and environment on metabolic expression of turmeric (Curcuma longa cv. Roma). *Indian Journal of Experimental Biology, 53*, pp. 406–411.

Santos-Sánchez, N.F., Salas-Coronado, R., Valadez-Blanco, R., Hernández-Carlos, B. and Guadarrama-Mendoza, P.C., 2017. Natural antioxidant extracts as food preservatives. *Acta Scientiarum Polonorum Technologia Alimentaria, 16*(4), pp. 361–370.

Sawicka, B. and Egbuna, C., 2020. Pests of agricultural crops and control measures. In *Natural remedies for pest, disease and weed control* (pp. 1–16). Academic Press.

Schmidt, M., Zannini, E., Lynch, K.M. and Arendt, E.K., 2019. Novel approaches for chemical and microbiological shelf life extension of cereal crops. *Critical Reviews in Food Science and Nutrition, 59*(21), pp. 3395–3419.

Shang, Z.P., Xu, L.L., Lu, Y.Y., Guan, M., Li, D.Y., Le, Z.Y., Bai, Z.L., Qiao, X. and Ye, M., 2019. Advances in chemical constituents and quality control of turmeric. *World Journal of Traditional Chinese Medicine, 5*(2), p. 116.

Sharma, R.K., Misra, B.P., Sarma, T.C., Bordoloi, A.K., Pathak, M.G. and Leclercq, P.A., 1997. Essential oils of Curcuma longa L. from Bhutan. *Journal of Essential Oil Research, 9*(5), pp. 589–592.

Sharma, S.K., Singh, S. and Tewari, S.K., 2019. Study of leaf oil composition from various accessions of Curcuma longa L. grown on partially reclaimed sodic soil. *International Journal of Plant and Environment, 5*(04), pp. 293–296.

Sikha, A. and Harini, A., 2015. Pharmacological activities of wild turmeric (Curcuma aromatica Salisb): A review. *Journal of Pharmacognosy and Phytochemistry, 3*(5), pp. 1–4.

Singh, G., Kapoor, I.P.S., Singh, P., de Heluani, C.S., de Lampasona, M.P. and Catalan, C.A., 2010. Comparative study of chemical composition and antioxidant activity of fresh and dry rhizomes of turmeric (Curcuma longa Linn.). *Food and Chemical Toxicology, 48*(4), pp. 1026–1031.

Singh, P., Singh, S., Kapoor, I.P.S., Singh, G., Isidorov, V. and Szczepaniak, L., 2013a. Chemical composition and antioxidant activities of essential oil and oleoresins from Curcuma zedoaria rhizomes, part-74. *Food Bioscience, 3*, pp. 42–48.

Singh, V., Jain, M., Misra, A., Khanna, V., Rana, M., Prakash, P., Malasoni, R., Dwivedi, A.K., Dikshit, M. and Barthwal, M.K., 2013b. Curcuma oil ameliorates hyperlipidaemia and associated deleterious effects in golden Syrian hamsters. *British Journal of Nutrition, 110*(3), pp. 437–446.

Soltys, D., Krasuska, U., Bogatek, R., Gniazdow, A., 2013. Allelochemicals asbio-herbicides
    -present and perspectives. In: Price, A.J., Kelton, J.A. (Eds.), *Herbicides-Current
    Research and Case Studies in Use. InTech, Croatia*, pp. 517–542.
Srinivasan, V., Thankamani, C.K., Dinesh, R., Kandiannan, K., Zachariah, T.J., Leela, N.K.,
    Hamza, S., Shajina, O. and Ansha, O., 2016. Nutrient management systems in turmeric:
    Effects on soil quality, rhizome yield and quality. *Industrial Crops and Products*, 85,
    pp. 241–250.
Stanojević, J.S., Stanojević, L.P., Cvetković, D.J. and Danilović, B.R., 2015. Chemical com-
    position, antioxidant and antimicrobial activity of the turmeric essential oil (Curcuma
    longa L.). *Advanced Technologies*, 4(2), pp. 19–25.
Tamta, A., Prakash, O., Punetha, H. and Pant, A.K., 2016. Chemical composition and in vitro
    antioxidant potential of essential oil and rhizome extracts of Curcuma amada Roxb.
    *Cogent Chemistry*, 2(1), p. 1168067.
Tawatsin, A., Wratten, S.D., Scott, R.R., Thavara, U. and Techadamrongsin, Y., 2001.
    Repellency of volatile oils from plants against three mosquito vectors. *Journal of
    Vector Ecology*, 26, pp. 76–82.
Tsai, S.Y., Huang, S.J., Chyau, C.C., Tsai, C.H., Weng, C.C. and Mau, J.L., 2011. Composition
    and antioxidant properties of essential oils from Curcuma rhizome. *Asian Journal of
    Arts and Sciences*, 2(1), pp. 57–66.
Ulbricht, C., Basch, E., Barrette, E.P., Boon, H., Chao, W., Costa, D., Higdon, E.R., Isaac, R.,
    Lynch, M., Papaliodis, G. and Grimes Serrano, J.M., 2011. Turmeric (Curcuma longa):
    An evidence-based systematic review by the natural standard research collaboration.
    *Alternative and Complementary Therapies*, 17(4), pp. 225–236.
Weiss, E.A., 2002. *Spice crops* (pp. 55–56). CABI Publishing.
Wilson, B., Abraham, G., Manju, V.S., Mathew, M., Vimala, B., Sundaresan, S. and Nambisan,
    B., 2005. Antimicrobial activity of Curcuma zedoaria and Curcuma malabarica tubers.
    *Journal of Ethnopharmacology*, 99(1), pp. 147–151.
Winter, C.A., Risley, E.A. and Nuss, G.W., 1962. Carrageenin-induced edema in hind paw
    of the rat as an assay for antiinflammatory drugs. *Proceedings of the Society for
    Experimental Biology and Medicine*, 111(3), pp. 544–547.
Yang, S., Liu, J., Jiao, J. and Jiao, L., 2020. Ar-turmerone exerts anti-proliferative and anti-
    inflammatory activities in HaCaT keratinocytes by inactivating hedgehog pathway.
    *Inflammation*, 43, pp. 478–486.
Yue, G.G., Cheng, S.W., Yu, H., Xu, Z.S., Lee, J.K., Hon, P.M., Lee, M.Y., Kennelly, E.J.,
    Deng, G., Yeung, S.K. and Cassileth, B.R., 2012. The role of turmerones on curcumin
    transportation and P-glycoprotein activities in intestinal Caco-2 cells. *Journal of
    Medicinal Food*, 15(3), pp. 242–252.
Yue, G.G.L., Jiang, L., Kwok, H.F., Lee, J.K.M., Chan, K.M., Fung, K.P., Leung, P.C. and
    Bik-San Lau, C., 2016. Turmeric ethanolic extract possesses stronger inhibitory activi-
    ties on colon tumour growth than curcumin – the importance of turmerones. *Journal of
    Functional Foods*, 22, pp. 565–577.
Zhang, L., Yang, Z., Wei, J., Su, P., Chen, D., Pan, W., Zhou, W., Zhang, K., Zheng, X., Lin,
    L. and Tang, J., 2017. Contrastive analysis of chemical composition of essential oil
    from twelve Curcuma species distributed in China. *Industrial Crops and Products*,
    108, pp. 17–25.
Zhao, J., Zhang, J.S., Yang, B., Lv, G.P. and Li, S.P., 2010. Free radical scavenging activity
    and characterization of sesquiterpenoids in four species of Curcuma using a TLC bio-
    autography assay and GC-MS analysis. *Molecules*, 15(11), pp. 7547–7557.

# 17 Pharmacological Aspects of Coriander Essential Oils

*Mohit Agrawal, Manmohan Singhal, Yash Jasoria,
Hema Chaudhary, and Bhupendra G. Prajapati*

## 17.1 INTRODUCTION

The use of herbs and plants in naturopathy is growing due to their low cost and lack of negative impacts. The herb coriander is one of them. Coriander (*Coriandrum sativum* Linn.), a member of the *Apiaceae* (*Umbelliferae*) family, is mostly grown from seeds all year (Momin et al., 2012). It is an annual herbaceous plant that is native to the Mediterranean region but is widely grown in North Africa, Central Europe, and Asia as a therapeutic and culinary herb. Additionally, it may be effectively cultivated under a variety of circumstances (Seidemann et al., 2005). The plant may grow to a height of 25 to 60 cm. It contains tiny, pinkish-white florets and alternating leaflets, as well as slender, spindle-shaped roots, an upright stalk, and a leafy plant. From June through July, the plant blooms, and two pericarps make up the spherical fruits that are produced (Burdock and Carabin, 2009). These very globular fruits have several longitudinal ridges on their surface, are practically ovate in shape, and have a mild, sweet, somewhat pungent flavor that tastes a bit like citrus with a note of sage. This fruit is 3 to 5 mm long, and when dried, it is often brown, though it may also be green, straw-colored, or white. Worldwide, the plant is widely cultivated for its seeds, spices, and essential oils. It is a well-known Ayurvedic medicinal plant in India called "Dhanya." Sausage flavoring is another application for it. The plant's entire body may be consumed, and its fresh leaves are frequently used in chutneys and salads as well as being used as a garnish (Bhat et al., 2014) In addition to being a component of pickling spices, the whole or ground seed (fruit) is also used to flavor a variety of commercial meals, most notably certain quick soups and stews, as well as numerous cakes, bread, and other pastries, alcoholic drinks, frozen dairy desserts, sweets, and puddings. Since ancient times, plants have played a significant role in sustaining human health and improving living conditions (Coşkuner and Karababa, 2007). Everywhere in the globe, coriander is used in a variety of traditional, ethnobotanical, and ethnomedical practices to treat a wide range of ailments. Due to its diaphoretic, diuretic, carminative, and stimulating properties, coriander is utilized in Indian traditional medicine to

DOI: 10.1201/9781003389774-17

treat digestive, respiratory, and urinary system diseases. Major research has been done recently on the chemical composition and biological effects of coriander seed and plant essential oils, including their antibacterial, antioxidant, hypoglycemic, hypolipidemic, anxiolytic, analgesic, anti-inflammatory, anti-convulsant, and other biological activities (Laribi et al., 2015). The high antioxidant activity of this plant, as well as its major constituent, linalool, may assist in regulating these effects. The biochemical composition of *Coriandrum sativum* L., its traditional and medical applications, its influence on ethnobotany and ethnomedicine, and its botanical characteristics (Sobhani et al., 2022).

## 17.2　HISTORY OF *CORIANDRUM SATIVUM* LINN

It is one of the oldest plants described in history, having been used for almost 5000 years. Since the second millennium BC, coriander appears to have been grown in Greece. "Herb of Happiness" was the name given to it in Egypt. The Chinese believed that coriander could be trusted and began using it in their medicinal practices around 207 BC (Pasha and Qureshi, 2017).

## 17.3　BOTANICAL DESCRIPTION OF *CORIANDRUM SATIVUM* LINN

- The Botanical Classification of *Coriandrum sativum* Linn (Sharma and Sharma, 2012)

**BOTANICAL CLASSIFICATION**

| | |
|---|---|
| **Division** | Angiospermae |
| **Series** | Calyciflorae |
| **Class** | Dicotyledonae |
| **Sub-class** | Polypetalae |
| **Order** | Umbellale (Apiales) |
| **Family** | Umbelliferae (Apiaceae) |
| **Genus** | Coriandrum |
| **Species** | Sativum |

- Several Alternate Names for *Coriandrum sativum* (Sharma and Sharma, 2012)

| | |
|---|---|
| Botanical Name | *Coriandrum sativum* Linn. |
| Common Name (English) | Coriander |
| Hindi Name | Dhaniya |
| Unani Name | Kishneez |
| Ayurvedic Name | Dhanyaka |
| Siddha Name | Kottumalli Vitai |

## 17.4   CHEMICAL COMPOSITION

Fresh herbage has a very distinct flavor and aroma to mature seeds. Linalool and certain other oxygenated monoterpenes and monoterpene hydrocarbons are significant ingredients in the oil separated from coriander fruit, but aliphatic aldehydes (mostly C10-C16 aldehydes) with fetid-like odors are prevalent in the fresh herb oil (Bhuiyan et al., 2009).

Essential oil and fatty oil are the components of coriander fruits that are essential. In comparison to the fatty oil content, which ranges from 9.9% to 27.7%, the essential oil content of dried coriander fruits varies from 0.03% to 2.6%. There is found a range of 0.1% to 0.36% essential oil concentration in the dried fruits from several accessions. The principal components in the oil of the coriander fruits farmed in Iran were found to include linalool (40.9% to 79.9%), neryl acetate (2.3% to 14.2%), γ-terpinene (0.1% to 13.6%), and α-pinene (1.2% to 7.1%) (Figure 17.1). According to an analysis of the essential oil content of *C. sativum* from Bulgaria, the three primary components were linalool (63.3%), α-pinene (6.1%), and p-cymene (5.0%) (Nejad Ebrahimi et al., 2010). Additionally, important components of the leaf oil include undecanoic acid (2.1%), 2-dodecanal (1.3%), 2-undecenal (3.9%), cyclododecane (2.5%), decamethylene glycol (1.2%), decanal (1.4%), and dodecanoic acid (2.6%). According to an assessment of Kenyan coriander leaves essential oil, the primary components were 2E-decenal (15.9%), decanal (14.3%), 2E-decen-1-ol (14.2%), and n-decanol (13.6%) (Matasyoh et al., 2009). Figure 17.1 shows some major constituents of coriander.

Multiple volatile components, including fatty acids, sterols, flavonoids, coumarins, catechins, terpenes, and polyphenols are abundant in coriander oil (Sriti et al., 2009; Al-Mofleh et al., 2006). Along with two other known isocoumarins, coriandrin and dihydrocoriandrin, two novel isocoumarins, coriandrone A and B, were isolated from the aerial sections of *Coriandrum sativum* Linn. (Baba et al., 1991). Coriandrones C, D, and E, three novel isocoumarins, were also isolated from entire *Coriandrum sativum* L. plants, and their properties were determined using spectrum and biochemical data (Taniguchi et al., 1996). The three main polyphenolic

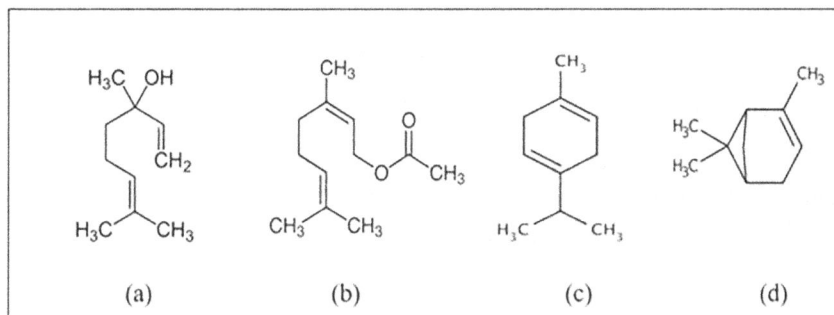

(a)          (b)          (c)          (d)

**FIGURE 17.1**   Major constituents of coriander (a) linalool, (b) neryl acetate, (c) γ-terpinene, and (d) α-pinene

compounds found in coriander aerial portions were identified as caffeic acid, protocatechin, and glycitin (de Almeida Melo et al., 2005).

## 17.5  TRADITIONAL AND MEDICINAL IMPORTANCE OF *CORIANDRUM SATIVUM* LINN IN ISLAMIC TRADITIONAL MEDICINE (ITM)

Coriander was one of the world's most ancient spice crops, with use dating back to about 1550 BC. It was employed as a stimulant, aromatic, and carminative in medicine. The primary therapeutic use of powdered fruit, fluid extract, and oil is as a flavoring to mask the taste of powerful purgatives and reduce patients' tendency to grumble (Al-Snafi et al., 2016). Coriander has been proven in Islamic Traditional Medicine to be helpful in treating a variety of ailments that have been subdivided into the following categories (Sobhani et al., 2022).

### 17.5.1  ORAL CAVITY

It is advised to use coriander leaves as a remedy for toothaches and bleeding gums.

### 17.5.2  EYE DISEASES

A coriander leaf cataplasm made with either dry bread or human milk is used to cure blindness, Ocular: blepharitis and conjunctivitis. Moreover, a leaf extract eye solution has been said to prevent measles and smallpox from emerging in this region.

### 17.5.3  SKIN DISEASES

The treatment of erysipelas, scrofula, itching, scabies, herpes, and heated inflammation is topical application of a combination of coriander leaves, dried bread, or barley and bean flour. Additionally, the seeds have been used topically to cure anthrax and hives. This treatment involves combining olive oil and honey with the seeds.

### 17.5.4  CARDIOVASCULAR DISEASES

Varicocele and warmed testicular vascular irritation can be alleviated by topically applying coriander seeds with olive oil and honey.

### 17.5.5  RESPIRATORY DISEASES

Respiratory symptoms such as cough and asthma can be improved with the use of leaf syrup.

### 17.5.6  GASTROINTESTINAL DISEASES

The migration of toxic humor from the stomach to the brain might result in headaches in ITM. The stomach can be tightened and this humor movement can be reduced by a cataplasm made from the seeds. Oral ingestion of coriander leaves with sugar is recommended as a sedative appetizer and a treatment for vomiting, nausea, and gastritis in several ancient medieval manuscripts.

## 17.6  PHARMACOLOGICAL ASPECTS OF *CORIANDRUM SATIVUM* LINN

### 17.6.1  ANXIOLYTIC

The current population is affected by anxiety, which has grown to be a huge topic of focus in neuroscience studies over the past decade. The use of complementary therapies and medicines made from plants that have "mind-altering" properties is becoming more popular. Motor tenseness, sympathetic hyperactivity, apprehension, and vigilance syndromes are symptoms of anxiety, which is a condition of extreme dread. In spite of its significant negative side effects, such as drowsiness, muscular relaxation, ataxia, forgetfulness, and ethanol and barbiturate potentiation and tolerance, benzodiazepines – the principal class of chemicals used in anxiety – remain the most often recommended therapy for anxiety (Mahendra and Bisht, 2011). The culinary and medical benefits of coriander are highly regarded. In the folkloric medicine systems of several cultures, all portions of this plant are used as flavoring agents and/ or as standard treatments for a variety of ailments, including anxiety, sleeplessness, convulsions, and dyspeptic symptoms (Sahib et al., 2013). The strong affinity of coriander flavonoids for central GABA receptors may result in an anxiolytic effect. The coriander seed's essential oil, aqueous extract, and hydroalcoholic extract all have sedative-hypnotic properties. They prolonged the period of time needed to fall asleep after taking phenobarbital (Emam and Heydari, 2006).

On the impact of linalool on the central nervous system, several investigations are addressed. Without affecting balance or body temperature, it has been demonstrated that this substance decreases locomotor activity (de Moura Linck et al., 2009). Inhaling linalool had an anti-anxiety impact and improved social relations while reducing offensive behavior. Coriander's sedation effects on newborn chicks were shown to be caused by linalool when it was administered intracerebrovascularly together with coriander essential oil (Gastón et al., 2016).

### 17.6.2  ANTIMICROBIAL

Another of coriander's most widely known biological properties is its antimicrobial activity. This property occurs in its seeds, leaves, extracts, and essential oils. Antimicrobial properties derived from plants offer a wide range of therapeutic applications; in addition to being successful in treating infectious disorders, they are also less likely to cause adverse effects that are frequently linked to antimicrobial chemicals. Furthermore, coriander seed extract shows powerful antimicrobial effects against Gram-positive bacteria (*Staphylococcus aureus* and *Bacillus*) and Gram-negative (*Escherichia coli*, *Klebsiella pneumonia*, *Pseudomonas aeruginosa*, *Proteus mirabilis*, and *Salmonella typhi*) (Zardini et al., 2012). It works mainly by damaging membranes, which results in cell death.

## 17.6.3 ANTICANCER

Globally, cancer is one of the most prevalent causes of death. Utilizing substances of natural origin, especially those derived from plants and their phytochemicals, in the treatment of cancer may alleviate the negative effects of standard therapy and may alter the immune response (Gomez-Flores et al., 2010). The growth of the HT 29 human colon cancer cell lines is inhibited by the ethanolic extract of *Coriandrum sativum*. As concentration rose, the cytotoxic impact became more pronounced. Concentration-dependent manner and cell-line-specific factors affected the cytotoxicity. It is abundantly obvious from this that the crude extract contains strong bioactive components that may serve as antiproliferative and anticancer agents. Despite the lack of a clear mechanism of action, it is known that the extract includes flavonoids and antioxidant polyphenolic chemicals. Free radicals are known to be scavenged by these substances, and they have a great deal of potential to help cancer cells. Consequently, adding *Coriandrum sativum* leaves to a healthy diet may help cure colon cancer (Nithya and Sumalatha, 2014). Coriander essential oil has a number of important constituents, linalool being one of them. This monoterpenoid substance has the potential to just slightly inhibit cell division. However, it's important to note that subtoxic doses of linalool augment DOX-induced cytotoxicity and pro-apoptotic effects in both cell lines. Linalool only modestly suppresses cell growth. In MCF7 AdrR cells, a strong synergism has been seen, which may be at least partially explained by Linalool's capacity to boost DOX accumulation and cause a drop in Bcl-xL levels. Linalool might consequently enhance anthracyclines' therapeutic index in the treatment of breast cancer, particularly in MDR tumors (Ravizza et al., 2008). We clarified the anticancer mechanism of the monoterpenoid alcohol linalool, which particularly promotes apoptosis in cancer cells via lipid peroxidation. Oxidative stress only manifested itself right away in cancer cells after treatment, according to electron spin resonance (ESR) spectroscopy, which makes it possible to see free radicals in living cells in real time. This showed that the naturally occurring substance linalool has an anticancer impact without having any negative side effects, and future ESR research may promote the use of linalool as a novel and affordable cancer treatment (Iwasaki et al., 2016).

## 17.6.4 ANTIFUNGAL

The inverted petriplate and food poisoning procedures were used to assess the antifungal properties of coriander oil and its oleoresin against eight fungi. The essential oil was found to be very effective against *Aspergillus terreus*, *Fusarium moniliforme*, *Fusarium oxysporum*, and *Curvularia palliscens* using the inverted petriplate method (Singh et al., 2006).

The antimicrobial peptide "Plantaricin CS" was recently discovered in coriander leaf extract and has demonstrated extremely potent antifungal activity against *Penicillium lilacinum* (MIC = 2.5 mg/ml) and *Aspergillus niger* (MIC = 2.3 mg/ml) (Zare-Shehneh et al., 2014).

For *C. albicans* strains, coriander oil and amphotericin B also had a synergistic impact, however for *C. tropicalis* strain, only an additive effect was seen. It has been demonstrated that coriander essential oil possesses a fungicidal effect against the investigated *Candida* strains with MLC values ranging from 0.05% to 0.4% (v/v), which are equal to the MIC value. The fungicidal effect is produced by the breakdown of the cytoplasmic membrane and subsequent liberation of intracellular materials, including DNA (Silva et al., 2011). *Candida albicans* isolates from individuals with periodontal disease's oral cavity were tested for resistance to extracts and essential oils from *Coriandrum sativum*. The chemical makeup of the essential oil and the amounts of 3-hexen-1-ol, 2-hexen-1-ol, and 1-decanol in *C. sativum* were determined (Furletti et al., 2011).

### 17.6.5 HYPOGLYCEMIC

The effects of coriander on carbohydrate metabolic activities led to an increase in the body's intake of glucose. Because of this herb, glycogenesis and glycolysis have risen along with the activities of hexokinase, phosphoglucomutase, and glucose-6-phosphate dehydrogenase. Due to coriander's ability to lower the activity of glucose-6-phosphatase and glycogen phosphorylase, glycogenolysis and gluconeogenesis are reduced (Chithra and Leelamma, 1999). In OHH-*Meriones shawi* rats, a single oral dose of CS extract (20 mg/kg) in sub-chronic administration of an aqueous coriander seed extract normalized glycemia and decreased the elevated IR (insulin resistant), levels of total cholesterol, LDL-cholesterol, and TG, without having a significant impact on BW (body weight), plasma urea, or creatinine and urea levels. Our findings also suggest that frequent ingestion of the comparatively safe coriander seeds may lower blood sugar levels and avoid or lessen cardiovascular problems brought on by dyslipidemia/hyperlipidemia in conditions including pre-diabetes, type 2 diabetes, and metabolic syndrome (Momin et al., 2012).

### 17.6.6 ANTIMIGRAINE

Headache is an exceedingly frequent symptom all over the world, and migraine is the second most commonly occurring kind of headache as the third most prevalent condition. Seventy-five percent of those who get migraines throughout their lives – or around 15% of the entire population – are women. For more than 90% of sufferers, migraine bouts can result in functional impairment (Kasmaei et al., 2016). The coriander seed oil contains the compound linalool, which has significant therapeutic benefits for treating illnesses of the CNS. Because oxidative damage produced by $A\beta(1-42)$ may be reduced with repeated exposure to coriander volatile oil, this may give neuroprotection. As a consequence, more preclinical research on coriander volatile oil as a possible therapy for AD cognitive impairment might be done (Cioanca et al., 2013). Linalool possesses analgesic and anti-inflammatory properties that relieve pain, which helps with migraines (Dussor and Cao, 2016). The ionotropic glutamate receptors AMPA, NMDA, and kainate may be responsible for the linalool's potent antinociception against glutamate-induced pain in mice (Peana et al., 2003). The TRPM8 channel may have a role in migraine, according to genome-wide association study. This channel is recognized as the sensor for cold temperature in cutaneous tissue and is mostly expressed on peripheral sensory neurons, is also present on deep visceral afferents, which are likely unlikely to be stimulated by cold

(Batista et al., 2008). According to Romero-Reyes et al., the expression of this gene has a role in the pathophysiology of migraines (Akerman et al., 2017), and linalool has been demonstrated to be an antagonist of this channel (Behrendt et al., 2004).

### 17.6.7 ANTISEIZURE

One percent of the population is thought to be affected by a neurological condition known as epilepsy (Sander et al., 2003). Epilepsy's onset and development are probably influenced by the oxidative stress caused by the excessive production of free radicals (Shin et al., 2011). As part of a thorough evaluation of any behavioral/psychiatric/learning co-morbidities, seizure providers will test for anxiousness and sadness (Reilly et al., 2011). The death of neurons and epileptic convulsions are influenced by oxidative stress and mitochondrial malfunction. In several animal seizure models, there is evidence that antioxidant treatment may lessen damages brought on by oxidative free radicals (Aguiar et al., 2012). Malondialdehyde (MDA) levels are decreased and total thiol content is increased by coriander extracts, which enhances the brain's antioxidant capability. *C. sativum* aerial portions work well as a preventative measure for seizures and PTZ-induced oxidative stress (Karami et al., 2015). In both PTZ and glutamate-related seizure models, it has been hypothesized that linalool, one of the primary components of coriander, has therapeutic effects. Glutamate, the primary excitatory neurotransmitter in the brain, accumulates more during seizures and epilepsies. By limiting L-[3H] glutamate binding, delaying the beginning of NMDA-induced seizures, decreasing cAMP levels, and avoiding convulsions caused by quinolinic acid, linalool can impede glutamatergic transmission (Elisabetsky et al., 1999). Similar to the majority of AEDs, linalool is hypothesized to affect voltage-gated ion channels (such as $Na^+$ and $Ca^{2+}$ channels) and $GABA_A$ receptors, respectively, to modulate excitatory and inhibitory neurotransmission (White et al., 2007). Linalool has an inhibitory action on both spontaneous activity and pentylenetetrazole-induced epileptiform activity at lower doses. These findings supported the inhibitory impact of linalool on $Na^+$ channels by raising the action potential threshold and decreasing the action potential rising phase. However, when administered directly to snail neurons at a high dose, it exhibits epileptogenic action (Vatanparast et al., 2017).

### 17.6.8 ANALGESIC

Pain is an uncomfortable feeling that is brought on by noxious stimuli that are harmful or have the potential to be harmful. In order to address a variety of human health issues, medicinal plants have frequently been regarded as one of the primary sources of medications. They are commonly employed to treat a variety of CNS conditions. In the proposed investigation, the analgesic qualities of various *C. sativum* aerial parts extracts were examined in relation to the effects of *Coriandrum sativum* on the CNS (Kazempor et al., 2015). Mice showed a 50% reduction in discomfort after receiving 200 mg/kg of coriander seed ethanol extract i.p. (Pathan et al., 2011). Utilizing the hot plate, tail flicking, and formalin procedures, the aqueous coriander seed extract was evaluated for its ability to reduce pain. A strong, dose-dependent analgesic effect of the aqueous extract was discovered. Linalool, which is a primary component of *C. sativum* seeds, contributes to their activity in part by acting through a painkiller mechanism (Taherian et al., 2012). Linalool significantly reduces glutamate-induced analgesia in mice, perhaps through pathways mediated by AMPA, NMDA, and kainate, which are ionotropic glutamate receptors (Batista et al., 2008) and shown that in experimental pain procedures, linalool complexed with β-cyclodextrin generates antinociceptive effects that are superior to those produced by linalool (Quintans-Júnior et al., 2013).

### 17.6.9 ANTI-INFLAMMATORY

Numerous illnesses progress in part due to inflammation, which when it becomes too severe increases the immune system's ability to attack healthy tissues and the body as a whole. When inflammation develops, a variety of pro-inflammatory mediators are overproduced, which causes a number of illnesses like rheumatism, diabetes, and cardiovascular conditions. The anti-inflammatory properties of coriander are evident in its fruits (Yuan et al., 2020). In the current study, the *in vivo* UV erythema test was used to examine the anti-inflammatory potential of coriander oil. A little anti-inflammatory effect was seen in this trial with the lipolotion containing coriander oil. When treating inflammatory skin conditions concurrently, this could be helpful (Reuter et al., 2008). Linalool and geranyl acetate, two bioactive chemicals found in abundance in coriander essential oil, have anti-inflammatory actions via a few molecular targets (Das et al., 2023). *Coriandrum sativum* hydroalcoholic extract and its essential oil have a preventive effect on rat models of acetic acid-induced acute colitis (Heidari et al., 2016).

### 17.6.10 NEUROPROTECTIVE

Neuro-degeneration is devastatingly influenced by oxidative stress, which causes free radical attacks on brain cells. Although oxygen is necessary for life, an unbalanced metabolism and excessive ROS production lead to a variety of ailments, including AD, PD, aging, and many other neurological conditions (Uttara et al., 2009). The neuroprotective action of coriander essential oils and their principal active component linalool against the neurotoxicity caused by Aβ(1–42), a critical basic factor in Alzheimer's disease (Caputo et al., 2021). Coriander is an effective treatment for AD due to its numerous benefits, including memory enhancement, cholesterol reduction, and anticholinesterase action in mice (Mani et al., 2011). The antioxidant activity of coriander (*Coriandrum sativum*) is what gives it its therapeutic benefits in brain ischemia-reperfusion damage. Additionally, it reduced calcium-induced neuronal damage (Vekaria et al., 2012).

### 17.6.11 CARDIOPROTECTIVE

Coriander extract has a preventative effect in isoproterenol-induced heart failure in Wistar rats. The considerable protection against heart failure offered by coriander extract may be related to its capacity to enhance left ventricular functions and baroreflex sensitivity, reduce lipid peroxidation, and regulate the expression of endothelin receptors (Dhyani et al., 2020). Myocardial infarction has been avoided by reducing myofibrillar damage with oral administration of methanol extract from coriander seeds. It could raise HDL levels while lowering levels of CK-MB, LDH, TG, LDL, and VLDL (Patel et al., 2012).

## 17.6.12 HEPATOPROTECTIVE

Numerous hepatic ailments have oxidative damage linked to their development. The antioxidant activity of extracts of *C. sativum* against $CCl_4$-induced oxidative stress in Wistar albino rats (Sreelatha et al., 2009). It is clear that the presence of phenolic compounds may be a contributing factor in the hepatoprotective effect of the plant *C. sativum* (Pandey et al., 2011). The number of hepatocytes that express TNF-α, NF-κB, and caspase-3 was shown to be lower in the *Coriandrum sativum* group compared to the ischemia/reperfusion injury (IRI) group. Kupffer cells were not stained in this group. The group treated with *Coriandrum sativum* showed a statistically significant decrease in the expression levels of the TNF-α, NF-κB, and caspase-3 groups (Kükner et al., 2021).

## 17.6.13 ANTIOXIDANT

Since coriander has a strong antioxidant activity, it is a rich source of phytochemicals and polyphenols. Oxidative stress can be caused by reactive oxygen species, which can damage tissues and biomolecules (Barros et al., 2012). Coriander's seeds and leaves will improve the food's antioxidant content and likely prevent food from oxidatively deteriorating. The antioxidant activity of coriander leaves was higher than that of the seeds. The coriander's ethyl acetate extract produced the most active result, including both the seeds and the leaves. Antioxidant action appears to be mediated by a number of distinct components (Wangensteen et al., 2004). The presence of the β-carotene component, which made up 61.14% of the carotenoids found in the extract, indicates that it plays a major role in the antioxidant activity of coriander. It is possible that the carotenoids work in concert because the crude extract has a stronger antioxidant effect than its component components (Guerra et al., 2005). When compared to a synthetic antioxidant (BHA 0.02%), coriander essential oil's antioxidant activity in butter cake was shown to be rather good (Darughe et al., 2012).

## 17.7  SAFETY CONSIDERATION

For medicinal and culinary purposes, coriander and its extracts were thought to be rather safe. As a result of the biological change of its primary component linalool, coriander seed essential oil did, however, demonstrate underlying oxidative tissue damage, necessitating more research into the product's safety limitations (Wei et al., 2019). The Algerian residents evaluated 22 elements in *Coriandrum sativum* Linn using the INAA procedure, including eight important nutrients (potassium, calcium, sodium, iron, zinc, chromium, cobalt, and selenium) and three hazardous elements (bromine, arsenic, and antimony) (Messaoudi and Begaa, 2019). This indicates that coriander seeds contained amounts significantly below the estimated allowed limits defined by FAO/WHO for human ingestion, both in terms of micro-nutrient components and potentially hazardous chemical elements (Messaoudi and Begaa, 2019).

## 17.8  FUTURE PERSPECTIVES

According to studies, *Coriandrum sativum* L. contains benefits that are anti-anxious, anticonvulsive, antioxidant, antispoilage, hypoglycemic, anti-inflammatory, diuretic, antihypertensive, hypolipidemic, antidepressant, and effective against Alzheimer's disease. Typically, polyphenols and linalool are responsible for the majority of these benefits (Benny and Thomas, 2019).

## 17.9  CONCLUSION

Since the beginning of time, people have seasoned food with spices and aromatic herbs in order to enhance flavor, increase food shelf life, and promote health. One of those wonder plants, coriander serves as both a spice and a natural remedy. *C. sativum* may be used as a possible medicinal plant and how its essential oil can be used as a natural cure for a variety of ailments. Although plants may be culti-vated all year, they are treated to increase flavor, profitability, and global commerce. The potential of *C. sativum* essential oil as a therapeutic plant is supported by a number of investigations on the chemical makeup and biological functions of its bioactive compounds found in the seed and herb of coriander. ITM recommends *C. sativum* essential oil for the treatment of inflammatory diseases such as inflam-mation, bleeding gums, and heated skin irritation. Coriander essential oil contains pharmacological properties that include, among others, antioxidant, antibacterial, antifungal, antidiabetic, hepatoprotective, and antihyperlipidemic effects based on its medicinal value. By keeping food from spoiling, the *C. sativum* essential oil is extremely important in preserving the shelf life of goods. Additionally, new devel-opments in the investigation of the bioactive components of coriander seeds and herbs in the pharma, beauty, agricultural, and culinary sectors have been noted. Coriander's safety has been endorsed by the FEMA and the US FDA, but further research is needed to determine its toxicity and potential side effects when ingested in greater quantities over extended periods of time. Importantly, the usage of cori-ander seed essential oil as a flavoring ingredient without any reports of hazardous consequences implies that this essential oil, and notably its primary component, linalool, should be regarded as generally harmless. Coriander essential oil's use as an antioxidant is perhaps its most significant and well-known quality. This plant is appropriately known as "the herb of happiness" due to its wide range of applications and preventive effects against many serious illnesses. This valuable knowledge of the bioactive components of coriander seeds and herbs, as well as their biological activities, may serve to increase enthusiasm for coriander by defining new clinical and pharmacological uses. As a result, it may be beneficial in the future to design new therapeutic preparations.

## REFERENCES

Aguiar CC, Almeida AB, Araújo PV, Abreu RN, Chaves EM, Vale OC, Macêdo DS, Woods DJ, Fonteles MM, Vasconcelos SM. Oxidative stress and epilepsy: Literature review. Oxidative Medicine and Cellular Longevity. 2012 Oct;2012.

Akerman S, Romero-Reyes M, Holland PR. Current and novel insights into the neurophysiology of migraine and its implications for therapeutics. Pharmacology & Therapeutics. 2017 Apr 1;172:151–170.

Al-Mofleh IA, Alhaider AA, Mossa JS, Al-Sohaibani MO, Rafatullah S, Qureshi S. Protection of gastric mucosal damage by *Coriandrum sativum* L. pretreatment in Wistar albino rats. Environmental Toxicology and Pharmacology. 2006 Jul 1;22(1):64–69.

Al-Snafi AE. A review on chemical constituents and pharmacological activities of Coriandrum sativum. IOSR Journal of Pharmacy. 2016 Jul;6(7):17–42.

Baba K, Xiao YQ, Taniguchi M, Ohishi H, Kozawa M. Isocoumarins from Coriandrum sativum. Phytochemistry. 1991 Jan 1;30(12):4143–4146.

Barros L, Duenas M, Dias MI, Sousa MJ, Santos-Buelga C, Ferreira IC. Phenolic profiles of in vivo and in vitro grown *Coriandrum sativum* L. Food Chemistry. 2012 May 15;132(2):841–848.

Batista PA, de Paula Werner MF, Oliveira EC, Burgos L, Pereira P, da Silva Brum LF, Dos Santos AR. Evidence for the involvement of ionotropic glutamatergic receptors on the antinociceptive effect of (–)-linalool in mice. Neuroscience Letters. 2008 Aug 8;440(3):299–303.

Batista PA, de Paula Werner MF, Oliveira EC, Burgos L, Pereira P, da Silva Brum LF, Dos Santos AR. Evidence for the involvement of ionotropic glutamatergic receptors on the antinociceptive effect of (–)-linalool in mice. Neuroscience Letters. 2008 Aug 8;440(3):299–303.

Behrendt HJ, Germann T, Gillen C, Hatt H, Jostock R. Characterization of the mouse cold-menthol receptor TRPM8 and vanilloid receptor type-1 VR1 using a fluorometric imaging plate reader (FLIPR) assay. British Journal of Pharmacology. 2004 Feb;141(4):737–745.

Benny A, Thomas J. Essential oils as treatment strategy for Alzheimer's disease: Current and future perspectives. Planta Medica. 2019 Feb;85(03):239–248.

Bhat S, Kaushal P, Kaur M, Sharma HK. Coriander (*Coriandrum sativum* L.): Processing, nutritional and functional aspects. African Journal of Plant Science. 2014 Jan;8(1):25–33.

Bhuiyan MN, Begum J, Sultana M. Chemical composition of leaf and seed essential oil of *Coriandrum sativum* L. from Bangladesh. Bangladesh Journal of Pharmacology. 2009 Dec 17;4(2):150–153.

Burdock GA, Carabin IG. Safety assessment of coriander (*Coriandrum sativum* L.) essential oil as a food ingredient. Food and Chemical Toxicology. 2009 Jan 1;47(1):22–34.

Caputo L, Piccialli I, Ciccone R, de Caprariis P, Massa A, De Feo V, Pannaccione A. Lavender and coriander essential oils and their main component linalool exert a protective effect against amyloid-β neurotoxicity. Phytotherapy Research. 2021 Jan;35(1):486–493.

Chithra V, Leelamma S. Coriandrum sativum – mechanism of hypoglycemic action. Food Chemistry. 1999 Nov 1;67(3):229–231.

Cioanca O, Hritcu L, Mihasan M, Hancianu M. Cognitive-enhancing and antioxidant activities of inhaled coriander volatile oil in amyloid β (1–42) rat model of Alzheimer's disease. Physiology & Behavior. 2013 Aug 15;120:193–202.

Coşkuner Y, Karababa E. Physical properties of coriander seeds (*Coriandrum sativum* L.). Journal of Food Engineering. 2007 May 1;80(2):408–416.

Darughe F, Barzegar M, Sahari MA. Antioxidant and antifungal activity of Coriander (*Coriandrum sativum* L.) essential oil in cake. International Food Research Journal. 2012;19(3):1253–1260.

Das S, Pradhan C, Pillai D. Dietary coriander (*Coriandrum sativum* L) oil improves anti-oxidant and anti-inflammatory activity, innate immune responses and resistance to Aeromonas hydrophila in Nile tilapia (Oreochromis niloticus). Fish & Shellfish Immunology. 2023 Jan 1;132:108486.

de Almeida Melo E, Mancini Filho J, Guerra NB. Characterization of antioxidant compounds in aqueous coriander extract (*Coriandrum sativum* L.). LWT-Food Science and Technology. 2005 Feb 1;38(1):15–19.

de Moura Linck V, da Silva AL, Figueiró M, Piato AL, Herrmann AP, Birck FD, Caramão EB, Nunes DS, Moreno PR, Elisabetsky E. Inhaled linalool-induced sedation in mice. Phytomedicine. 2009 Apr 1;16(4):303–307.

Dhyani N, Parveen A, Siddiqi A, Hussain ME, Fahim M. Cardioprotective efficacy of *Coriandrum sativum* (L.) seed extract in heart failure rats through modulation of endo-thelin receptors and antioxidant potential. Journal of Dietary Supplements. 2020 Jan 2;17(1):13–26.

Dussor G, Cao YQ. TRPM8 and migraine. Headache: The Journal of Head and Face Pain. 2016 Oct;56(9):1406–1417.

Elisabetsky E, Brum LS, Souza DO. Anticonvulsant properties of linalool in glutamate-related seizure models. Phytomedicine. 1999 May 1;6(2):107–113.

Emam GM, Heydari HG. Sedative-hypnotic activity of extracts and essential oil of coriander seeds. (2006): 22–27.

Furletti VF, Teixeira IP, Obando-Pereda G, Mardegan RC, Sartoratto A, Figueira GM, Duarte RM, Rehder VL, Duarte MC, Höfling JF. Action of *Coriandrum sativum* L. essential oil upon oral Candida albicans biofilm formation. Evidence-Based Complementary and Alternative Medicine. 2011 Oct;2011.

Gastón MS, Cid MP, Vázquez AM, Decarlini MF, Demmel GI, Rossi LI, Aimar ML, Salvatierra NA. Sedative effect of central administration of *Coriandrum sativum* essential oil and its major component linalool in neonatal chicks. Pharmaceutical Biology. 2016 Oct 2;54(10):1954–1961.

Gomez-Flores R, Hernández-Martínez H, Tamez-Guerra P, Tamez-Guerra R, Quintanilla-Licea R, Monreal-Cuevas E, Rodríguez-Padilla C. Antitumor and immunomodu-lating potential of Coriandrum sativum. Journal of Natural Products Volume 3 .2010;3:54–63.

Guerra NB, de Almeida Melo E, Mancini Filho J. Antioxidant compounds from coriander (*Coriandrum sativum* L.) etheric extract. Journal of Food Composition and Analysis. 2005 Mar 1;18(2–3):193–199.

Heidari B, Sajjadi SE, Minaiyan M. Effect of *Coriandrum sativum* hydroalcoholic extract and its essential oil on acetic acid-induced acute colitis in rats. Avicenna Journal of Phytomedicine. 2016 Mar;6(2):205.

Iwasaki K, Zheng YW, Murata S, Ito H, Nakayama K, Kurokawa T, Sano N, Nowatari T, Villareal MO, Nagano YN, Isoda H. Anticancer effect of linalool via cancer-specific hydroxyl radical generation in human colon cancer. World Journal of Gastroenterology. 2016 Nov 11;22(44):9765.

Karami R, Hosseini M, Mohammadpour T, Ghorbani A, Sadeghnia HR, Rakhshandeh H, Vafaee F, Esmaeilizadeh M. Effects of hydroalcoholic extract of *Coriandrum sativum* on oxidative damage in pentylenetetrazole-induced seizures in rats. Iranian Journal of Neurology. 2015 Apr 4;14(2):59.

Kasmaei HD, Ghorbanifar Z, Zayeri F, Minaei B, Kamali SH, Rezaeizadeh H, Amin G, Ghobadi A, Mirzaei Z. Effects of *Coriandrum sativum* syrup on migraine: A random-ized, triple-blind, placebo-controlled trial. Iranian Red Crescent Medical Journal. 2016 Jan;18(1).

Kazempor SF. The analgesic effects of different extracts of aerial parts of *Coriandrum sati-vum* in mice. International Journal of Biomedical Science: IJBS. 2015 Mar;11(1):23.

Kükner A, Soyler G, Toros P, Dede G, Meriçli F, Işık S, Edebal O, Özoğul C. Protective effect of *Coriandrum sativum* extract against inflammation and apoptosis in liver ischaemia/reperfusion injury. Folia Morphologica. 2021;80(2):363–371.

Laribi B, Kouki K, M'Hamdi M, Bettaieb T. Coriander (*Coriandrum sativum* L.) and its bioactive constituents. Fitoterapia. 2015 Jun 1;103:9–26.

Mahendra P, Bisht S. Anti-anxiety activity of *Coriandrum sativum* assessed using different experimental anxiety models. Indian Journal of Pharmacology. 2011 Sep;43(5):574.

Mani V, Parle M, Ramasamy K, Abdul Majeed AB. Reversal of memory deficits by *Coriandrum sativum* leaves in mice. Journal of the Science of Food and Agriculture. 2011 Jan 15;91(1):186–192.

Matasyoh JC, Maiyo ZC, Ngure RM, Chepkorir R. Chemical composition and antimicrobial activity of the essential oil of Coriandrum sativum. Food Chemistry. 2009 Mar 15;113(2):526–529.

Messaoudi M, Begaa S. Dietary intake and content of some micronutrients and toxic elements in two algerian spices (*Coriandrum sativum* L. and Cuminum cyminum L.). Biological Trace Element Research. 2019 Apr;188(2):508–513.

Momin AH, Acharya SS, Gajjar AV. Coriandrum sativum-review of advances in phytopharmacology. International Journal of Pharmaceutical Sciences and Research. 2012 May 1;3(5):1233.

Nejad Ebrahimi S, Hadian J, Ranjbar H. Essential oil compositions of different accessions of *Coriandrum sativum* L. from Iran. Natural Product Research. 2010 Sep 10;24(14):1287–1294.

Nithya TG, Sumalatha D. Evaluation of in vitro anti-oxidant and anticancer activity of *Coriandrum sativum* against human colon cancer HT-29 cell lines. International Journal of Pharmacy and Pharmaceutical Sciences. 2014;6(2):421–424.

Pandey A, Bigoniya P, Raj V, Patel KK. Pharmacological screening of *Coriandrum sativum* Linn. for hepatoprotective activity. Journal of Pharmacy and Bioallied Sciences. 2011 Jul;3(3):435.

Pasha H, Qureshi HJ. Pharmacological Effects of Coriander Coriandrum sativum. Esculapio. 2017;13(1):1–4.

Patel DK, Desai SN, Gandhi HP, Devkar RV, Ramachandran AV. Cardio protective effect of *Coriandrum sativum* L. on isoproterenol induced myocardial necrosis in rats. Food and Chemical Toxicology. 2012 Sep 1;50(9):3120–3125.

Pathan AR, Kothawade KA, Logade MN. Anxiolytic and analgesic effect of seeds of *Coriandrum sativum* Linn. INTERNATIONAL JOURNAL OF RESEARCH IN PHARMACY AND CHEMISTRY. 2011;1(4):1087–1099.

Peana AT, Paolo SD, Chessa ML, Moretti MD, Serra G, Pippia P. (–)-Linalool produces antinociception in two experimental models of pain. European Journal of Pharmacology. 2003 Jan 26;460(1):37–41.

Quintans-Júnior LJ, Barreto RS, Menezes PP, Almeida JR, Viana AF, Oliveira RC, Oliveira AP, Gelain DP, de Lucca Júnior W, Araújo AA. β-Cyclodextrin-complexed (–)-linalool produces antinociceptive effect superior to that of (–)-linalool in experimental pain protocols. Basic & Clinical Pharmacology & Toxicology. 2013 Sep;113(3):167–172.

Ravizza R, Gariboldi MB, Molteni R, Monti E. Linalool, a plant-derived monoterpene alcohol, reverses doxorubicin resistance in human breast adenocarcinoma cells. Oncology Reports. 2008 Sep 1;20(3):625–630.

Reilly C, Agnew R, Neville BG. Depression and anxiety in childhood epilepsy: A review. Seizure. 2011 Oct 1;20(8):589–597.

Reuter J, Huyke C, Casetti F, Theek C, Frank U, Augustin M, Schempp C. Anti-inflammatory potential of a lipolotion containing coriander oil in the ultraviolet erythema test. JDDG: Journal der Deutschen Dermatologischen Gesellschaft. 2008 Oct;6(10):847–851.

Sahib NG, Anwar F, Gilani AH, Hamid AA, Saari N, Alkharfy KM. Coriander (*Coriandrum sativum* L.): A potential source of high-value components for functional foods and nutraceuticals-A review. Phytotherapy Research. 2013 Oct;27(10):1439–1456.

Sander JW. The epidemiology of epilepsy revisited. Current Opinion in Neurology. 2003 Apr 1;16(2):165–170.

Seidemann J. *World spice plants*. Berlin, Heidelberg: Springer; 2005.

Sharma MM, Sharma RK. Coriander. In KV Peter (Ed.), *Handbook of herbs and spices* (pp. 216–249). Cambridge: Woodhead Publishing; 2012.

Shin EJ, Jeong JH, Chung YH, Kim WK, Ko KH, Bach JH, Hong JS, Yoneda Y, Kim HC. Role of oxidative stress in epileptic seizures. Neurochemistry International. 2011 Aug 1;59(2):122–137.

Silva F, Ferreira S, Duarte A, Mendonca DI, Domingues FC. Antifungal activity of *Coriandrum sativum* essential oil, its mode of action against Candida species and potential synergism with amphotericin B. Phytomedicine. 2011 Dec 15;19(1):42–47.

Singh G, Maurya S, De Lampasona MP, Catalan CA. Studies on essential oils, Part 41. Chemical composition, antifungal, antioxidant and sprout suppressant activities of coriander (Coriandrum sativum) essential oil and its oleoresin. Flavour and Fragrance Journal. 2006 May;21(3):472–479.

Sobhani Z, Mohtashami L, Amiri MS, Ramezani M, Emami SA, Simal-Gandara J. Ethnobotanical and phytochemical aspects of the edible herb *Coriandrum sativum* L. Journal of Food Science. 2022 Apr;87(4):1386–1422.

Sreelatha S, Padma PR, Umadevi M. Protective effects of *Coriandrum sativum* extracts on carbon tetrachloride-induced hepatotoxicity in rats. Food and Chemical Toxicology. 2009 Apr 1;47(4):702–708.

Sriti J, Talou T, Wannes WA, Cerny M, Marzouk B. Essential oil, fatty acid and sterol composition of Tunisian coriander fruit different parts. Journal of the Science of Food and Agriculture. 2009 Aug 15;89(10):1659–1664.

Taherian AA, Vafaei AA, Ameri J. Opiate system mediate the antinociceptive effects of *Coriandrum sativum* in mice. Iranian Journal of Pharmaceutical Research: IJPR. 2012;11(2):679.

Taniguchi M, Yanai M, Xiao YQ, Kido TI, Baba K. Three isocoumarins from Coriandrum sativum. Phytochemistry. 1996 Jun 1;42(3):843–846.

Uttara B, Singh AV, Zamboni P, Mahajan R. Oxidative stress and neurodegenerative diseases: A review of upstream and downstream antioxidant therapeutic options. Current Neuropharmacology. 2009 Mar 1;7(1):65–74.

Vatanparast J, Bazleh S, Janahmadi M. The effects of linalool on the excitability of central neurons of snail Caucasotachea atrolabiata. Comparative Biochemistry and Physiology Part C: Toxicology & Pharmacology. 2017 Feb 1;192:33–39.

Vekaria RH, Patel MN, Bhalodiya PN, Patel V, Desai TR, Tirgar PR. Evaluation of neuroprotective effect of *Coriandrum sativum* linn. against ischemic-reperfusion insult in brain. International Journal of Phytopharmacology. 2012;2:186–193.

Wangensteen H, Samuelsen AB, Malterud KE. Antioxidant activity in extracts from coriander. Food Chemistry. 2004 Nov 1;88(2):293–297.

Wei JN, Liu ZH, Zhao YP, Zhao LL, Xue TK, Lan QK. Phytochemical and bioactive profile of *Coriandrum sativum* L. Food Chemistry. 2019 Jul 15;286:260–267.

White HS, Smith MD, Wilcox KS. Mechanisms of action of antiepileptic drugs. International Review of Neurobiology. 2007 Jan 1;81:85–110.

Yuan R, Liu Z, Zhao J, Wang QQ, Zuo A, Huang L, Gao H, Xu Q, Khan IA, Yang S. Novel compounds in fruits of coriander (Coşkuner & Karababa) with anti-inflammatory activity. Journal of Functional Foods. 2020 Oct 1;73:104145.

Zardini HZ, Tolueinia B, Momeni Z, Hasani Z, Hasani M. Analysis of antibacterial and anti-fungal activity of crude extracts from seeds of Coriandrum sativum. Gomal Journal of Medical Sciences. 2012 Dec 31;10(2).

Zare-Shehneh M, Askarfarashah M, Ebrahimi L, Kor NM, Zare-Zardini H, Soltaninejad H, Hashemian Z, Jabinian F. Biological activities of a new antimicrobial peptide from Coriandrum sativum. International Journal of Biosciences. 2014;4(6):89–99.

# 18 Nigella Sativa L. – A Note on Phytochemistry, Extraction, Pharmacological Activities, and Therapeutic Utility

*Prasanna Srinivasan Ramalingam,*
*Rudra Awdhesh Kumar Mishra,*
*Janaki Ramaiah Mekala,*
*Kodiveri Muthukaliannan Gothandam,*
*and Sivakumar Arumugam*

## 18.1 ETHNOBOTANY AND PHARMACOGNOSTICAL CHARACTERISTICS

*Nigella sativa* L. belonging to the Ranunculaceae family is an annual flowering plant native to Middle East countries and India. *N. sativa* is widely cultivated in India, Egypt, Iran, Turkey, and Saudi Arabia (Tiji et al. 2021). It is also known as black cumin and its seeds have been used in several traditional medicinal practices such as Traditional Arabic and Islamic Medicine (TAIM), folk medicine, and Indian traditional practices such as Ayurveda, Siddha, and Unani due to their versatile medicinal properties to treat various diseases and ailments (Dalli et al. 2021). The taxonomic classification of *Nigella sativa* (Taxonomic Serial No: 506592) was retrieved from the Integrated Taxonomic Information System database and provided in Table 18.1.

The *N. sativa* (black cumin) seeds are heavily reported to treat various diseases such as asthma, diarrhea, bronchitis, headache, anorexia, hypertension, paralysis, inflammation, cough, amenorrhea, and skin infections. It is also used to protect renal, cardio, hepatic, and immune systems (Kooti et al. 2016; Amin and Hosseinzadeh 2016). The black cumin seeds are also reported to possess versatile pharmacological activities such as antibacterial, antifungal, antiviral, anticancer, antioxidant, anti-inflammatory, anti-diabetic, anti-obesity, analgesic, antipyretic, antiproliferative, antihypertensive, and anti-insecticidal activities (Hannan et al. 2021; Yimer et al. 2019; Ali and Blunden

DOI: 10.1201/9781003389774-18

---

**TABLE 18.1**

**Taxonomic Classification of *Nigella sativa* L.**

| Taxonomy | Nomenclature |
|---|---|
| Kingdom | Plantae |
| Phylum | Tracheophyta |
| Class | Magnoliopsida |
| Order | Ranunculales |
| Family | Ranunculaceae |
| Genus | Nigella |
| Species | Sativa |

---

2003). In addition, it is also used to treat snake bites and insect bites, and its seed essential oil is used as a local anesthetic and antiseptic agent during treatments (Tariq 2008).

## 18.2   USAGE IN TRADITIONAL MEDICINAL PRACTICES

In several traditional medicinal practices, black cumin is used to treat various ailments and diseases (Hannan et al. 2021). The father of early modern medicine Avicenna stated that this cumin is used to treat depression-related disorders and fatigue, and is also able to stimulate the energy of the human body in his book entitled *The Canon of Medicine* (Ahmad et al. 2013). In Egypt, due to the potential antimicrobial activity of the black cumin seeds, it is used in the process of mummification. In southeastern Morocco, cumin seeds are used to treat diabetes mellitus, hypertension, and cardiovascular diseases (Salehi et al. 2021). In South Asian countries, it is used to treat asthma and bronchitis, and other inflammatory-related diseases. In Indian traditional practices such as Ayurveda, Siddha, and Unani, black cumin is used to treat digestion-related disorders and is also stated to provide hepatoprotective activities. Additionally, it is also used in several dishes of Indian cuisine (Yimer et al. 2019).

## 18.3   PHYTOCHEMISTRY OF *NIGELLA SATIVA*

*Nigella sativa* possesses versatile pharmacological activities due to the potential phytoconstituents present in it, especially in its seeds. Comparatively, the black cumin seeds have high phytoconstituents composition, comprising 37% essential oils followed by 31% carbohydrates, 16% proteins, 2.3% minerals, and 6.5% dietary fibers (El-Naggar et al. 2017; Tiruppur Venkatachallam et al. 2010). Generally, cumin seeds consist of alkaloids, terpenes, polyphenols, flavonoids, saponins, tannins, carboxylic acids, and coumarins. The terpenes, alkaloids, and polyphenols including flavonoids are predominant phytoconstituents of black cumin seeds and are heavily reported to possess various pharmacological activities. The 2D structures of predominant terpenes and terpenoids such as thymoquinone (TQ), thymohydroquinone, alpha-copaene, myrcene, α-pinene, p-cymene, thymohydroquinone dimethyl ether, sabinene, terpinolene, camphene, longifolene, 1,8-cineole/eucalyptol, limonene, zonarene, linalool, carvacrol, thymol, davanone, carvone, and tagetenone; predominant polyphenols such as kaempferol, quercetin, patuletin, quercitrin, luteolin, apigenin, myricetin, isoquercetin, fisetin, rutin, chicoric acid, caffeic acid, 4-hydroxycinnamic acid, sinapic acid, and ferulic acid; and predominant alkaloids such as nigellidine, nigellamine C, nigellicine, and nigellamine D are shown in Figure 18.1, Figure 18.2, and Figure 18.3 respectively. The phytoconstituents class, extraction and isolation techniques, and the biological activities of the aforementioned phytochemicals are provided in Table 18.2.

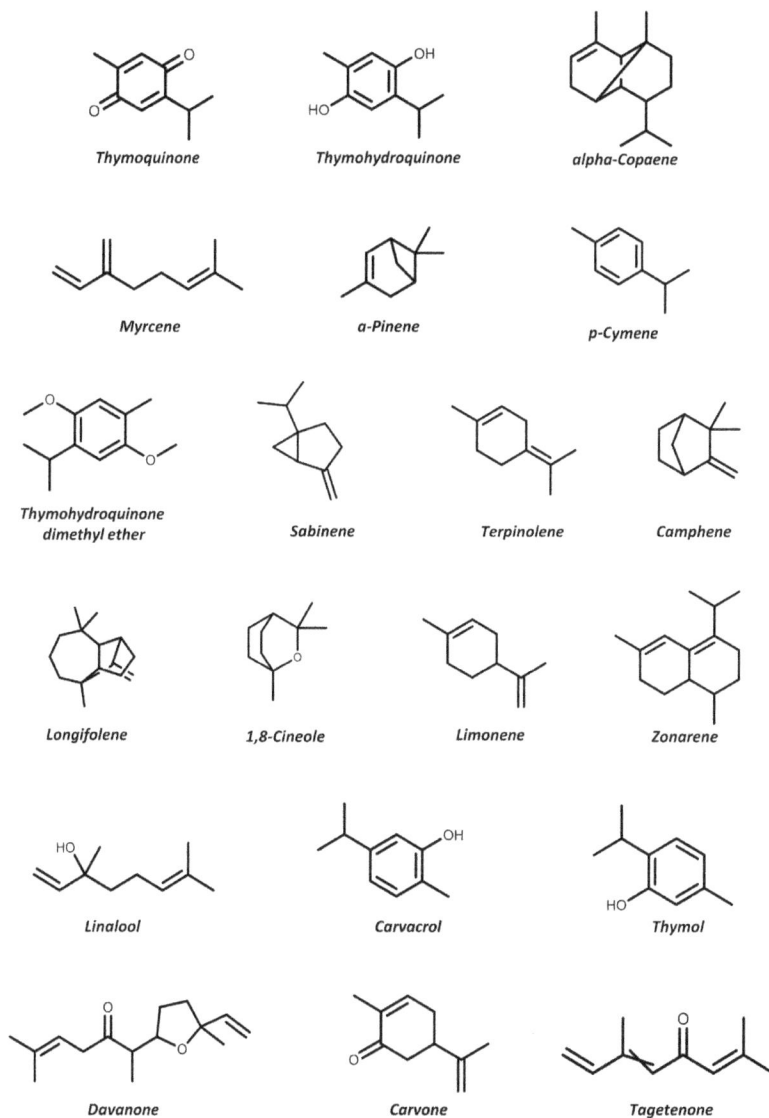

**FIGURE 18.1** 2D structures of terpenes and terpenoids of *Nigella sativa*.

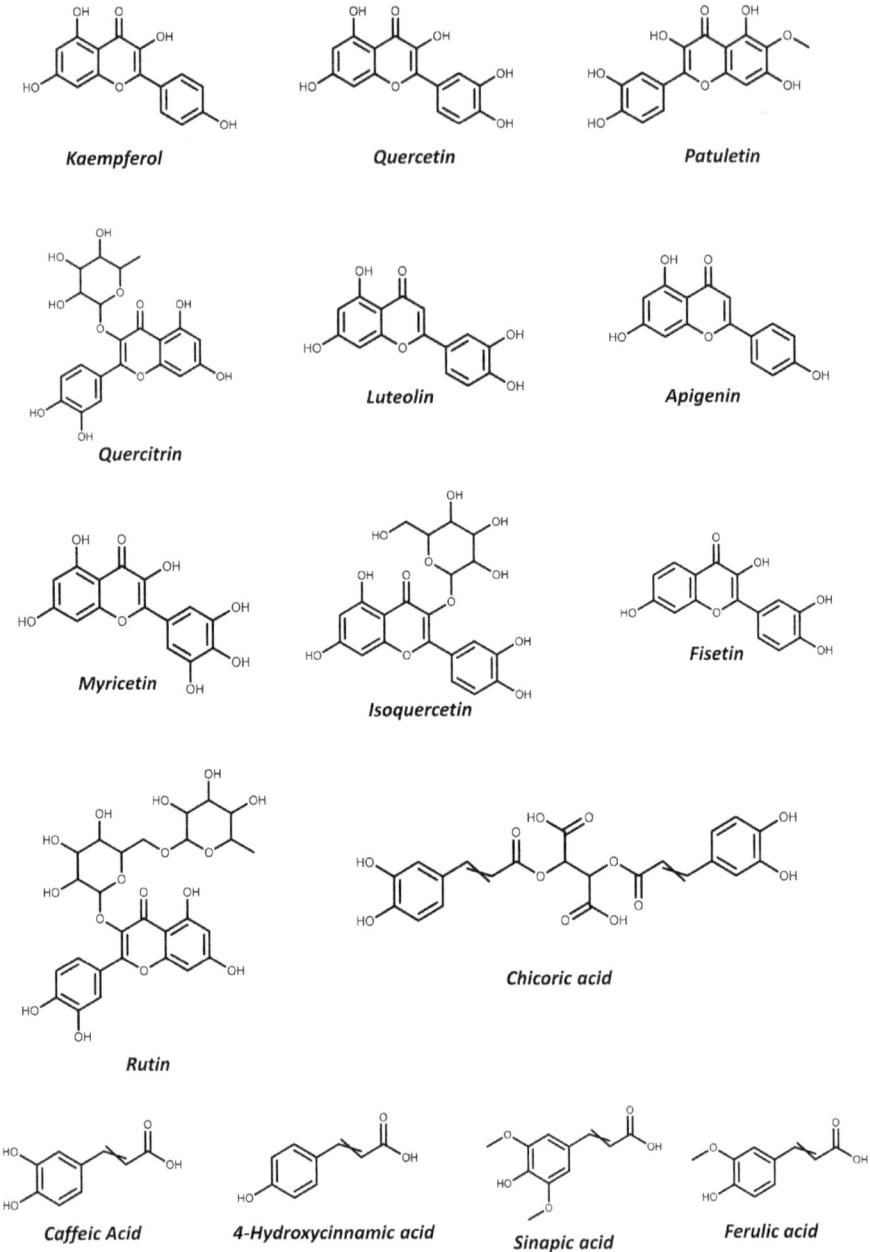

**FIGURE 18.2**   2D structures of polyphenols of *Nigella sativa*.

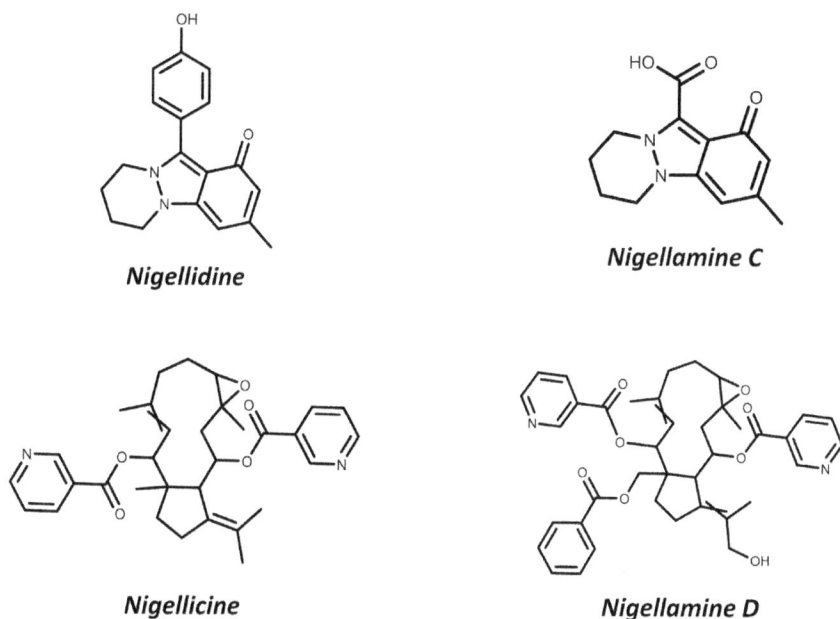

**FIGURE 18.3** 2D structures of alkaloids of *Nigella sativa*.

Black cumin seeds contain nearly 30% of thymoquinone (TQ) (2-isopropyl-5-methylbenzo-1,4-quinone), a predominant monoterpenoid that is highly reported to have potential pharmacological activities such as antimicrobial, anticancer, antioxidant, anti-inflammatory, hepatoprotective, and immunomodulatory properties (Rahim et al. 2022). TQ satisfies Lipinski's drug-likeness properties and due to its hydrophilicity and low molecular weight it shows high gastrointestinal absorption, blood-brain barrier permeability, and bioavailability properties (Salehi et al. 2021).

## 18.4 EXTRACTION, ISOLATION, AND CHARACTERIZATION STRATEGIES

Solvent extraction and cold-press extraction are the most used extraction techniques for the isolation of essential oils of *Nigella sativa* seeds. Apart from the aforementioned extraction method, depending upon the phytochemical class versatile extraction techniques such as maceration, distillation, Soxhlet's extraction, ultrasound and microwave-assisted extractions, supercritical fluid extraction, solid-phase extraction, simultaneous distillation–extraction, and pressurized liquid extraction can be used (Zaky, Shim, and Abd El-Aty 2021). The isolated compounds/phytoconstituents/phytochemicals can be characterized by gas chromatography-mass spectrometry, normal and reverse phase-high performance liquid chromatography, column chromatography, and high-performance counter-current chromatography (Dalli et al. 2021). The detailed extraction strategies along with the biological activities for the predominant phytoconstituents of *Nigella sativa* seeds are given in Table 18.2.

**TABLE 18.2**

**Extraction/isolation methods and biological activities of phytoconstituents of *Nigella sativa***

| Phytoconstituent Name | Phytoconstituent Class | Extraction/Isolation Methods | Biological Activity |
|---|---|---|---|
| Thymoquinone | Monoterpenoid | SE, MAE (Iqbal, Ahmad, and Pandey 2018) | Anticancer, anti-inflammatory, antimicrobial, hepatoprotective (Rahim et al. 2022) |
| Thymohydroquinone | Monoterpenoid | LLE (Rani At et al. 2022) | Antiviral, anticancer, anti-inflammatory (Esharkawy, Almalki, and Hadda 2022) |
| α-Copaene | Sesquiterpene | SFME (Erkan et al. 2012) | Antioxidant, antibacterial (Erkan et al. 2012) |
| Myrcene | Monoterpenoid | HD, SAE (Surendran et al. 2021) | Antinociceptive, neuroprotective, anti-ageing (Surendran et al. 2021) |
| α-Pinene | Bicyclic monoterpenoid | SFE, MAE (Karimkhani et al. 2022) | Antioxidant, antibacterial, anticancer (Karimkhani et al. 2022) |
| p-Cymene | Monoterpene | SPE (Marchese et al. 2017) | Antimicrobial, antinociceptive, anti-inflammatory, anxiolytic, anticancer (Marchese et al. 2017) |
| Thymohydroquinone dimethyl ether | Monoterpene | HD (Rani At et al. 2022) | Antiviral, anticancer, anti-inflammatory (Wajs-Bonikowska et al. 2021) |
| Sabinene | Bicyclic monoterpenoid | HS-SPME (Cozzolino et al. 2022) | Antioxidant, anti-inflammatory, antifungal, anticancer (Cozzolino et al. 2022) |
| Terpinolene | Cyclic monoterpene | SDE (Menezes et al. 2021) | Larvicidal, insecticidal (Menezes et al. 2021) |
| Camphene | Bicyclic monoterpenoid | SFE (Wong et al. 2001) | Antioxidant, anticancer (Girola et al. 2015) |
| Longifolene | Sesquiterpenoid | KD (Grover et al. 2022) | Anticancer, antimicrobial (Grover et al. 2022) |
| 1,8-Cineole/ Eucalyptol | Monoterpenoid | ATPE (Dang et al. 2010) | Antiseptic, anti-inflammatory, insecticidal (Dang et al. 2010) |
| Limonene | Monoterpene | LLE, PLE (Morsi 2000) | Antibacterial, antioxidant (Morsi 2000) |
| Zonarene | Sesquiterpenoid | HD, SFE (Noriega et al. 2019) | Anti-leishmanial, antioxidant, antimicrobial (Noriega et al. 2019) |
| Linalool | Noncyclic monoterpenoid | HD (Elsharif, Banerjee, and Buettner 2015) | Anti-lipoperoxidant, sedative, anxiolytic, analgesic, anticonvulsant (Elsharif, Banerjee, and Buettner 2015) |
| Carvacrol | Monoterpene | HD (Suntres, Coccimiglio, and Alipour 2015) | Vasorelaxant, hepatoprotective, spasmolytic (Suntres, Coccimiglio, and Alipour 2015) |

**TABLE 18.2** (*Continued*)
**Extraction/isolation methods and biological activities of phytoconstituents of *Nigella sativa***

| Phytoconstituent Name | Phytoconstituent Class | Extraction/Isolation Methods | Biological Activity |
|---|---|---|---|
| Thymol | Monoterpene | PLE, MAE (Marchese et al. 2016) | Antiseptic, local anesthetic, antinociceptive, cicatrizing (Marchese et al. 2016) |
| Davanone | Bicyclic sesquiterpenoid | SFC (Coleman et al. 2007) | Antimicrobial, antioxidant (Coleman et al. 2007) |
| Carvone | Monoterpene | UAE, SPE (Bouyahya et al. 2021) | antidiabetic, antiarthritic, anticonvulsant, antiparasitic, neurological (Bouyahya et al. 2021) |
| Tagetenone | Acyclic monoterpenoid | HD, SFE (Salehi et al. 2018) | Antimicrobial, anticancer, insecticidal (Salehi et al. 2018) |
| Kaempferol | Flavonol | SE, SFE (Cid-Ortega and Monroy-Rivera 2018) | Anti-lipoperoxidant, anticancer, antimicrobial, antioxidant (Cid-Ortega and Monroy-Rivera 2018) |
| Quercetin | Hydroxyflavone | SAE, UAE (Zhu et al. 2019) | Gastroprotective, antioxidant, antimicrobial, immunomodulatory (J.K. Kim and Park 2018) |
| Patuletin | Trimethoxyflavone | SAE, HPCCC (Wei et al. 2011) | Antioxidant, antimicrobial (Wei et al. 2011) |
| Quercitrin | Flavonol | SAE, ATPE (Adeniyi et al. 2022) | Anti-sickling, DNA topoisomerase I inhibition, immunomodulatory (Adeniyi et al. 2022) |
| Luteolin | Flavone | SE, UAE, MC (Abidin et al. 2014) | Antimicrobial, antimalarial, anti-inflammatory, anticancer (Abidin et al. 2014) |
| Apigenin | Flavone | MC, SAE (Salehi et al. 2019) | Anti-amyloidogenic, neuroprotective, cognition enhancement, COX-2 inhibition (Salehi et al. 2019) |
| Myricetin | Flavonol | SPME (Kumar, Malik, and Tewary 2009) | Antioxidant, anti-inflammatory, anticancer (Kumar, Malik, and Tewary 2009) |
| Isoquercetin | Hydroxyflavone | UAE, HD (Mbikay and Chrétien 2022) | Anticoagulant, antioxidant, immunomodulatory (Mbikay and Chrétien 2022) |
| Fisetin | Hydroxyflavonol | HD, MC (S.H. Kim and Huh 2022) | Antioxidant, antimicrobial, anticancer (S.H. Kim and Huh 2022) |
| Rutin | Flavonol | UAE, MAE (Chahyadi and Elfahmi 2020) | Antimalarial, insecticidal, neuroprotective (Chahyadi and Elfahmi 2020) |

(*Continued*)

**TABLE 18.2 (*Continued*)**
**Extraction/isolation methods and biological activities of phytoconstituents of *Nigella sativa***

| Phytoconstituent Name | Phytoconstituent Class | Extraction/Isolation Methods | Biological Activity |
|---|---|---|---|
| Chicoric acid | Phenylpropanoid | SE, HD (Lee and Scagel 2013) | Anti-HIV, glucose and lipid homeostasis, neuroprotection (Lee and Scagel 2013) |
| Caffeic acid | Phenylpropanoid | SE, MC (Pyne and Paria 2022) | Antioxidant, anticancer, neuroprotective (Pyne and Paria 2022) |
| 4-Hydroxycinnamic acid | Phenylpropanoid | SE (Gołaswska et al. 2023) | Cardioprotective, antioxidant, anticancer (Gołaswska et al. 2023) |
| Sinapic acid | Phenylpropanoid | LLE, SAE (Chadni et al. 2021) | Antimutagenic, antihyperglycemic, neuroprotective (Chadni et al. 2021) |
| Ferulic acid | Phenylpropanoid | SAE (Zduńska et al. 2018) | Anti-arrhythmic, antithrombotic, antidiabetic (Zduńska et al. 2018) |
| Nigellidine | Indazole alkaloid | CC (Z. Ali et al. 2008) | Antioxidant, anti-inflammatory, hepatoprotective, immunomodulatory (Maiti et al. 2022) |
| Nigellamine C | Dolabellane-type diterpene alkaloids | RP-HPLC (Morikawa et al. 2004) | Antimicrobial, lipid metabolism (Morikawa et al. 2004) |
| Nigellicine | Pyridazinoindazole alkaloid | MC (Dalli et al. 2021) | Antibacterial, antioxidant (Dalli et al. 2021) |
| Nigellamine D | Dolabellane-type diterpene alkaloids | RP-HPLC (Morikawa et al. 2004) | Immunomodulatory (Morikawa et al. 2004) |

*Note:* Soxhlet extraction (SE), Liquid-liquid extraction (LLE), Solvent-free microwave extraction (SFME), Maceration (MC), Hydro distillation (HD), Microwave-assisted extraction (MAE), Ultrasound-assisted extraction (UAE), Steam distillation (SD), Accelerated solvent extraction (ASE), Reverse phase-high performance liquid chromatography (RP-HPLC), Column chromatography (CC), High-performance counter-current chromatography (HPCCC), Solvent-assisted extraction (SAE), Supercritical fluid extraction (SFE), Solid-phase extraction (SPE), Simultaneous distillation–extraction (SDE), Kugelrohr distillation (KD), Aqueous two-phase extraction (ATPE), Solid phase micro-extraction (SPME), Headspace solid phase micro-extraction (HS-SPME), Supercritical fluid chromatography (SFC), Liquid-liquid extraction (LLE), Pressurized liquid extraction (PLE).

## 18.5   PHARMACOLOGY

### 18.5.1   ANTIOXIDANT ACTIVITY

The supplementation of rats with *Nigella sativa* (NS) seeds led to an increase in the activity of the antioxidant enzyme catalase (CAT) and the overall antioxidant activity, as compared to the control group (Mahmoud et al. 2021). In a clinical study involving healthy individuals, a daily intake of NS seed extract resulted in a non-significant decrease in the level of the oxidative stress marker MDA after five days, along with a non-significant increase in the activity of the antioxidant enzyme super-oxide dismutase (SOD) and a significant increase in the level of the antioxidant mol-ecule glutathione GSH. In rats, the administration of NS oil (NSO) or thymoquinone (TQ), the active compound in NS seeds, led to an increase in the activity of the antioxidant enzyme ceruloplasmin and a reduction in lipid peroxidation and oxida-tive stress in renal tissues exposed to radiation (Alkis et al. 2021). Similarly, in rats with STZ-induced diabetes, NS ethanolic extract was found to protect against DNA damage and lipid peroxidation, while also increasing SOD activity. Black cumin oils also exhibited antioxidant activity by reducing MDA, oxidizing glutathione levels, and increasing hydrogen donor capacity in rats. These findings support the antioxi-dant properties of NS seeds and their potential as a protective agent against oxidative stress-related diseases (Pop et al. 2020).

### 18.5.2 ANTI-INFLAMMATORY AND IMMUNOMODULATORY ACTIVITY

The effects of black cumin on inflammation and immunity have been studied in various experiments. Injection of NSO at different doses to rats with carrageenan-induced edema in the hind paw resulted in a significant reduction of edema, likely due to inhibition of eicosanoid and lipid generation. NS has also been found to improve animal weight and increase the size of the spleen in rats, which is responsible for clearing harmful particles from the body. This effect is attributed to the plant's immune-stimulant activity, because it increases the production of IL-12, TNF-$\alpha$, IF-$\gamma$, and CD8 in the spleen (Gholamnezhad, Boskabady, and Hosseini 2021). Acute treatment with black cumin oil has shown anti-inflammatory effects, while sub-acute treatment did not. TQ, a component of black cumin, has been found to protect against chronic periodontitis by inhibiting the production of TNF-$\alpha$. The hydroalco-holic extract of black cumin has been shown to decrease the expression of NFK and IKK mRNAs, indicating that the plant's anti-inflammatory effect is associated with a reduction in the expression of these genes (Pop et al. 2020). The high-dose group of NS oils significantly increased the levels of IL-2, IL-4, and IL-6 in the serum of mice, decreased the level of TNF-$\alpha$, and regulated the level of cytokines to exert immunomodulatory effects. This effect is attributed to the up-regulation of PI3K protein expression and down-regulation of PTEN expression, increasing antioxidant enzyme activity, and decreasing ROS and TNF-$\alpha$. By activating the PI3K signaling pathway and regulating the FoxO1 factor, the immunomodulatory effect is exerted by decreasing the expression of PTEN, inhibiting TLR4/NF-B, and the expression of pro-inflammatory cytokines, while increasing the release of anti-inflammatory factors (Liang et al. 2021).

### 18.5.3 ANTIBACTERIAL ACTIVITY

The methanolic extract of NS has demonstrated significant antibacterial activ-ity against various strains, including *Staphylococcus aureus*, *Escherichia coli*, and *Pseudomonas aeruginosa*, as well as multi-drug resistant bacteria like

*Staphylococcus saprophyticus* and *Staphylococcus epidermis*. Furthermore, the NS oils obtained using cold press techniques have a synergistic effect when combined with antibiotics, particularly with Augmentin, and are effective against methicillin-resistant *S. aureus* (MRSA) (Al-Khalifa et al. 2021). The aqueous extract of NS seeds obtained by decoction also exhibits antibacterial potential against both Gram-positive and Gram-negative bacteria (Sangi et al. 2015). The n-hexane extract of NS has shown promising antibacterial activity against clinical *S. aureus* and MTCC bacteria, such as *S. aureus* and *Salmonella typhi*. The use of NSO is effective against bacterial infections in *Oreochromis niloticus* after an intraperitoneal injection of *Aeromonas hydrophila* and *Pseudomonas fluorescens*. This treatment was associated with a decrease in the expression of cytochrome P450 1 A (CYP1A), which normally increases in response to oxidative stress and for detoxification of the organism during an infection (Sangi et al. 2015). Essential oils added to stored boiler meat also proved to be effective in reducing the total number of bacteria, including cold-resistant bacteria, while maintaining the nutritional value of the meat. It led to a significant decrease in *Bacillus spp.* This bacterium was found to be highly sensitive to both the EO and NS powder (Al-Khalifa et al. 2021).

### 18.5.4 ANTIFUNGAL ACTIVITY

The methanolic extract of *Nigella* was found to possess antifungal activity against various strains, such as *Trichophyton sp.*, *Candida albicans*, *Candida tropicalis*, *Candida krusei*, *Penicillium sp.*, and *Aspergillus niger*, with MIC values of 25 mg/mL and 12.5 mg/mL against *Candida albicans* and *Candida parapsilosis*, respectively. Additionally, the aqueous extract exhibited effective antifungal activity against different mucor fungal species, with inhibition percentages ranging from 30% to 70% (Sangi et al. 2015). An isolated peptide from nigella seeds, nigellothionines, was found to exhibit antifungal activity against *A. flavus*, *A. fumigatus*, and *A. oryzae*. The n-butanol extract demonstrated antifungal activity against *Candida albicans*, *Candida krusei*, and *Candida parapsilosis*, with a MIC of 0.125 and 0.5 µL/mL. The terpenoid compounds and fatty acids present in nigella may be responsible for the observed antifungal effects (Barashkova et al. 2021). Various fractions obtained by fractionation of the methanolic extract of nigella were tested for antifungal activity against *Fusarium oxysporum* and *Macrophomina phaseolina*. The therapeutic potential of black cumin was evaluated in a study conducted on female rats that were inoculated with *Candida albicans*, which showed a potent reduction in the number of fungal colonies following treatment with NS extract at a dosage of 6.6 mL/kg (Dalli et al. 2021).

### 18.5.5 CARDIO-PROTECTIVE AND ANTIHYPERTENSIVE ACTIVITY

Rat models, pre-treated with NSO for 14 days, showed a significant decrease in aspartate aminotransferase levels after acute-induced myocardial infarction (Gholamnezhad, Boskabady, and Hosseini 2021). In a patient study setting, *Nigella sativa* oil was administered for eight weeks and showed a significant decrease in systolic and diastolic blood pressure levels. Another human study revealed that 2 g of NS supplementation showed a decrease in systolic blood pressure but did not affect diastolic blood pressure (Al Asoom LI 2021). In the study, IGF-I levels were elevated only in the exercise group, and no significant difference was observed in the "NS + exercise" group. This suggests that NS may induce the intervention of another IGF-I analog in cardiac hypertrophy mediated by the GH-IGF I-PI3P-Akt pathway (Al Asoom LI 2021).

### 18.5.6 ANTIVIRAL ACTIVITY

A study was conducted to investigate the therapeutic potential of black cumin oil on patients with mild COVID-19 symptoms. The results showed that a dose of 500 mg/kg of NSO was able to significantly improve the average number of days to cure compared to the control group (Koshak et al. 2021). Computational studies have also been carried out to investigate the antiviral activity of black cumin against SARS-CoV-2 which showed that TQ may exhibit inhibitory activity against SARS-CoV-2 protease and can protect cells by modulating endosomal pH and inhibits the interaction of viral proteins (Kadil, Mouhcine, and Filali 2021). Nigellamine is reported to block the entry of SARS-CoV-2 through inhibitory activity on ACE2 and shows good binding affinity towards RNA-dependent RNA polymerase and can inhibit TMPRSS2, which facilitates the endocytosis of the virus. Nigellone, nigellidine, and kaempferol, present in black cumin, also showed a high affinity with COVID-19 C19MP proteases (Mir et al. 2022).

### 18.5.7 ANTIDIABETIC ACTIVITY

The hydroacetone extract of NS can inhibit $\alpha$-amylase, and consumption of 5 g/day of black cumin for six months has been found to decrease glycated hemoglobin. In rats with streptozotocin-induced diabetes, the hydroalcoholic extract (50%) was found to reduce fasting blood glucose levels (Bin Jardan et al. 2021). The combination of TQ and metformin (50/200 mg/kg) resulted in a decrease in blood glucose level by 41.3%. However, some adverse effects, such as diarrhea and abdominal pain, were observed in volunteers who received the combination of TQ (50 or 100 mg) with metformin (1000 mg) (Alaaeldin et al. 2021). A hydroalcoholic combination of *Morinda citrifolia*, *Trigonella foenum-graecum*, and *Nigella sativa* was studied for its inhibited activity on pancreatic $\alpha$-amylase at different doses, with the most effective dose being 140/70/140 mg/kg. *In vivo* studies confirmed the results obtained in vitro, showing that all three doses were able to decrease blood glucose levels, with the second dose being the most effective (Hannan et al. 2021).

### 18.5.8 ANTICANCER ACTIVITY

The *Nigella sativa* seed oil extracts were reported to possess significant anticancer properties against various cancer types such as lung, colon, breast, and pancreatic adenocarcinoma. In addition to its antioxidant activity, a combination of NS extract and honey was found to inhibit the growth of ovarian cancer cells (PA-1) in a dose-dependent manner (Barashkova et al. 2021). Aqueous NS extract containing α-hederin showed potential anticancer activity in different cancers. In another study TQ induced P38 activated cell death and ERK elevation in SK-Hep 1 liver cancer cells. Also, the ferulic acid and thymoquinone combination showed potential anticancer properties against various cancers with minimum IC50 values (Zaoui et al. 2002).

### 18.5.9 ANTI-OBESITY AND DYSLIPIDEMIC ACTIVITY

The hydroalcoholic extract of NS reduced cholesterol, TG, and LDL, while increasing HDL. It also improved the vasodilatory response and prevented the VCAM-1 elevation. The combination of black cumin seeds and fenugreek administered to overweight individuals showed a significant decrease in LDL, TG, VLDL, and atherogenicity index (Rao et al. 2020), and a significant decrease in total cholesterol, LDL, MDA, triglycerides, and an increase in HDL. Supplementation of NSO at 2 g/day increased HDL levels and decreased LDL levels and atherogenicity index (Chaieb et al. 2011).

## 18.6 TOXICOLOGY

Although the *Nigella sativa* showed tremendous pharmacological properties, it also offers some toxicological properties. Numerous studies have confirmed the safety of *Nigella sativa*, with no reported toxic effects. One study administered NSO orally at a dose of 2 mg/kg for 12 weeks and found an LD50 of 28.8 mL/kg body weight, while intraperitoneal administration showed an LD50 of 2.06 mL/kg body weight (Zaoui et al. 2002). However, TQ administration to albino mice at a dose of 870 mg/kg body weight was found to be highly toxic, with an LD50 value of 794 mg/kg body weight in rats. Nevertheless, a subacute treatment with TQ for 90 days did not cause any physiological changes (Zaoui et al. 2002).

## 18.7 THYMOQUINONE: A PROMISING THERAPEUTIC AGENT

Thymoquinone (TQ) possesses significant medicinal properties and pharmacological activities such as antimicrobial, antidiabetic, antihypertension, and anticancer properties. TQ exerted significant antimicrobial activities against several human pathogenic organisms such as *Staphylococcus aureus*, *Staphylococcus epidermidis*, *Streptococcus salivarius*, *Streptococcus oralis*, *Streptococcus mutans*, and *Enterococcus faecalis*, and prevents biofilm formation (Al-Khalifa et al. 2021; Chaieb et al. 2011). In streptozotocin-induced diabetic male Wistar rats, TQ reduced glucose levels in the serum and showed potential antidiabetic activity (Sangi et al. 2015). TQ exerts antidiabetic properties through various mechanisms including increased insulin secretion, decreased insulin resistance, activation of beta-cell production, reduced levels of gluconeogenesis, and activation of AMPK and PPAR-γ pathways (Maideen 2021). TQ was reported to have antihypertensive properties by decreasing total cholesterol levels, inhibiting the HMG-CoA reductase levels, decrease in serum aldosterone, altering angiotensin-converting enzyme levels,

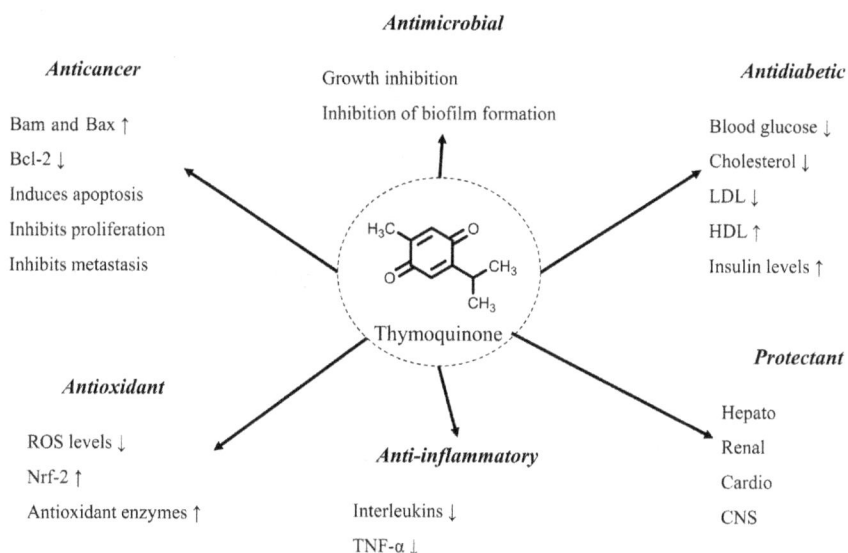

**FIGURE 18.4** Pharmacological properties of thymoquinone.

possessing antioxidant properties, and preventing renal damage (Khattab and Nagi 2007). TQ was heavily reported for its anticancer properties against various cancers such as lung, breast, colon, and pancreatic adenocarcinomas. It exerts various anticancer mechanisms by involving in signaling pathways such as MAPK pathway, PI3K-mTOR pathway, Wnt pathway, and JAK-STAT signaling pathways and also plays a crucial role in the cancer cell cycle (Farooqi, Attar, and Xu 2022). TQ induces apoptosis by downregulating anti-apoptotic proteins like Bcl-2 and Bcl-xL and upregulating pro-apoptotic proteins like Bam and Bax; induces the expression and production of executioner caspases; reduces the production of intracellular ROS levels; and increases the p53 activity in cancer cells (Homayoonfal, Asemi, and Yousefi 2022). Several preclinical and clinical trials reported the versatile therapeutic potential of TQ. The clinical trials employed to study the therapeutic effects of *Nigella sativa* and thymoquinone against various diseases were retrieved from the *clinicaltrial.gov* database and their study data are provided in Table 18.3 (accessed on 28 March 2023).

## 18.8 COMMERCIAL USAGE OF *NIGELLA SATIVA* ESSENTIAL OILS

Due to the valuable medicinal value of black cumin seed oils, it has a great market value. The seed oils and the TQ have been manufactured and produced by various industries all over the world as capsules and health supplements. Some of the companies, namely Simple Life Nutrition, Activation Products, Gaia Herbs, Amazing Herbs, MAJU, and Sakoon Nutrition that produce black cumin seed oil supplements along with their market proposition value, are compiled and provided in Table 18.4.

**TABLE 18.3**

**Clinical Trials on Thymoquinone and *Nigella sativa***

| NCT Number | Phase | Study Title | Condition | Intervention | Study Design | Status |
|---|---|---|---|---|---|---|
| NCT04852510 | Phase 2/3 | Amelioration of Polycystic Ovary Syndrome Related Disorders by Supplementation of Thymoquinone and Metformin | Polycystic Ovary Syndrome (PCOS) | Metformin and Metformin + TQ combination | Randomized, Open Label, and Parallel Assignment | Completed |
| NCT05497895 | Early Phase 1 | The Assessment of Clinical Efficacy of Topical Application of 5% Thymoquinone Gel for Gingivitis Patients | Gingivitis | TQ gel 5% | Randomized, Triple Masked, and Parallel Assignment | Not yet recruiting |
| NCT03208790 | Phase 2 | Clinical and Immunohisochemical [sic] Evaluation of Chemopreventive Effect of Thymoquinone on Oral Potentially Malignant Lesions | Premalignant Lesion | 10 mg *Nigella sativa* buccal tablets | Randomized, Triple Masked, and Parallel Assignment | Completed |
| NCT04686461 | NA | Effect of Thymoquinone Extracted from *Nigella sativa* in the Treatment of Arsenical Keratosis | Keratotic Nodular Size | *N. sativa* seeds extract | Open Label and Single Group Assignment | Unknown |
| NCT03776448 | NA | The Effect of 2 Grams Daily Supplementation of Sativa Nigra Oil on Blood Glucose Levels of Adults | Diabetes Mellitus | | Randomized, Double Masked, and Parallel Assignment | Unknown |
| NCT04553705 | Phase 2/3 | Omega-3, *Nigella sativa*, Indian Costus, Quinine, Anise Seed, Deglycyrrhizinated Licorice, Artemisinin, Febrifugine on Immunity of Patients with (COVID-19) | Covid-19, Immunodeficiency | | Randomized, Double Masked, and Sequential Assignment | Completed |
| NCT04292314 | Phase 2/3 | Hydroxy Urea, Omega 3, *Nigella sativa*, Honey on Oxidative Stress and Iron Chelation in Pediatric Major Thalassemia | Iron Overload, Oxidative Stress, Thalassemia Major | | Randomized, Double Masked, and Parallel Assignment | Completed |

**TABLE 18.4**
**Black Cumin Products and Supplements in the Market**

| Product Name | Quantity | Market Value (in USD) | Company Name | Country Name | Source |
|---|---|---|---|---|---|
| Black Seed Capsules | 500 mg | 17.95 | Simple Life Nutrition | USA | https://simplelifenutrition.com/ |
| Black Cumin Oil | 250 mL | 49 | Activation Products | USA | https://shop.activationproducts.com/ |
| Black Seed Oil | 60 capsules | 23.71 | Gaia Herbs | USA | www.gaiaherbs.com/ |
| Whole Spectrum Black Seed | 100 capsules | 18 | Amazing Herbs | Turkey | www.amazingherbs.com/ |
| Cold Pressed Black Seed Oil | 60 capsules | 22.49 | MAJU | Indonesia | https://majusuperfoods.com/products/majus-black-seed-oil-gelcaps |
| Black Seed Oil Gummies | 60 gummies | 22.46 | Sakoon Nutrition | USA | https://sakoonnutrition.com/ |

## 18.9   CONCLUSION AND FUTURE PERSPECTIVES

*Nigella sativa* (black cumin) is a traditionally important medicinal plant and especially its seeds are heavily used to treat various diseases and ailments because of their potential pharmacological activities and significant biological properties. In the present chapter, we have highlighted the extraction, isolation, and characterization of predominant phytoconstituents of *Nigella sativa* seeds. Also, their versatile pharmacological activities have been discussed with more importance to the monoterpene thymoquinone (TQ), which has unique therapeutic potential against different modalities. In addition, we have listed some of the products produced from black cumin for the enrichment of human welfare. Even though we have unlocked several pieces of knowledge about black cumin, still more research is needed for the enhancement of complementary and alternative medicine and the development of precision medicine in the near future.

## FUNDING

This research received no external funding.

## ACKNOWLEDGMENTS

The authors would like to thank the Vellore Institute of Technology (VIT), Vellore, India, and KL University for providing the necessary facilities to carry out this work.

## CONFLICTS OF INTEREST

The authors declare no conflict of interest.

## REFERENCES

Abidin, Lubna, Mohd Mujeeb, Showkat Rasool Mir, Shah Alam Khan, and Aftab Ahmad. 2014. "Comparative Assessment of Extraction Methods and Quantitative Estimation of Luteolin in the Leaves of Vitex Negundo Linn. by HPLC." *Asian Pacific Journal of Tropical Medicine* 7S1 (September): S289–S293. https://doi.org/10.1016/S1995-7645(14)60248-0.

Adeniyi, Olayemi, Rafael Baptista, Sumana Bhowmick, Alan Cookson, Robert J Nash, Ana Winters, Jianying Shen, and Luis A J Mur. 2022. "Isolation and Characterisation of Quercitrin as a Potent Anti-Sickle Cell Anaemia Agent from Alchornea Cordifolia." *Journal of Clinical Medicine* 11 (8). https://doi.org/10.3390/jcm11082177.

Ahmad, Aftab, Asif Husain, Mohd Mujeeb, Shah Alam Khan, Abul Kalam Najmi, Nasir Ali Siddique, Zoheir A Damanhouri, and Firoz Anwar. 2013. "A Review on Therapeutic Potential of *Nigella sativa*: A Miracle Herb." *Asian Pacific Journal of Tropical Biomedicine* 3 (5): 337–352. https://doi.org/10.1016/S2221-1691(13)60075-1.

Al Asoom, Lubna Ibrahim. 2021. "Molecular Mechanisms of *Nigella sativa*- and *Nigella sativa* Exercise-Induced Cardiac Hypertrophy in Rats." *Evidence-Based Complementary and Alternative Medicine ECAM* 2021: 5553022. https://doi.org/10.1155/2021/5553022.

Al-Khalifa, Khalifa S, Rasha AlSheikh, Moahmmed T Al-Hariri, Hosam El-Sayyad, Maher S Alqurashi, Saqib Ali, and Amr S Bugshan. 2021. "Evaluation of the Antimicrobial Effect of Thymoquinone against Different Dental Pathogens: An In Vitro Study." *Molecules (Basel, Switzerland)* 26 (21). https://doi.org/10.3390/molecules26216451.

Alaaeldin, Rania, Iman A M Abdel-Rahman, Heba Ali Hassan, Nancy Youssef, Ahmed E Allam, Sayed F Abdelwahab, Qing-Li Zhao, and Moustafa Fathy. 2021. "Carpachromene Ameliorates Insulin Resistance in HepG2 Cells via Modulating IR/IRS1/PI3k/Akt/GSK3/FoxO1 Pathway." *Molecules (Basel, Switzerland)* 26 (24). https://doi.org/10.3390/molecules26247629.

Ali, B H, and Gerald Blunden. 2003. "Pharmacological and Toxicological Properties of *Nigella sativa*." *Phytotherapy Research : PTR* 17 (4): 299–305. https://doi.org/10.1002/ptr.1309.

Ali, Zulfiqar, Daneel Ferreira, Paulo Carvalho, Mitchell A Avery, and Ikhlas A Khan. 2008. "Nigellidine-4-O-Sulfite, the First Sulfated Indazole-Type Alkaloid from the Seeds of *Nigella sativa*." *Journal of Natural Products* 71 (6): 1111–1112. https://doi.org/10.1021/np800172x.

Alkis, Hilal, Elif Demir, Mehmet Resit Taysi, Suleyman Sagir, and Seyithan Taysi. 2021. "Effects of *Nigella sativa* Oil and Thymoquinone on Radiation-Induced Oxidative Stress in Kidney Tissue of Rats." *Biomedicine & Pharmacotherapy = Biomedecine & Pharmacotherapie* 139 (July): 111540. https://doi.org/10.1016/j.biopha.2021.111540.

Amin, Bahareh, and Hossein Hosseinzadeh. 2016. "Black Cumin (*Nigella sativa*) and Its Active Constituent, Thymoquinone: An Overview on the Analgesic and Anti-Inflammatory Effects." *Planta Medica* 82 (1–2): 8–16. https://doi.org/10.1055/s-0035-1557838.

Barashkova, Anna S, Vera S Sadykova, Victoria A Salo, Sergey K Zavriev, and Eugene A Rogozhin. 2021. "Nigellothionins from Black Cumin (*Nigella sativa L.*) Seeds Demonstrate Strong Antifungal and Cytotoxic Activity." *Antibiotics (Basel, Switzerland)* 10 (2). https://doi.org/10.3390/antibiotics10020166.

Bouyahya, Abdelhakim, Hamza Mechchate, Taoufiq Benali, Rokia Ghchime, Saoulajan Charfi, Abdelaali Balahbib, Pavel Burkov, Mohammad Ali Shariati, Jose M Lorenzo, and Nasreddine El Omari. 2021. "Health Benefits and Pharmacological Properties of Carvone." *Biomolecules* 11 (12). https://doi.org/10.3390/biom11121803.

Chadni, Morad, Amandine L Flourat, Valentin Reungoat, Louis M M Mouterde, Florent Allais, and Irina Ioannou. 2021. "Selective Extraction of Sinapic Acid Derivatives from Mustard Seed Meal by Acting on PH: Toward a High Antioxidant Activity Rich Extract." *Molecules (Basel, Switzerland)* 26 (1). https://doi.org/10.3390/molecules26010212.

Chahyadi, Agus, and Elfahmi. 2020. "The Influence of Extraction Methods on Rutin Yield of Cassava Leaves (Manihot Esculenta Crantz)." *Saudi Pharmaceutical Journal : SPJ : The Official Publication of the Saudi Pharmaceutical Society* 28 (11): 1466–1473. https://doi.org/10.1016/j.jsps.2020.09.012.

Chaieb, Kamel, Bochra Kouidhi, Hanene Jrah, Kacem Mahdouani, and Amina Bakhrouf. 2011. "Antibacterial Activity of Thymoquinone, an Active Principle of *Nigella sativa* and Its Potency to Prevent Bacterial Biofilm Formation." *BMC Complementary and Alternative Medicine* 11 (April): 29. https://doi.org/10.1186/1472-6882-11-29.

Cid-Ortega, Sandro, and José Alberto Monroy-Rivera. 2018. "Extraction of Kaempferol and Its Glycosides Using Supercritical Fluids from Plant Sources: A Review." *Food Technology and Biotechnology* 56 (4): 480–493. https://doi.org/10.17113/ftb.56.04.18.5870.

Coleman, William Monroe 3rd, Michael Frances Dube, Mehdi Ashraf-Khorassani, and Larry Thomas Taylor. 2007. "Isomeric Enhancement of Davanone from Natural Davana Oil Aided by Supercritical Carbon Dioxide." *Journal of Agricultural and Food Chemistry* 55 (8): 3037–3043. https://doi.org/10.1021/jf062652y.

Cozzolino, Rosaria, José S Câmara, Livia Malorni, Giuseppe Amato, Ciro Cannavacciuolo, Milena Masullo, and Sonia Piacente. 2022. "Comparative Volatilomic Profile of Three Finger Lime (Citrus Australasica) Cultivars Based on Chemometrics Analysis of HS-SPME/GC-MS Data." *Molecules (Basel, Switzerland)* 27 (22). https://doi.org/10.3390/molecules27227846.

Dalli, Mohammed, Oussama Bekkouch, Salah-Eddine Azizi, Ali Azghar, Nadia Gseyra, and Bonglee Kim. 2021. "*Nigella sativa L.* Phytochemistry and Pharmacological Activities: A Review (2019–2021)." *Biomolecules* 12 (1). https://doi.org/10.3390/biom12010020.

Dang, Yuan-Ye, Xiao-Cen Li, Qing-Wen Zhang, Shao-Ping Li, and Yi-Tao Wang. 2010. "Preparative Isolation and Purification of Six Volatile Compounds from Essential Oil of Curcuma Wenyujin Using High-Performance Centrifugal Partition Chromatography." *Journal of Separation Science* 33 (11): 1658–1664. https://doi.org/10.1002/jssc.200900453.

El-Naggar, Tarek, María Emilia Carretero, Carmen Arce, and María Pilar Gómez-Serranillos. 2017. "Methanol Extract of *Nigella sativa* Seed Induces Changes in the Levels of Neurotransmitter Amino Acids in Male Rat Brain Regions." *Pharmaceutical Biology* 55 (1): 1415–1422. https://doi.org/10.1080/13880209.2017.1302485.

Elsharif, Shaimaa A, Ashutosh Banerjee, and Andrea Buettner. 2015. "Structure-Odor Relationships of Linalool, Linalyl Acetate and Their Corresponding Oxygenated Derivatives." *Frontiers in Chemistry* 3: 57. https://doi.org/10.3389/fchem.2015.00057.

Erkan, Naciye, Zhou Tao, H P Vasantha Rupasinghe, Burcu Uysal, and Birsen S Oksal. 2012. "Antibacterial Activities of Essential Oils Extracted from Leaves of Murraya Koenigii by Solvent-Free Microwave Extraction and Hydro-Distillation." *Natural Product Communications* 7 (1): 121–124.

Esharkawy, Eman R, Faisal Almalki, and Taibi Ben Hadda. 2022. "In Vitro Potential Antiviral SARS-CoV-19- Activity of Natural Product Thymohydroquinone and Dithymoquinone from *Nigella sativa*." *Bioorganic Chemistry* 120 (March): 105587. https://doi.org/10.1016/j.bioorg.2021.105587.

Farooqi, Ammad Ahmad, Rukset Attar, and Baojun Xu. 2022. "Anticancer and Anti-Metastatic Role of Thymoquinone: Regulation of Oncogenic Signaling Cascades by

Thymoquinone." *International Journal of Molecular Sciences* 23 (11). https://doi.org/10.3390/ijms23116311.

Gholamnezhad, Zahra, Mohammad Hossein Boskabady, and Mahmoud Hosseini. 2021. "The Effect of Chronic Supplementation of *Nigella sativa* on Splenocytes Response in Rats Following Treadmill Exercise." *Drug and Chemical Toxicology* 44 (5): 487–492. https://doi.org/10.1080/01480545.2019.1617301.

Girola, Natalia, Carlos R Figueiredo, Camyla F Farias, Ricardo A Azevedo, Adilson K Ferreira, Sarah F Teixeira, Tabata M Capello, et al. 2015. "Camphene Isolated from Essential Oil of Piper Cernuum (Piperaceae) Induces Intrinsic Apoptosis in Melanoma Cells and Displays Antitumor Activity in Vivo." *Biochemical and Biophysical Research Communications* 467 (4): 928–934. https://doi.org/10.1016/j.bbrc.2015.10.041.

Gołmwska, Sylwia, Iwona Łukasik, Adrian Arkadiusz Chojnacki, and Grzegorz Chrzanowski. 2023. "Flavonoids and Phenolic Acids Content in Cultivation and Wild Collection of European Cranberry Bush Viburnum Opulus L." *Molecules (Basel, Switzerland)* 28 (5). https://doi.org/10.3390/molecules28052285.

Grover, Madhuri, Tapan Behl, Tarun Virmani, Mohit Sanduja, Hafiz A Makeen, Mohammed Albratty, Hassan A Alhazmi, Abdulkarim M Meraya, and Simona Gabriela Bungau. 2022. "Exploration of Cytotoxic Potential of Longifolene/Junipene Isolated from Chrysopogon Zizanioides." *Molecules (Basel, Switzerland)* 27 (18). https://doi.org/10.3390/molecules27185764.

Hannan, Md Abdul, Md Ataur Rahman, Abdullah Al Mamun Sohag, Md Jamal Uddin, Raju Dash, Mahmudul Hasan Sikder, Md Saidur Rahman, et al. 2021. "Black Cumin (*Nigella sativa* L.): A Comprehensive Review on Phytochemistry, Health Benefits, Molecular Pharmacology, and Safety." *Nutrients* 13 (6). https://doi.org/10.3390/nu13061784.

Homayoonfal, Mina, Zatollah Asemi, and Bahman Yousefi. 2022. "Potential Anticancer Properties and Mechanisms of Thymoquinone in Osteosarcoma and Bone Metastasis." *Cellular & Molecular Biology Letters* 27 (1): 21. https://doi.org/10.1186/s11658-022-00320-0.

Iqbal, Mohammed Shariq, Ausaf Ahmad, and Brijesh Pandey. 2018. "Solvent Based Optimization for Extraction and Stability of Thymoquinone from *Nigella sativa* Linn. and Its Quantification Using RP-HPLC." *Physiology and Molecular Biology of Plants : An International Journal of Functional Plant Biology* 24 (6): 1209–1219. https://doi.org/10.1007/s12298-018-0593-5.

Jardan, Yousef A Bin, Abdul Ahad, Mohammad Raish, Mohd Aftab Alam, Abdullah M Al-Mohizea, and Fahad I Al-Jenoobi. 2021. "Effects of Garden Cress, Fenugreek and Black Seed on the Pharmacodynamics of Metoprolol: An Herb-Drug Interaction Study in Rats with Hypertension." *Pharmaceutical Biology* 59 (1): 1088–1097. https://doi.org/10.1080/13880209.2021.1961817.

Kadil, Youness, Mohammed Mouhcine, and Houda Filali. 2021. "In Silico Investigation of the SARS CoV2 Protease with Thymoquinone, the Major Constituent of *Nigella sativa*." *Current Drug Discovery Technologies* 18 (4): 570–573. https://doi.org/10.2174/1570163817666200712164406.

Karimkhani, Mohammad Mahdi, Mahmoud Nasrollahzadeh, Mehdi Maham, Abdollah Jamshidi, Mohammad Saeed Kharazmi, Danial Dehnad, and Seid Mahdi Jafari. 2022. "Extraction and Purification of α-Pinene; a Comprehensive Review." *Critical Reviews in Food Science and Nutrition*, November, 1–26. https://doi.org/10.1080/10408398.2022.2140331.

Khattab, Mahmoud M, and Mahmoud N Nagi. 2007. "Thymoquinone Supplementation Attenuates Hypertension and Renal Damage in Nitric Oxide Deficient Hypertensive Rats." *Phytotherapy Research : PTR* 21 (5): 410–414. https://doi.org/10.1002/ptr.2083.

Kim, Jae Kwang, and Sang Un Park. 2018. "Quercetin and Its Role in Biological Functions: An Updated Review." *EXCLI Journal* 17: 856–863. https://doi.org/10.17179/excli2018-1538.

Kim, Su-Hwan, and Chang-Ki Huh. 2022. "Isolation and Identification of Fisetin: An Antioxidative Compound Obtained from Rhus Verniciflua Seeds." *Molecules (Basel, Switzerland)* 27 (14). https://doi.org/10.3390/molecules27144510.

Kooti, Wesam, Zahra Hasanzadeh-Noohi, Naim Sharafi-Ahvazi, Majid Asadi-Samani, and Damoon Ashtary-Larky. 2016. "Phytochemistry, Pharmacology, and Therapeutic Uses of Black Seed (Nigella Sativa)." *Chinese Journal of Natural Medicines* 14 (10): 732–745. https://doi.org/10.1016/S1875-5364(16)30088-7.

Koshak, Abdulrahman E, Emad A Koshak, Abdullah F Mobeireek, Mazen A Badawi, Siraj O Wali, Husam M Malibary, Ali F Atwah, Meshari M Alhamdan, Reem A Almalki, and Tariq A Madani. 2021. "*Nigella sativa* for the Treatment of COVID-19: An Open-Label Randomized Controlled Clinical Trial." *Complementary Therapies in Medicine* 61 (September): 102769. https://doi.org/10.1016/j.ctim.2021.102769.

Kumar, Ashwini, Ashok Kumar Malik, and Dhananjay Kumar Tewary. 2009. "A New Method for Determination of Myricetin and Quercetin Using Solid Phase Microextraction-High Performance Liquid Chromatography-Ultra Violet/Visible System in Grapes, Vegetables and Red Wine Samples." *Analytica Chimica Acta* 631 (2): 177–181. https://doi.org/10.1016/j.aca.2008.10.038.

Lee, Jungmin, and Carolyn F Scagel. 2013. "Chicoric Acid: Chemistry, Distribution, and Production." *Frontiers in Chemistry* 1: 40. https://doi.org/10.3389/fchem.2013.00040.

Liang, Qiongxin, Jing Dong, Senye Wang, Wenjing Shao, Adel F Ahmed, Yan Zhang, and Wenyi Kang. 2021. "Immunomodulatory Effects of *Nigella sativa* Seed Polysaccharides by Gut Microbial and Proteomic Technologies." *International Journal of Biological Macromolecules* 184 (August): 483–496. https://doi.org/10.1016/j.ijbiomac.2021.06.118.

Mahmoud, Hany Salah, Amani A Almallah, Heba Nageh Gad El-Hak, Tahany Saleh Aldayel, Heba M A Abdelrazek, and Howayda E Khaled. 2021. "The Effect of Dietary Supplementation with *Nigella sativa* (Black Seeds) Mediates Immunological Function in Male Wistar Rats." *Scientific Reports* 11 (1): 7542. https://doi.org/10.1038/s41598-021-86721-1.

Maideen, Naina Mohamed Pakkir. 2021. "Antidiabetic Activity of *Nigella sativa* (Black Seeds) and Its Active Constituent (Thymoquinone): A Review of Human and Experimental Animal Studies." *Chonnam Medical Journal* 57 (3): 169–175. https://doi.org/10.4068/cmj.2021.57.3.169.

Maiti, Smarajit, Amrita Banerjee, Aarifa Nazmeen, Mehak Kanwar, and Shilpa Das. 2022. "Active-Site Molecular Docking of Nigellidine with Nucleocapsid-NSP2-MPro of COVID-19 and to Human IL1R-IL6R and Strong Antioxidant Role of *Nigella sativa* in Experimental Rats." *Journal of Drug Targeting* 30 (5): 511–521. https://doi.org/10.1080/1061186X.2020.1817040.

Marchese, Anna, Carla Renata Arciola, Ramona Barbieri, Ana Sanches Silva, Seyed Fazel Nabavi, Arold Jorel Tsetegho Sokeng, Morteza Izadi, et al. 2017. "Update on Monoterpenes as Antimicrobial Agents: A Particular Focus on p-Cymene." *Materials (Basel, Switzerland)* 10 (8). https://doi.org/10.3390/ma10080947.

Marchese, Anna, Ilkay Erdogan Orhan, Maria Daglia, Ramona Barbieri, Arianna Di Lorenzo, Seyed Fazel Nabavi, Olga Gortzi, Morteza Izadi, and Seyed Mohammad Nabavi. 2016. "Antibacterial and Antifungal Activities of Thymol: A Brief Review of the Literature." *Food Chemistry* 210 (November): 402–414. https://doi.org/10.1016/j.foodchem.2016.04.111.

Mbikay, Majambu, and Michel Chrétien. 2022. "Isoquercetin as an Anti-Covid-19 Medication: A Potential to Realize." *Frontiers in Pharmacology* 13: 830205. https://doi.org/10.3389/fphar.2022.830205.

Menezes, Isis Oliveira, Jackelyne Roberta Scherf, Anita Oliveira Brito Pereira Bezerra Martins, Andreza Guedes Barbosa Ramos, Jullyana de Souza Siqueira Quintans, Henrique Douglas Melo Coutinho, Jaime Ribeiro-Filho, and Irwin Rose Alencar de Menezes. 2021. "Biological Properties of Terpinolene Evidenced by in Silico, in Vitro and in Vivo Studies: A Systematic Review." *Phytomedicine : International Journal of Phytotherapy and Phytopharmacology* 93 (December): 153768. https://doi.org/10.1016/j.phymed.2021.153768.

Mir, Shabir Ahmad, Ahmad Firoz, Mohammed Alaidarous, Bader Alshehri, Abdul Aziz Bin Dukhyil, Saeed Banawas, Suliman A Alsagaby, et al. 2022. "Identification of SARS-CoV-2 RNA-Dependent RNA Polymerase Inhibitors from the Major Phytochemicals of *Nigella sativa*: An in Silico Approach." *Saudi Journal of Biological Sciences* 29 (1): 394–401. https://doi.org/10.1016/j.sjbs.2021.09.002.

Morikawa, Toshio, Fengming Xu, Kiyofumi Ninomiya, Hisashi Matsuda, and Masayuki Yoshikawa. 2004. "Nigellamines A3, A4, A5, and C, New Dolabellane-Type Diterpene Alkaloids, with Lipid Metabolism-Promoting Activities from the Egyptian Medicinal Food Black Cumin." *Chemical & Pharmaceutical Bulletin* 52 (4): 494–497. https://doi.org/10.1248/cpb.52.494.

Morsi, N M. 2000. "Antimicrobial Effect of Crude Extracts of *Nigella sativa* on Multiple Antibiotics-Resistant Bacteria." *Acta Microbiologica Polonica* 49 (1): 63–74.

Noriega, Paco, Alessandra Guerrini, Gianni Sacchetti, Alessandro Grandini, Edwin Ankuash, and Stefano Manfredini. 2019. "Chemical Composition and Biological Activity of Five Essential Oils from the Ecuadorian Amazon Rain Forest." *Molecules (Basel, Switzerland)* 24 (8). https://doi.org/10.3390/molecules24081637.

Pop, Raluca Maria, Octavia Sabin, Șoimița Suciu, Stefan Cristian Vesa, Sonia Ancuța Socaci, Veronica Sanda Chedea, Ioana Corina Bocsan, and Anca Dana Buzoianu. 2020. "*Nigella sativa*'s Anti-Inflammatory and Antioxidative Effects in Experimental Inflammation." *Antioxidants (Basel, Switzerland)* 9 (10). https://doi.org/10.3390/antiox9100921.

Pyne, Smritikana, and Kishalay Paria. 2022. "Optimization of Extraction Process Parameters of Caffeic Acid from Microalgae by Supercritical Carbon Dioxide Green Technology." *BMC Chemistry* 16 (1): 31. https://doi.org/10.1186/s13065-022-00824-y.

Rahim, Muhammad Abdul, Aurbab Shoukat, Waseem Khalid, Afaf Ejaz, Nizwa Itrat, Iqra Majeed, Hyrije Koraqi, et al. 2022. "A Narrative Review on Various Oil Extraction Methods, Encapsulation Processes, Fatty Acid Profiles, Oxidative Stability, and Medicinal Properties of Black Seed (*Nigella sativa*)." *Foods (Basel, Switzerland)* 11 (18). https://doi.org/10.3390/foods11182826.

Rani At, Jeeja, Asha Thomas, Mathew Kuruvilla, Muhammed Arshad, and Abraham Joseph. 2022. "The Co-Adsorption of Thymohydroquinone Dimethyl Ether (THQ) and Coumarin Present in the Aqueous Extract of Ayapana Triplinervis on Mild Steel and Its Protection in Hydrochloric Acid up to 323 K: Computational and Physicochemical Studies." *RSC Advances* 12 (23): 14328–14341. https://doi.org/10.1039/d2ra02109a.

Rao, Amit S, Shyamala Hegde, Linda M Pacioretty, Jan DeBenedetto, and John G Babish. 2020. "*Nigella sativa* and Trigonella Foenum-Graecum Supplemented Chapatis Safely Improve HbA1c, Body Weight, Waist Circumference, Blood Lipids, and Fatty Liver in Overweight and Diabetic Subjects: A Twelve-Week Safety and Efficacy Study." *Journal of Medicinal Food* 23 (9): 905–919. https://doi.org/10.1089/jmf.2020.0075.

Salehi, Bahare, Cristina Quispe, Muhammad Imran, Iahtisham Ul-Haq, Jelena Živković, Ibrahim M Abu-Reidah, Surjit Sen, et al. 2021. "Nigella Plants – Traditional Uses, Bioactive Phytoconstituents, Preclinical and Clinical Studies." *Frontiers in Pharmacology* 12: 625386. https://doi.org/10.3389/fphar.2021.625386.

Salehi, Bahare, Marco Valussi, Maria Flaviana Bezerra Morais-Braga, Joara Nalyda Pereira Carneiro, Antonio Linkoln Alves Borges Leal, Henrique Douglas Melo Coutinho, Sara Vitalini, et al. 2018. "Tagetes Spp. Essential Oils and Other Extracts: Chemical Characterization and Biological Activity." *Molecules (Basel, Switzerland)* 23 (11). https://doi.org/10.3390/molecules23112847.

Salehi, Bahare, Alessandro Venditti, Mehdi Sharifi-Rad, Dorota Kręgiel, Javad Sharifi-Rad, Alessandra Durazzo, Massimo Lucarini, et al. 2019. "The Therapeutic Potential of Apigenin." *International Journal of Molecular Sciences* 20 (6). https://doi.org/10.3390/ijms20061305.

Sangi, Sibghatullah Muhammad Ali, Mansour Ibrahim Sulaiman, Mohammed Fawzy Abd El-Wahab, Elsamoual Ibrahim Ahmedani, and Soad Shaker Ali. 2015. "Antihyperglycemic Effect of Thymoquinone and Oleuropein, on Streptozotocin-Induced Diabetes Mellitus in Experimental Animals." *Pharmacognosy Magazine* 11 (Suppl 2): S251–S257. https://doi.org/10.4103/0973-1296.166017.

Suntres, Zacharias E, John Coccimiglio, and Misagh Alipour. 2015. "The Bioactivity and Toxicological Actions of Carvacrol." *Critical Reviews in Food Science and Nutrition* 55 (3): 304–318. https://doi.org/10.1080/10408398.2011.653458.

Surendran, Shelini, Fatimah Qassadi, Geyan Surendran, Dash Lilley, and Michael Heinrich. 2021. "Myrcene-What Are the Potential Health Benefits of This Flavouring and Aroma Agent?" *Frontiers in Nutrition* 8: 699666. https://doi.org/10.3389/fnut.2021.699666.

Tariq, Mohammad. 2008. "*Nigella sativa* Seeds: Folklore Treatment in Modern Day Medicine." *Saudi Journal of Gastroenterology : Official Journal of the Saudi Gastroenterology Association*. India. https://doi.org/10.4103/1319-3767.41725.

Tiji, Salima, Yahya Rokni, Ouijdane Benayad, Nassima Laaraj, Abdeslam Asehraou, and Mostafa Mimouni. 2021. "Chemical Composition Related to Antimicrobial Activity of Moroccan *Nigella sativa* L. Extracts and Isolated Fractions." *Evidence-Based Complementary and Alternative Medicine : ECAM* 2021: 8308050. https://doi.org/10.1155/2021/8308050.

Tiruppur Venkatachallam, Suresh Kumar, Hajimalang Pattekhan, Soundar Divakar, and Udaya Sankar Kadimi. 2010. "Chemical Composition of *Nigella sativa L.* Seed Extracts Obtained by Supercritical Carbon Dioxide." *Journal of Food Science and Technology* 47 (6): 598–605. https://doi.org/10.1007/s13197-010-0109-y.

Wajs-Bonikowska, Anna, Janusz Malarz, Łukasz Szoka, Paweł Kwiatkowski, and Anna Stojakowska. 2021. "Composition of Essential Oils from Roots and Aerial Parts of Carpesium Cernuum and Their Antibacterial and Cytotoxic Activities." *Molecules (Basel, Switzerland)* 26 (7). https://doi.org/10.3390/molecules26071883.

Wei, Yun, Qianqian Xie, Derek Fisher, and Ian A Sutherland. 2011. "Separation of Patuletin-3-O-Glucoside, Astragalin, Quercetin, Kaempferol and Isorhamnetin from Flaveria Bidentis (L.) Kuntze by Elution-Pump-out High-Performance Counter-Current Chromatography." *Journal of Chromatography. A* 1218 (36): 6206–6211. https://doi.org/10.1016/j.chroma.2011.01.058.

Wong, Victor, S Grant Wyllie, Charles P Cornwell, and Deidre Tronson. 2001. "Supercritical Fluid Extraction (SFE) of Monoterpenes from the Leaves of Melaleuca Alternifolia (Tea Tree)." *Molecules : A Journal of Synthetic Chemistry and Natural Product Chemistry*. https://doi.org/10.3390/60100092.

Yimer, Ebrahim M, Kald Beshir Tuem, Aman Karim, Najeeb Ur-Rehman, and Farooq Anwar. 2019. "*Nigella sativa* L. (Black Cumin): A Promising Natural Remedy for Wide Range of Illnesses." *Evidence-Based Complementary and Alternative Medicine : ECAM* 2019: 1528635. https://doi.org/10.1155/2019/1528635.

Zaky, Ahmed A, Jae-Han Shim, and A M Abd El-Aty. 2021. "A Review on Extraction, Characterization, and Applications of Bioactive Peptides From Pressed Black Cumin Seed Cake." *Frontiers in Nutrition* 8: 743909. https://doi.org/10.3389/fnut.2021.743909.

Zaoui, A, Y Cherrah, N Mahassini, K Alaoui, H Amarouch, and M Hassar. 2002. "Acute and Chronic Toxicity of *Nigella sativa* Fixed Oil." *Phytomedicine : International Journal of Phytotherapy and Phytopharmacology* 9 (1): 69–74. https://doi.org/10.1078/0944-7113-00084.

Zduńska, Kamila, Agnieszka Dana, Anna Kolodziejczak, and Helena Rotsztejn. 2018. "Antioxidant Properties of Ferulic Acid and Its Possible Application." *Skin Pharmacology and Physiology* 31 (6): 332–336. https://doi.org/10.1159/000491755.

Zhu, Yingpeng, Jiangliu Yu, Chunyan Jiao, Jinfeng Tong, Lei Zhang, Yan Chang, Weina Sun, Qing Jin, and Yongping Cai. 2019. "Optimization of Quercetin Extraction Method in Dendrobium Officinale by Response Surface Methodology." *Heliyon* 5 (9): e02374. https://doi.org/10.1016/j.heliyon.2019.e02374.

# 19 An Update of Anticancer Application of Essential Oils

*Mohit Agrawal, Manmohan Singhal,*
*Amit Kumar Nayak, and Shailendra Bhatt*

## 19.1 INTRODUCTION

The disease cancer is a rapid acting health problem in the whole world and the second acting cause of death after heart diseases. According to an upcoming report by the International Agency for Research on Cancer (IARC) in the year 2008 there were around 12 million new cases of cancer in the whole world. In the present time more than 10 million cases of cancer per year are occurring which involves a group of more than 100 diseases as cancer of liver, cancer of lungs, cancer of stomach and many more (Reddy L. et al., 2003). The most examining way in affecting carcinogenesis is by hindering with modulating steps as well as by the associated signal transduction pathways. There are many physiological and biochemical carcinogenics, such as ultraviolet radiations, ionizing radiations, infections by virus, bacteria, and parasites, and contamination of food through mycotoxins. There are other kinds of cancer which are due to oxygen-centered free radicals and other reactive species due to over-production of these free radicals which can cause oxidative damage to the biological molecules. There is not any completely effective drug available on the market for treating most types of cancers. There is a normal call for new drugs which are highly effective with low toxicity and a very much lesser environmental impact. There are some novel natural products which have opportunities in the area of innovation for drug discovery (Surh YJ, 2003). As we know natural products show a major role in prevention and treatment of cancer. A certain amount of anti-tumor agents of natural origin are used currently in the clinic. Over half of all anticancer prescription drugs were approved on international ground between the year 1940 and 2006. The natural compounds taken from medicinal plants which have a high source of novel anticancer activity are drawing major interest (Luk JM et al., 2007). The traditional medicinal herbs used in the areas of pharmaceutical and dietary therapy for many years in East Africa, China, Japan, India, and many others are used commonly in the cancer therapy. The early investigations tell that an average of 35% in the total human cancer-related mortality was due to diet. Much evidence from population and also from lab studies has shown an inverse relation between the sufficient consumption of fruits and vegetables and the risks of certain types of cancers; that is, a diet high in fruits, vegetables, and whole

DOI: 10.1201/9781003389774-19

grains is linked with lower risk of cancer. The protective anticancer effects from these dietary compounds are known to be due to the induction of the cellular defense system, which includes detoxification and antioxidant enzymes, along with inhibiting the cell cycle arrest and cell death-promoting antioxidant, anti-inflammatory, and anti-cell growth signalling pathways (Fresco P et al., 2006). It is thought that more than 5000 individual phytochemicals are being identified in fruits, vegetables, grains, and other plants which are classified on the basis of phenolics.

## 19.2 CHEMICAL CLASSIFICATION, USES, AND THERAPEUTIC POTENTIAL OF EOS AND THEIR CONSTITUENTS

Aromatic plants produce the concentrated hydrophobic liquids with a characteristic odor known as EOs. These secondary metabolites, often known as volatile or ethereal oils, are found in varying degrees in different plant sections. The elements of the EOs determine their makeup and other biological characteristics. Terpenes, aromatic compounds, and other molecules with different sources may all be components. Based on their chemical compositions, the components of EOs have been categorized (Gómez RC et al., 2007). EOs are thought to be more powerful than their individual components because of their synergistic and more focused action. Additionally, the content of EOs produced by plants in various situations varies, and as a result, they have distinct applications. Since ancient times, EOs and their components have been employed for their distinct fragrances in perfumery and as flavoring ingredients in culinary products. A general classification based on chemical structures is described in EOs along with samples. Due to their calming and stimulating qualities, EOs are frequently utilized in aromatherapy to enhance health. With active compounds that are being employed in medicine, EOs are used for massage, baths, and inhalation as relaxants and therapy choices as aromatherapies for a variety of disorders. These EOs are lipophilic, which makes it simple for them to penetrate cell membranes and enter the cell. EOs are thought to have strong antioxidant properties that may have anticancer implications (Tabor E 2007).

## 19.3 EOS AND CONSTITUENTS AS ANTICANCER AGENTS

One of the most important plant products, EOs are employed in complementary and alternative medicine. EOs and their constituents are currently being investigated for their positive effects on various malignancies (Lee JY et al., 2007). The National Institutes of Health's online database may be searched for "cancer-essential oils" as of February 2014: of all 135 research papers, 117 – or a substantial rise in the number of publications in this field – were released after 2005. It has been shown that EOs from many plants have anticancer potential against mouth, breast, lung, prostate, liver, colon, and brain cancer, and even leukemia (Shiotani A et al., 2005). Not only EOs, but also some of their constituents, have been shown to have cytotoxic effects on cancer cell lines and in *in vivo* studies, including carvacrol, limonene, geraniols, myrcene, perillyl alcohol (POH), humulene, caryophyllene, thymol, and Phase I and Phase II clinical trials in cancer patients have been conducted on several of these, such as POH. Terpinen-4-ol is one of several terpene analogues that have been shown to cause apoptosis and have anticancer effects. The existing studies demonstrating the anticancer properties of EOs from various plants and their constituents have been meticulously gathered and reported in the current review. Several tables have been created to organize the entire body of literature.

## 19.4  MECHANISM OF ACTION OF EOS

The cancer cell is the target of drugs used to treat cancer by causing apoptosis or cell cycle arrest. Therefore, natural substances that induce apoptosis in cancer cells are important tools in the fight against the disease. EOs with therapeutic potential have the ability to inhibit cancer and avoid chemotherapy (Groopman JD et al., 1996). The activation of detoxifying enzymes, modification of DNA repair signals, and anti-metastatic and antiangiogenetic activities are some of the mechanisms involved in cancer treatment (Cai Y et al., 2004). The antiproliferative activity of EOs in cancer cells is mediated by a variety of routes, and EOs are even successful at shrinking tumors in animal models, depicting several EOs' potential targets for preventing cancer (Efferth T et al., 2007). Due to their lack of noticeable effects on normal cells, EOs are effective anticancer agents. The EOs in this section have been studied to see if they can impede the growth of cancer cells in different ways.

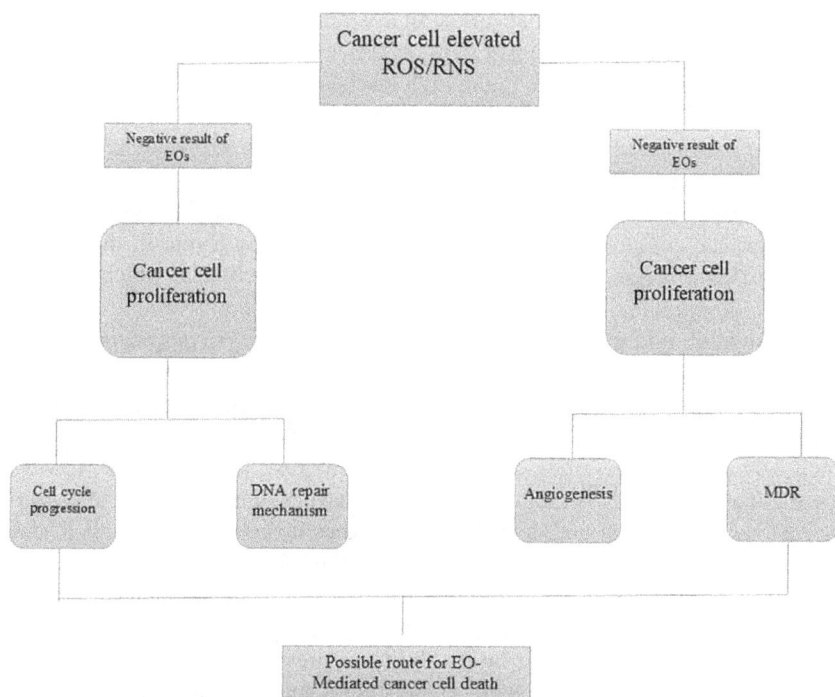

**FIGURE 19.1**   To prevent cancer: Multi-targeted roles of essential oils.

## 19.5 ANTICANCER MECHANISMS OF ESSENTIAL OIL

### 19.5.1 ANTIOXIDANT

Antioxidant activity is one of the areas of essential oil research that has drawn the most attention because oxidation harms various biological substances and subsequently causes many diseases, including cancer, liver disease, Alzheimer's disease, ageing, joint problems, swelling, diabetes, vascular dementia, atherosclerosis, and AIDS (Doll R et al, 1981). Hence, in order to prevent oxidative damage, antioxidants have been utilized to treat a range of diseases. Several scientists have been studying the antioxidant capacities of various essential oils in recent years in an effort to discover risk-free natural antioxidants. As a result, many studies have shown that essential oils are the best naturally occurring sources of antioxidants currently accessible. Hydrogen peroxide and superoxide anions combine to create hydroxyl radicals in eukaryotes, which are very damaging to mitochondrial DNA. Reactive oxygen species (ROS) are produced as a result of damaged mitochondrial DNA that hinders the production of the electron transport protein (Greenwald P, 1996). The reactive phenoxy radicals that are created when an injured mitochondrial membrane produces free radicals mix with essential oil to limit further damage. Thyme essential oil showed the strongest antioxidant properties of the essential oils evaluated in one study, followed by clove leaf, cinnamon leaf, basil, eucalyptus, and chamomile. Antioxidant qualities have been discovered in the essential oils of basil, cumin, juniper, eucalyptus, and coriander. *Thymus spathulifolius* contains high levels of thymol (36.5%) and carvacrol (29.8%), which gave the essential oil in that plant antioxidant capabilities. Egyptian maize silk essential oil displayed significant antioxidant activity due to the high levels of thymol (20.5%) and carvacrol (58.1%) (Kwon KH, et.al, 2007). Essential oils from the plants *Salvia cryptantha* and *Salvia multicaulis* have more antioxidant power than ascorbic acid or butylated hydroxytoluene (BHT). Furthermore, it was found that the essential oil from *Curcuma zedoaria* was a potent radical scavenger. Terpenes and terpenoids, among other fragrance components, have been suggested to play a role in the essential oils' antioxidant action. One of these ingredients is 1,8-cineole, which is present in *Mentha aquatic*, *Mentha longifolia*, and *Mentha piperita*, as well as menthone, linalool, thymol, and eugenol. The essential oils of *Thymus caespititius*, *Thymus camphorates*, and *Thymus mastichina* contained high quantities of linalool and 1,8-cineole, which had antioxidant activity similar to that of vitamin E (Adorjan B and Buchbauer G, 2010). The essential oil of lemon balm (*Melissa officinalis* L.), which contains neral/geranial, citronellal, isomenthone, and menthone, has been shown to have strong antioxidant action. There have also been reports of essential oils' *in vivo* antioxidant activity. The rabbits' diet included oregano oil to delay lipid oxidation. When turkeys were given the same oil, a reduction in lipid oxidation impact was observed that was comparable to that of alpha-tocopheryl acetate The hydroxyl radical scavenging abilities of *Achillea millefolium* subsp. *millefolium* essential oil were demonstrated by its ability to prevent the non-enzymatic lipid peroxidation of rat liver homogenate. These studies suggest that using essential oils can help prevent a number of degenerative diseases because they are strong natural antioxidant sources (Figure 19.2).

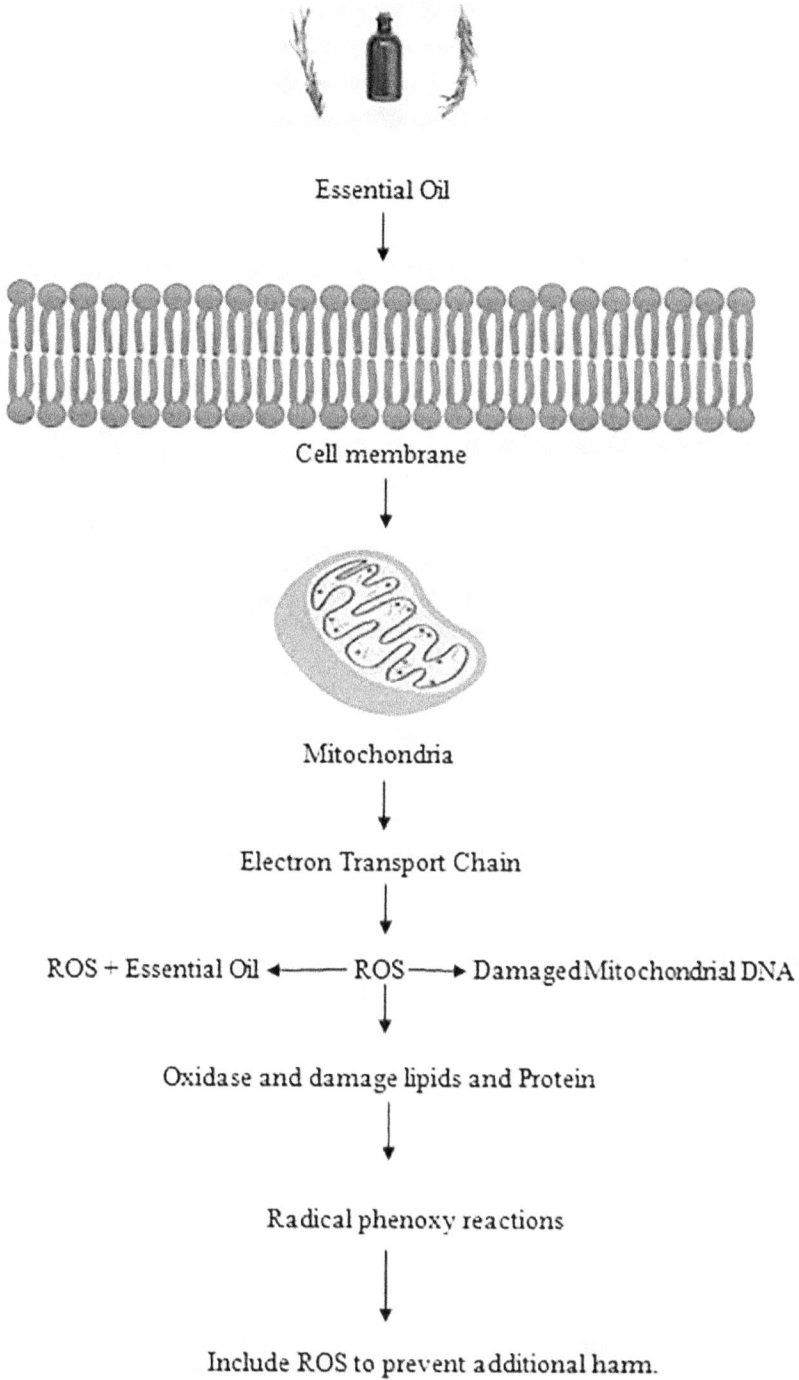

FIGURE 19.2 Essential oil mechanism of antioxidant action.

## 19.5.2 ANTIMUTAGEN

Antimutagenicity is a characteristic of essential oils that is demonstrated by various mechanisms, including inhibition of the mutagen's penetration inside the cell, inactivation of the mutagen directly, capture of antioxidant radicals produced by the mutagen, activation of antioxidant enzymes, and inhibition of the pro-mutagens' conversion to the mutagens by P450 metabolites (Giaginis C and Theocharis S, 2011). The antimutagenic substances work by encouraging error-free DNA repair. As far as is known, no research has been done on the sort of antimutagenicity that involves *E. coli* DNA being repaired by terpene and phenolic chemicals derived from essential oils. Alpha-terpinene, alpha-terpineol, 1,8-cineole, camphor, and citral are a few chemical compounds derived from aromatic plants that alter hepatic monooxygenase activity by interacting with pro-mutagen xenobiotic bio-transformation. It is well established that using essential oils can lessen cell death and mitochondrial damage in the yeast *Saccharomyces cerevisiae* (Figure 19.3) (Abdolmohammadi et.al, 2010).

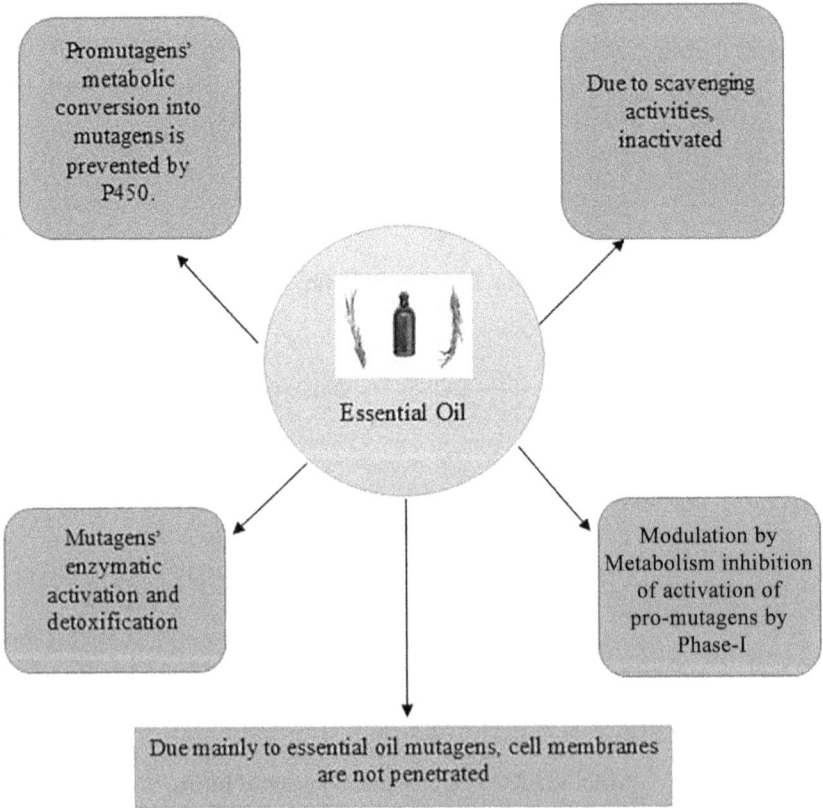

**FIGURE 19.3** Mechanism of antimutagenic essential oil.

### 19.5.3 Antiproliferation

The antiproliferative activities of *Satureja hortensis*, *Satureja montana*, *Salvia officinalis*, *Lavandula officinalis*, *Thymus vulgaris*, etc. was tested on human erythroleukemia K562 cells. It is found that the essential oils which are taken from *S. montana* (IC50 value 56 µm/ml) and *M. arvensis* (IC50 value 85 µm/ml) has shown many good biological activities in inhibition of cell growth of K562 cell line. The common active constituents pinene, gamma-terpinene, 4-terpineol, etc., have shown antiproliferative activity between IC50 value 329 to 98 µm/ml. As shown in other different studies the active compound eugenol from clove, nutmeg, basil, etc., have shown many antiproliferative activities against many cancer cell lines and animal models (Hardin A et al., 2010). It is also reported that there is apoptosis-mediated proliferation inhibition of human colon cancer cells with the volatile constituents of *Citrus aurantifolia*. When this oil was used at a concentration of 100 g/ml for 48 hours, human colon cancer cells (SW-480) were inhibited by 78%. After 24 and 48 hours, respectively, lime volatile oil exhibited DNA fragmentation and an up to 1.8 and 2-fold increase of caspase-3, which may indicate that apoptosis was involved. Lime volatile oil's ability to induce apoptosis was further supported by analysis of the expression of apoptosis-related proteins, which also revealed that lime volatile oil may be useful in preventing colon cancer (Halliwell B and Gutteridge J, 1990). In the volatile oils of *Thymus vulgaris*, *Carum copticum*, *Origanum*, and oregano, carvacro, one of the phenolic monoterpenes, can be found. The antiproliferative effects of carvacrol in metastatic breast cancer cells (MDA-MB231) were based on the activation of the classical apoptosis response, which includes a reduction in mitochondrial membrane potential and an increase in cytochrome c released from mitochondria, a reduction in the Bcl-2/Bax ratio, an increase in caspase activity, and cleavage of poly (ADP-ribose) polymerase (PARP). *Astrodaucus orientalis* has been shown to have antiproliferative effects on the T47D human breast cancer cell line (Paz-Elizur T, et al., 2008).

## 19.6   ENHANCEMENT OF IMMUNE FUNCTIONS AND SURVEILLANCE

When particular elements are taken into account, such as stress reduction, supporting good intestinal bacteria, and fostering improved blood and lymph quality, immune system-improving mechanisms are effective. Aromatherapy is an approach that has largely been successful. According to Cristina Proano-Carrion (thearomablog.com/essential-oils-for-the-immune-system), aromatherapy is the use of essential oils through a variety of methods to enhance immune function (Preedy V, et al., 1998). It is crucial for improving immune system performance. It functions in a number of ways, including regulating the hormones released by the adrenal glands, which reduces stress, enhancing the immune system by assisting the lymphatic system in removing toxins, promoting the generation of immune-stimulating cells, and destroying hazardous microorganisms. One study examined the impact of aromatherapy on human immunological function using

*Citrus limonum* and *Lavandula angustifolia*. It was discovered that inhaling lemon essential oil improved mood and increased norepinephrine release; however other immunological data acquired did not support either essential oil's efficacy. Inflammation is a common feature of many diseases, including those of arthritis, asthma, multiple sclerosis, inflammatory bowel disease, and atherosclerosis. It is a reaction to harm brought on by noxious physical or chemical stimuli (Moreira PI, et al., 2005). The reactive oxygen species (ROS), lipid mediators, proteases, and cytokines are some of the soluble mediators of inflammation that are released during this often-acute phase response, which can also become chronic. Additionally, macrophage cells are crucial in the beginning and development of a number of inflammatory disorders, including those brought on by septic shock and persistent inflammatory illnesses. In LPS-stimulated murine macrophages, researchers identified a nedocromil from *Curcuma heyneana* that inhibits iNOS, COX-2, and pro-inflammatory cytokines by downregulating the NF-B pathway (Figure 19.4) (Liu J and Mori A, 2005).

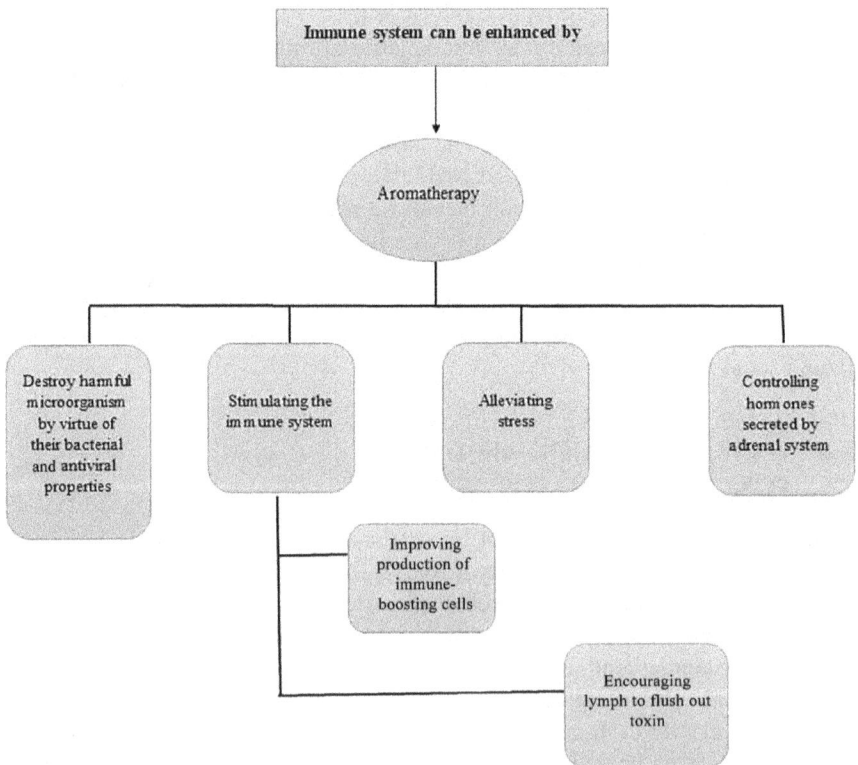

**FIGURE 19.4**  Process through which essential oils boost immune system performance by helping lymph to remove toxins.

## 19.7 MODULATION OF MULTIDRUG RESISTANCE

As a result of increased drug efflux by energy-dependent drug transporters from the ABC (ATP-binding cassette) superfamily, many tumors have been reported to have multidrug resistant (MDR) phenotypes, which typically involve reduced intracellular drug accumulation and/or impairment of one or more steps of the apoptotic signaling cascades (Čolak E, 2008). In MCF7 WT and MCF7 Adr (Adriamycin-resistant) human breast cancer cell lines, linalool overcomes doxo-rubicin resistance. Lavender (*Lavandula officinalis*), coriander seeds, and other aromatic plants' essential oils include linalool, an acyclic monoterpene alcohol. The para-benzoquinone reportedly appeared in another research study. To assess the *in vitro* antitumoral efficacy of tea tree oil, human melanoma M14 wild type (WT) cells and their drug-resistant counterparts, M14 Adriamycin-resistant (ADR) cells, were utilized (Naito Y et al., 2008). Tea tree oil and its main constituent terpinen-4-ol appear to be less effective at preventing the proliferation of human M14 melanoma cells than the drug-selected resistant cell line M14 ADR, which expresses high levels of P-gp in the plasma membrane. Gamma-linolenic acid (GLA) is known to have a specific tumor-killing action. Moreover, it has been hypothesized that GLA might increase some cancer cells' receptivity to chemotherapy's lethal effects (Jain SK, 2006). Human melanoma M14 wild type (WT) cells and their drug-resistant counterparts, M14 Adriamycin-resistant (ADR) cells, selected by prolonged exposure to doxorubicin, were used to assess the *in vitro* antitumoral activity of tea tree oil. Tea tree oil and its primary component, terpinen-4-ol, do not appear to be as successful at stopping the proliferation of human M14 melanoma cells as the drug-selected resistant cell line M14 ADR, which expresses high levels of P-gp in the plasma membrane (Beal MF, 2006). Tea tree oil and its primary component, terpinen-4-ol, do not appear to be as successful at stopping the proliferation of human M14 melanoma cells as the drug-selected resistant cell line M14 ADR, which expresses high levels of P-gp in the plasma membrane.

## 19.8 CONCLUSION

Despite their direct impact on tumor cells, essential oils have been found to have favorable chemical effects on the immune system. The activity of white blood cells is increased by essential oils, making them more effective at removing bacteria and other objects from the body. It is believed that small molecules control the activity of the essential oil's primary constituents. As a result, essential oils function at various stages for numerous diseases, including cancer, just as many plant-based medications. More innovative essential oils and unidentified compounds should be tested for their anticancer abilities. In addition, individual molecules must be synthetically modified for their increased activity. Overall, the outlook for using essential oils to treat cancer is quite encouraging, and the scientific and medical organizations agree that more research is necessary to create successful treatment regimens for this gravely debilitating disease.

## REFERENCES

Abdolmohammadi, M.; Fouladdel, S.; Shafiee, A.; Amin, G.; Ghaffari, S.; Azizi, E. Antiproliferative and apoptotic effect of Astrodaucus orientalis (L.) drude on T47D human breast cancer cell line potential mechanisms of action. Afr J Biotechnol, **2010**, 8.

Adorjan, B.; Buchbauer, G. Biological properties of essential oils: An updated review. Flavour Fragr J, **2010**, 25, 407–426.

Beal, M.F. Mitochondria, oxidative damage, and inflammation in Parkinson's disease. Annals New York Acad Sci, **2006**, 991, 120–131.

Cai, Y.; Luo, Q.; Sun, M.; Corke, H. Antioxidant activity and phenolic compounds of 112 traditional Chinese medicinal plants associated with anticancer. Life Sci, **2004**, 74, 2157–2184.

Čolak, E. New markers of oxidative damage to macromolecules. J Med Biochem, **2008**, 27, 1–16.

Doll, R.; Peto, R. The causes of cancer: quantitative estimates of avoidable risks of cancer in the United States today. J Natl Cancer Inst, **1981**, 66, 1192–1308.

Efferth, T.; Li, P.C.H.; Konkimalla, V.S.B.; Kaina, B. From traditional Chinese medicine to rational cancer therapy. Trends Mol Med, **2007**, 13, 353–361.

Fresco, P.; Borges, F.; Diniz, C.; Marques, M. New insights on the anticancer properties of dietary polyphenols. Med Res Rev, **2006**, 26, 747–766.

Giaginis, C.; Theocharis, S. Current evidence on the anticancer potential of Chios Mastic Gum. Nutr Cancer, **2011**, 63, 1174–1184.

Gómez, R.C.; De, Castro, C.J. González, B.M.; Causes of lung cancer: Smoking, environmental tobacco smoke exposure, occupational and environmental exposures and genetic predisposition. Med Clin, **2007**, 128, 390–396.

Greenwald, P. Chemoprevention of cancer. Sci Am, **1996**, 275, 96–100.

Groopman, J.D.; Wang, J.S.; Scholl, P. Molecular biomarkers for aflatoxins: From adducts to gene mutations to human liver cancer. Can J Physiol Pharm, **1996**, 74, 203–209.

Halliwell, B.; Gutteridge, J. The antioxidants of human extracellular fluids. Arch Biochem Biophys, **1990**, 280, 1.

Hardin, A.; Crandall, P.G.; Stankus, T. Essential oils and antioxidants derived from citrus by-products in food protection and medicine: An introduction and review of recent literature. J of Agric & Food Inform, **2010**, 11, 99–122.

Jain, S.K. Superoxide dismutase overexpression and cellular oxidative damage in diabetes a commentary on: Overexpression of mitochondrial superoxide dismutase in mice protects the retina from diabetes-induced oxidative stress. Free Radic Biol Med, **2006**, 41, 1187–1190.

Kwon, K.H.; Barve, A.; Yu, S.; Huang, M.T.; Kong, A.N.T. Cancer chemoprevention by phytochemicals: Potential molecular targets, biomarkers and animal models1. Acta Pharmacol Sin, **2007**, 28, 1409–1421.

Lee, J.Y.; Li, J.; Yeung, E.S. Single-molecule detection of surface-hybridized human papilloma virus DNA for quantitative clinical screening. Anal Chem, **2007**, 79, 8083–8089.

Liu, J.; Mori, A. Oxidative damage hypothesis of stress-associated aging acceleration: Neuroprotective effects of natural and nutritional antioxidants. Res Commun Biol Psychol Psychiat Neurosc, **2005**, 30, 103.

Luk, J.M.; Wang, X.; Liu, P.; Wong, K.F.; Chan, K.L.; Tong, Y.; Hui, C.K.; Lau, G.K.; Fan, S.T. Traditional Chinese herbal medicines for treatment of liver fibrosis and cancer: From laboratory discovery to clinical evaluation. Liver Int, **2007**, 27, 879–890.

Moreira, P.I.; Smith, M.A.; Zhu, X.; Honda, K.; Lee, H.; Aliev, G.; Perry, G. Oxidative damage and Alzheimer's disease: Are antioxidant therapies useful. Drug News Perspect, **2005**, 18, 13–19.

Naito, Y.; Uchiyama, K.; Aoi, W.; Hasegawa, G.; Nakamura, N.; Yoshida, N.; Maoka, T.; Takahashi, J.; Yoshikawa, T. Prevention of diabetic nephropathy by treatment with astaxanthin in diabetic db/db mice. BioFactors, **2008**, 20, 49–59.

Patil, J.R.; Jayaprakasha, G.; Chidambara Murthy, K.; Tichy, S.E.; Chetti, M.B.; Patil, B.S. Apoptosis-mediated proliferation inhibition of human colon cancer cells by volatile principles of Citrus aurantifolia. Food Chem, **2009**, 114, 1351–1358.

Paz-Elizur, T.; Sevilya, Z.; Leitner-Dagan, Y.; Elinger, D.; Roisman, L.C.; Livneh, Z. DNA repair of oxidative DNA damage in human carcinogenesis: Potential application for cancer risk assessment and prevention. Cancer Lett, **2008**, 266, 60–72.

Poulsen, H.E.; Prieme, H.; Loft, S. Role of oxidative DNA damage in cancer initiation and promotion. Eur J Cancer Prev, **1998**, 7, 9–16.

Preedy, V.; Reilly, M.; Mantle, D.; Peters, T. Oxidative damage in liver disease. J Intern Fed Clin Chem, **1998**, 10, 16–20.

Reddy, L.; Odhav, B.; Bhoola, K.; Natural products for cancer prevention: A global perspective. Pharmacol Ther, **2003**, 99, 1–13.

Surh, Y.J. Cancer chemoprevention with dietary phytochemicals. Nat Rev Cancer, **2003**, 3, 768–780.

Tabor, E. Pathogenesis of hepatitis B virus-associated hepatocellular carcinoma. Hepatol Res, **2007**, 37, S110–S114.

# Index

For Product Safety Concerns and Information please contact our EU
representative GPSR@taylorandfrancis.com
Taylor & Francis Verlag GmbH, Kaufingerstraße 24, 80331 München, Germany